Neonatal Gastroenterology: Challenges, Controversies, and Recent Advances

Editor

SUDARSHAN R. JADCHERLA

CLINICS IN PERINATOLOGY

www.perinatology.theclinics.com

Consulting Editor
LUCKY JAIN

June 2020 • Volume 47 • Number 2

ELSEVIER

1600 John F. Kennedy Boulevard ● Suite 1800 ● Philadelphia, Pennsylvania, 19103-2899

http://www.theclinics.com

CLINICS IN PERINATOLOGY Volume 47, Number 2
June 2020 ISSN 0095-5108, ISBN-13: 978-0-323-72078-6

Editor: Kerry Holland
Developmental Editor: Casey Potter

Clinics in Perinatology (ISSN 0095-5108) is published quarterly by Elsevier Inc., 360 Park Avenue South, New York, NY 10010-1710. Months of issue are March, June, September, and December. Business and Editorial Offices: 1600 John F. Kennedy Blvd., Ste. 1800, Philadelphia, PA 19103-2899. Customer Service Office: 3251 Riverport Lane, Maryland Heights, MO 63043. Periodicals postage paid at New York, NY and additional mailing offices. Subscription prices are $312.00 per year (US individuals), $610.00 per year (US institutions), $365.00 per year (Canadian individuals), $747.00 per year (Canadian institutions), $435.00 per year (international individuals), $747.00 per year (international institutions), $100.00 per year (US and Canadian students), and $195.00 per year (International students). International air speed delivery is included in all Clinics subscription prices. All prices are subject to change without notice. **POSTMASTER:** Send address changes to *Clinics in Perinatology*, Elsevier Health Sciences Division, Subscription Customer Service, 3251 Riverport Lane, Maryland Heights, MO 63043. **Customer Service: Telephone: 1-800-654-2452** (U.S. and Canada); **1-314-447-8871** (outside U.S. and Canada). **Fax: 1-314-447-8029. E-mail: journalscustomerservice-usa@elsevier.com** (for print support); **journalsonlinesupport-usa@elsevier.com** (for online support).

Reprints. For copies of 100 or more, of articles in this publication, please contact the Commercial Reprints Department, Elsevier Inc., 360 Park Avenue South, New York, NY 10010-1710. Tel. 212-633-3874; Fax: 212-633-3820; E-mail: reprints@elsevier.com.

Clinics in Perinatology is also published in Spanish by McGraw-Hill Interamericana Editores S.A., P.O. Box 5-237, 06500 Mexico D.F., Mexico.

Clinics in Perinatology is covered in *MEDLINE/PubMed (Index Medicus) Current Contents, Excepta Medica, BIOSIS and ISI/BIOMED.*

Contributors

CONSULTING EDITOR

LUCKY JAIN, MD, MBA
George W. Brumley Jr Professor and Chair, Emory University School of Medicine,
Department of Pediatrics, Chief Academic Officer, Children's Healthcare of Atlanta,
Executive Director, Emory and Children's Pediatric Institute, Atlanta, Georgia, USA

EDITOR

SUDARSHAN R. JADCHERLA, MD, FRCP (Ireland), DCH, AGAF, FAAP
Professor of Pediatrics and Associate Division Chief of Neonatology, Academics,
Divisions of Neonatology, Pediatric Gastroenterology, Hepatology and Nutrition, Director,
The Neonatal and Infant Feeding Disorders Program, Principal Investigator, Innovative
Feeding Disorders Research Program, Center for Perinatal Research, Abigail Wexner
Research Institute, Nationwide Children's Hospital, Department of Pediatrics, College of
Medicine, The Ohio State University College of Medicine, Columbus, Ohio, USA

AUTHORS

LEONOR ADRIANA MASSIEU, RD, LD, CNSC
Department of Clinical Nutrition Services, Texas Children's Hospital, Houston, Texas, USA

HANY ALY, MD, MSHS
Department of Neonatology, Cleveland Clinic Children's, Cleveland Clinic Lerner College
of Medicine, Cleveland, Ohio, USA

DIANE M. ANDERSON, PhD, RD, LD
Division of Neonatology, Department of Pediatrics, Baylor College of Medicine, Texas
Children's Hospital, Houston, Texas, USA

ANKUR CHUGH, MD
Pediatric Gastroenterology, Medical College of Wisconsin, Milwaukee, Wisconsin, USA

STACEY DALGLEISH, RN, MN, NNP
Neonatal Nurse Practitioner, Department of Pediatrics, Neonatal Intensive Care Unit,
Alberta Health Services, Cumming School of Medicine, Alberta Children's Hospital,
Calgary, Alberta, Canada

ISABELLE G. DE PLAEN, MD
Department of Pediatrics, Ann & Robert H. Lurie Children's Hospital of Chicago,
Northwestern University, Feinberg School of Medicine, Chicago, Illinois, USA

MOLLY C. DIENHART, MD
Assistant Professor of Clinical Pediatrics, Division of Gastroenterology, Hepatology and
Nutrition, The Ohio State University College of Medicine, Center for Intestinal Rehabilitation
and Nutrition Support, Nationwide Children's Hospital, Columbus, Ohio, USA

STEVEN H. ERDMAN, MD
Professor of Clinical Pediatrics, Division of Gastroenterology, Hepatology and Nutrition, Nationwide Children's Hospital, The Ohio State University College of Medicine, Columbus, Ohio, USA

GANGA GOKULAKRISHNAN, MD, MS
Division of Neonatology, Department of Pediatrics, Baylor College of Medicine, Texas Children's Hospital, Houston, Texas, USA

ISH K. GULATI, MD
Innovative Infant Feeding Disorders Research Program, Assistant Professor of Pediatrics, Division of Neonatology, Center for Perinatal Research, Abigail Wexner Research Institute, Nationwide Children's Hospital, Department of Pediatrics, College of Medicine, The Ohio State University College of Medicine, Columbus, Ohio, USA

SHABIH U. HASAN, MD
Professor, Department of Pediatrics, Alberta Health Services, Cumming School of Medicine, Health Sciences Centre, Calgary, Alberta, Canada

KATHRYN A. HASENSTAB, BS, BME
Innovative Infant Feeding Disorders Research Program, Nationwide Children's Hospital, Center for Perinatal Research, Abigail Wexner Research Institute, Columbus, Ohio, USA

EMILY HOLLISTER, PhD
Diversigen, Inc, Vice President, Information Technology and Analytics, Houston, Texas, USA

SUDARSHAN R. JADCHERLA, MD, FRCP (Ireland), DCH, AGAF, FAAP
Professor of Pediatrics and Associate Division Chief of Neonatology, Academics, Divisions of Neonatology, Pediatric Gastroenterology, Hepatology and Nutrition, Director, The Neonatal and Infant Feeding Disorders Program, Principal Investigator, Innovative Feeding Disorders Research Program, Center for Perinatal Research, Abigail Wexner Research Institute, Nationwide Children's Hospital, Department of Pediatrics, College of Medicine, The Ohio State University College of Medicine, Columbus, Ohio, USA

ABHAY K. LODHA, MD
Associate Professor, Department of Pediatrics, Alberta Health Services, Cumming School of Medicine, Foothills Medical Centre, Calgary, Alberta, Canada

AKHIL MAHESHWARI, MD
Department of Pediatrics, Johns Hopkins School of Medicine, Baltimore, Maryland, USA

ETHAN A. MEZOFF, MD
Assistant Professor of Clinical Pediatrics, Center for Intestinal Rehabilitation and Nutrition Support, Division of Gastroenterology, Hepatology and Nutrition, Nationwide Children's Hospital, The Ohio State University College of Medicine, Columbus, Ohio, USA

PETER C. MINNECI, MD
Professor, Department of Surgery, The Ohio State University College of Medicine, Center for Surgical Outcomes Research, Abigail Wexner Research Institute, Nationwide Children's Hospital, Columbus, Ohio, USA

JOSEF NEU, MD
Professor, Director, Neonatal-Perinatal Medicine Fellowship Program, Section of Neonatology, Department of Pediatrics, University of Florida, Gainesville, Florida, USA

MOHAN PAMMI, MD, PhD
Associate Professor, Section of Neonatology, Department of Pediatrics, Baylor College of Medicine, Texas Children's Hospital, Houston, Texas, USA

RAVI MANGAL PATEL, MD, MSc
Associate Professor of Pediatrics, Division of Neonatology, Department of Pediatrics, Emory University School of Medicine, Children's Healthcare of Atlanta, Atlanta, Georgia, USA

CAROL JEAN POTTER, MD
Associate Professor of Clinical Pediatrics, Nationwide Children's Hospital, The Ohio State University, Columbus, Ohio, USA

MURALIDHAR H. PREMKUMAR, MBBS, DCH, DNB, MRCPCH, MS
Division of Neonatology, Department of Pediatrics, Baylor College of Medicine, Texas Children's Hospital, Houston, Texas, USA

RADHIKA RASTOGI, MD, MPH
Cleveland Clinic Lerner College of Medicine, Cleveland, Ohio, USA

SHANTANU RASTOGI, MD, MMM
Newborn Services, George Washington University Hospital and Children's National Medical Center, Washington, DC, USA

ALLISON THOMAS ROSE, MD
Fellow, Division of Neonatology, Department of Pediatrics, Emory University School of Medicine, Children's Healthcare of Atlanta, Atlanta, Georgia, USA

VIVEK SAROHA, MD, PhD
Assistant Professor of Pediatrics, Division of Neonatology, Department of Pediatrics, Emory University School of Medicine, Children's Healthcare of Atlanta, Atlanta, Georgia, USA

JONATHAN L. SLAUGHTER, MD, MPH
Principal Investigator, Center for Perinatal Research, Abigail Wexner Research Institute, Nationwide Children's Hospital, Assistant Professor, Department of Pediatrics, College of Medicine, Division of Epidemiology, College of Public Health, The Ohio State University, Columbus, Ohio, USA

ZAKIA SULTANA, BA
Innovative Infant Feeding Disorders Research Program, Center for Perinatal Research, Abigail Wexner Research Institute, Nationwide Children's Hospital, Columbus, Ohio, USA

SREEKANTH VISWANATHAN, MD, MS
Division of Neonatology, Department of Pediatrics, Nemours Children's Hospital, Associate Professor of Pediatrics, University of Central Florida College of Medicine, Orlando, Florida, USA

KENT C. WILLIAMS, MD
Associate Professor of Clinical Pediatrics, Division of Gastroenterology, Hepatology and Nutrition, Nationwide Children's Hospital, The Ohio State University College of Medicine, Columbus, Ohio, USA

MIRA YOUNIS, MD
Department of Neonatology, Cleveland Clinic Children's, Cleveland Clinic Lerner College
of Medicine, Cleveland, Ohio, USA

KAMRAN YUSUF, MD
Associate Professor, Department of Pediatrics, Alberta Health Services, Cumming School
of Medicine, Health Sciences Centre, Calgary, Alberta, Canada

Contents

> Aerodigestive disorders, those affecting the upper and lower airway or upper gastrointestinal tract, are interrelated anatomically during fetal development and functionally after birth. Successful respiration and feeding requires careful coordination to promote effective swallowing and prevent aspiration. I describe the epidemiology, including the prevalence of the most common aerodigestive disorders. The ability of an infant to feed by mouth at discharge, without a surgically placed feeding tube, is an important neurodevelopmental marker. Therefore, aerodigestive disorders have a high potential for lifelong morbidities and health care expenditures. When available, published research on related medical costs for these disorders is provided.

> Development of enteral and oral feeding milestones in infants is intricately linked to physiologic maturation of the gastrointestinal tract and its complex interplay with cardiorespiratory and central nervous system control and coordination. Assessment of an infant's developmental skills and maturation can guide us with targeted management approaches and prediction of feeding outcomes. In this article, we review and summarize the developmental aspects of oral feeding and swallowing physiology, and current understanding of the pathophysiological changes associated with feeding difficulties in infants.

> Gastroesophageal reflux (GER) is considered physiologic and is a normal process; whereas, when aerodigestive consequences are associated, it is often interpreted as GER disease (GERD). However, the distinction between them remains a challenge in infants in the NICU. Reflux-type of symptoms are heterogeneous, and often managed with changes in diet, feeding methods, and acid-suppressive therapy; all these empiric therapies lack objectivity; hence, practice variation is universal. We clarify the

current controversies, explain the potential role of GERD in causing symptoms and complications, and highlight current advances. The evidence basis for the diagnostic strategies is discussed.

Ish K. Gulati, Zakia Sultana, and Sudarshan R. Jadcherla

Deglutition disorders (DD) can be transient and considered as physiologic during normal maturation. However, when oral feeding milestones are impaired and bothersome symptoms and aerodigestive consequences are associated, it is interpreted as DD with varying specific entities, such as feeding difficulties, swallowing disorders, aerodigestive illness, and aspiration syndromes. Symptoms related to DD are heterogeneous and managed empirically. This article clarifies current controversies, explains the potential role of safe feeding and physiologic and pathophysiologic perspectives, and highlights current advances in the field. Evidence basis for diagnostic strategies is discussed, and involves evaluation for structure and function tests, and nutrition and feeding assessment.

Shabih U. Hasan, Abhay K. Lodha, Kamran Yusuf, and Stacey Dalgleish

In the United States, preterm birth rates have steadily increased since 2014. Despite the recent advances in neonatal-perinatal care, more than 40% of very low-birth-weight infants develop chronic lung disease (CLD) and almost 25% have feeding difficulties resulting in delayed achievement of full oral feeds and longer hospital stay. Establishment of full oral feeds, a major challenge for preterm infants, becomes magnified among those on respiratory support and/or with CLD. The strategies to minimize aerodigestive disorders include supporting nonnutritive sucking, developing infant-directed feeding protocols, sensory oromotor stimulation, and early introduction of oral feeds.

Mira Younis, Radhika Rastogi, Ankur Chugh, Shantanu Rastogi, and Hany Aly

Early diagnosis of diarrhea is critical to prevent disease progression. Diarrhea in newborns can be congenital or acquired; acquired diarrheas are the major cause in infants. Congenital diarrheal diseases are rare and include defects in digestion, absorption, and transport of nutrients, and electrolytes; disorders of enterocyte differentiation and polarization; defects of enteroendocrine cell differentiation; dysregulation of the intestinal immune response; and dysfunction of the immune system. This review discusses the clinical approach that may help in early identification and management of different congenital diarrheal diseases.

Ethan A. Mezoff, Peter C. Minneci, and Molly C. Dienhart

Pediatric intestinal failure occurs when gut function is insufficient to meet the nutrient and hydration needs of the growing child. The commonest cause is short bowel syndrome with maldigestion and malabsorption following massive bowel loss. The remnant bowel adapts during the process of intestinal rehabilitation. Management promotes the achievement of enteral autonomy while mitigating the risk of comorbid disease. The future of care is likely to see expansion of pharmacologic methods for augmenting bowel adaptation, tissue engineering techniques enabling immune suppression–free autologous bowel transplant, and the development of electronic health record tools for efficient, collaborative study and care improvement.

Liver dysfunction is a common problem in the sick premature infant. The dysfunction is usually multifactorial and often underlies a combination of liver immaturity, comorbidities, and/or the presence of primary liver disease. The liver of the preterm infant has a paucity of bile ducts, low levels of many hepatic enzymes and transporters, and a small bile acid pool. Many other organ systems are immature as well and do not respond to stress the way they would later in infancy. This articles discusses how prematurity affects the liver, how it responds to secondary insults, and approaches to evaluation.

Human milk is the most optimal source of nutrition for preterm and term infants. However, in most preterm infants, breast milk fails to meet the energy needs of the newborn infant. Overwhelming evidence supports the fortification of breast milk in preterm infants to facilitate better short-term outcomes. Several single-nutrient and multinutrient breast milk supplements and fortifiers are used to improve the macronutrient and micronutrient content of breast milk. An individualized fortification strategy has the potential to offer better results compared with standard fortification strategies. Human milk–derived fortification is promising, but the benefits in exclusively human milk–fed preterm infants are unclear.

The causes of neonatal gut injury are multifactorial and include ischemia, tissue hypoxia due to anemia, excessive inflammation, deficiency of growth factors, and food protein sensitivity. The developing intestinal microbiome plays a role in some of these forms of intestinal injury but knowledge of its relative role in each remains poorly understood. Commensal bacteria are required for normal immune development and immune tolerance. Dysbiosis in the neonatal gut that alters the patterns of commensal and pathogenic bacteria may accentuate gut injury.

PROGRAM OBJECTIVE

The goal of *Clinics in Perinatology* is to keep practicing perinatologists, neonatologists, obstetricians, practicing physicians and residents up to date with current clinical practice in perinatology by providing timely articles reviewing the state of the art in patient care.

TARGET AUDIENCE

Perinatologists, neonatologists, obstetricians, practicing physicians, residents and healthcare professionals who provide patient care utilizing findings from *Clinics in Perinatology*.

LEARNING OBJECTIVES

Upon completion of this activity, participants will be able to:

1. Review the physiology and pathophysiology of the aerodigestive and gastrointestinal systems in the premature infant.
2. Discuss evidence-based diagnostic strategies and potential opportunities for further research and novel therapies in neonatal gastroenterological problems.
3. Recognize key principles of providing cutting-edge, evidence-based, optimal nutrition into clinical practice.

ACCREDITATION

The Elsevier Office of Continuing Medical Education (EOCME) is accredited by the Accreditation Council for Continuing Medical Education (ACCME) to provide continuing medical education for physicians.

The EOCME designates this journal-based CME activity for a maximum of 13 *AMA PRA Category 1 Credit(s)*™. Physicians should claim only the credit commensurate with the extent of their participation in the activity.

All other health care professionals requesting continuing education credit for this enduring material will be issued a certificate of participation.

DISCLOSURE OF CONFLICTS OF INTEREST

The EOCME assesses conflict of interest with its instructors, faculty, planners, and other individuals who are in a position to control the content of CME activities. All relevant conflicts of interest that are identified are thoroughly vetted by EOCME for fair balance, scientific objectivity, and patient care recommendations. EOCME is committed to providing its learners with CME activities that promote improvements or quality in healthcare and not a specific proprietary business or a commercial interest.

The planning committee, staff, authors and editors listed below have identified no financial relationships or relationships to products or devices they or their spouse/life partner have with commercial interest related to the content of this CME activity:

Hany Aly, MD; Diane M. Anderson, PhD, RD, LD; Ankur Chugh, MD; Stacey Dalgleish, RN, MN, NNP; Isabelle G. De Plaen, MD; Molly C. Dienhart, MD; Steven H. Erdman, MD; Ganga Gokulakrishnan, MD, MS; Ish K. Gulati, MD; Shabih U. Hasan, MD; Kathryn A. Hasenstab, BS, BME; Kerry Holland; Emily Hollister, PhD; Sudarshan Jadcherla, MD; Lucky Jain; Marilu Kelly, MSN, RN, CNE, CHCP; Abhay K. Lodha, MD; Akhil Maheshwari, MD; L. Adriana Massieu, RD, LD, CNSC; Ethan A. Mezoff, MD; Peter C. Minneci, MD; Swaminathan Nagarajan; Josef Neu, MD; Mohan Pammi, MD, PhD; Ravi Mangal Patel, MD, MSc; C.J. Potter, MD; Radhika Rastogi, BA; Shantanu Rastogi, MD; Allison Thomas Rose, MD; Vivek Saroha, MD, PhD; Jonathan L. Slaughter, MD, MPH; Zakia Sultana, BA; Sreekanth Viswanathan, MD, MS; Kent C. Williams, MD; Mira Younis, MD; Kamran Yusuf, MD

The planning committee, staff, authors and editors listed below have identified financial relationships or relationships to products or devices they or their spouse/life partner have with commercial interest related to the content of this CME activity:

Muralidhar H. Premkumar, MBBS, DCH, DNB, MRCPCH, MS: consultant/advisor for Fresenius Kabi Deutschland GmbH

UNAPPROVED/OFF-LABEL USE DISCLOSURE

The EOCME requires CME faculty to disclose to the participants:

1. When products or procedures being discussed are off-label, unlabelled, experimental, and/or investigational (not US Food and Drug Administration [FDA] approved); and
2. Any limitations on the information presented, such as data that are preliminary or that represent ongoing research, interim analyses, and/or unsupported opinions. Faculty may discuss information about

pharmaceutical agents that is outside of FDA-approved labelling. This information is intended solely for CME and is not intended to promote off-label use of these medications. If you have any questions, contact the medical affairs department of the manufacturer for the most recent prescribing information.

TO ENROLL
To enroll in the *Clinics in Perinatology* Continuing Medical Education program, call customer service at 1-800-654-2452 or sign up online at http://www.theclinics.com/home/cme. The CME program is available to subscribers for an additional annual fee of USD 245.00.

METHOD OF PARTICIPATION
In order to claim credit, participants must complete the following:
1. Complete enrolment as indicated above.
2. Read the activity.
3. Complete the CME Test and Evaluation. Participants must achieve a score of 70% on the test. All CME Tests and Evaluations must be completed online.

CME INQUIRIES/SPECIAL NEEDS
For all CME inquiries or special needs, please contact elsevierCME@elsevier.com.

CLINICS IN PERINATOLOGY

SERIES OF RELATED INTEREST

Obstetrics and Gynecology Clinics of North America
https://www.obgyn.theclinics.com/

THE CLINICS ARE AVAILABLE ONLINE!
Access your subscription at:
www.theclinics.com

Foreword

Why Our Gastrointestinal Tract Is So Important

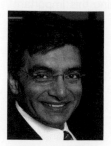

Lucky Jain, MD
Consulting Editor

It is hard to overstate the importance of our gut and the multiple physiologic functions it manages, particularly in the neonatal period. In fact, long-term outcomes are directly connected to optimal nutrition and gut function in the first few years after birth.[1] In a Foreword written several years ago, I had quoted Anthelme Brillat-Savarin's words of wisdom from nearly 300 years ago, *"Tell me what you eat and I will tell you what you are."*[2] Science continues to validate the truth and science behind this statement with an open challenge to us all: *"If we are what we eat, then our babies are what we feed them!"*[2]

Separating the contributions of the *food* and *feeding* has been difficult. Proponents of breast-feeding claim that it is not just the breast milk, but also the act of feeding at the breast that has significant effects on mental/behavioral health and cognition of the growing infant, even though underlying neurobiological mechanisms are difficult to elucidate.[3] This issue is further complicated by the fact that babies with neurologic problems to begin with have a hard time establishing oral feeds. Feeding difficulties and dysphagia are often the first signs of significant neurologic injury. Regardless, studies show that successful breast-feeding experience in early life is associated with improved intelligence, language skills, and memory.[4,5] Consistent with these findings, maternal separation has been shown to be associated with neonatal intestinal injury.[6]

There is also considerable new evidence supporting the existence of a gut-brain axis and the role intestinal dysbiosis plays in pathogenesis of inflammatory bowel disease, obesity, and neurodevelopmental disorders in adults.[7] The presence of such a link is intertwined with multiple events at birth and involves a complex interaction of microbiome, the hypothalamic-pituitary axis, and the autonomic nervous system.

Indeed, as you will read in this issue of the *Clinics in Perinatology*, high-risk neonates encounter considerable feeding difficulties once they emerge from their initial

Clin Perinatol 47 (2020) xv–xvi
https://doi.org/10.1016/j.clp.2020.04.003
0095-5108/20/© 2020 Published by Elsevier Inc.

perinatology.theclinics.com

challenges of prematurity, birthing issues, or surgical complications. These include poor coordination of sucking and swallowing, gastroesophageal reflux disease, malabsorption syndromes, and necrotizing enterocolitis to name just a few.

These topics have been covered in great depth in this issue of the *Clinics in Perinatology* edited by Dr Jadcherla. Authors also point to the need for more research into feeding dynamics and physiology of the developing gastrointestinal tract. As always, I am grateful to the publishing staff at Elsevier, including Kerry Holland, Casey Potter, and Nicholas Henderson, for their support in bringing this important publication to you.

Lucky Jain, MD
Emory University School of Medicine, and Children's Healthcare of Atlanta
2015 Uppergate Drive NE
Atlanta, GA 30322, USA

E-mail address:
ljain@emory.edu

REFERENCES

1. Geogieff MK, Ramel SE, Cusick SE. Nutritional influences on brain development. Acta Paediatr 2018;107:1310–21.
2. Jain L. Our babies are what we feed them. Clin Perinatol 2014;41:xv–xvii.
3. Krol KM, Grossmann T. Psychological effects of breastfeeding on children and mothers. Bundesgesundheitsbl 2018;61:977–85.
4. Mortensen EL, Michaelsen KF, Sanders SA, et al. The association between duration of breastfeeding and adult intelligence. JAMA 2002;287:2365–71.
5. Raju TN. Breastfeeding is a dynamic biologic process—not simply a meal at the breast. Breastfeeding Med 2011;6:257–9.
6. Li B, Yu FZ, Munich A, et al. Neonatal intestinal injury induced by maternal separation: pathogenesis and pharmacological targets. Can J Physiol Pharmacol 2019; 97:193–6.
7. Sherman MP, Zaghouani H, Niklas V. Gut microbiota, the immune system, and diet influence the neonatal gut-brain axis. Pediatr Res 2015;77:127–35.

Preface

Neonatal Gastroenterology: Challenges, Controversies, and Recent Advances

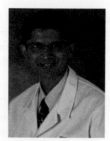

Sudarshan R. Jadcherla, MD, FRCP (Ireland), DCH, AGAF, FAAP
Editor

Neonatal research has clearly shown that diagnostic precision and rational management of neonatal feeding and gastroenterologic issues improve long-term growth and development of neonatal intensive care unit (NICU) survivors. The application of technological advances has and will continue to improve survival rates among neonates, albeit with the consequences of prolonged hospitalization, chronic morbidities, parental stress, and increased health care burden. A major determinant of long-term morbidity and function in infants is their aerodigestive quality of life, which defines the overall quality of life not only in these infants but also in their parents. This is now a global problem (ie, not only multisystemic, but also a growing worldwide concern).

Maturational pathophysiology changes rapidly, thereby challenging us to develop innovative management strategies. Providing optimal nutrition is a complex process and cutting-edge research is now informing ways to implement these principles into clinical practice. Although new evidence is emerging, overcoming myths and controversies is a challenging task. In this issue of the *Clinics in Perinatology*, we bring to forefront current controversies in this field and discuss evidence-based diagnostic strategies and potential opportunities for further research and novel therapies. We clarify the physiology and pathophysiology of the aerodigestive and gastrointestinal systems and their inextricable interrelationships in the premature infant.

Given this setting, this issue of the *Clinics in Perinatology* highlights the pathophysiologic basis of the commonly confronted neonatal gastroenterologic problems in the NICU. We clarified myths and developed potentially implementable "best practices" so that they are readily available to our readers. Each of the authors is eminent in their

Clin Perinatol 47 (2020) xvii–xviii
https://doi.org/10.1016/j.clp.2020.04.002
0095-5108/20/© 2020 Published by Elsevier Inc.

field, and their expertise in their respective clinically aligned topics will bring forth the latest and the best in this issue.

Finally, it is relevant to note that the current practices in the care of convalescing infants with aerodigestive and gastrointestinal problems require the neonatologist to be the team leader directing personalized and well-coordinated interdisciplinary care, rather than the multitude of consultants and experts driving multiple care plans in parallel. To this effect, the authors have done a tremendous job in discussing physiology, pathophysiology, and objective-evidence basis for treatment, all of which can be helpful at disseminating knowledge at cribside rounds. In that way, vertical transfer of true knowledge will happen at a faster pace.

I dedicate this issue *to my parents*, Mrs Kamala B. Jadcherla and Mr Rameshwar R. Jadcherla, for instilling in me to teach what has been taught to me, and *to my mentors*, Professors Brendan Drumm, Thomas N. Hansen, Carol Lynn Berseth, Reza Shaker, and Sree Aswath, for giving me the opportunity to learn and create new knowledge and look for innovative opportunities in serving others.

Sudarshan R. Jadcherla, MD, FRCP (Ireland), DCH, AGAF, FAAP
Divisions of Neonatology, Pediatric
Gastroenterology, and Nutrition
The Neonatal and Infant
Feeding Disorders Program
Innovative Feeding Disorders
Research Program
Center for Perinatal Research
WB 5211
The Research Institute at
Nationwide Children's Hospital
575 Children's Cross Roads
Columbus, OH 43215, USA

E-mail address:
Sudarshan.Jadcherla@Nationwidechildrens.org

Neonatal Aerodigestive Disorders
Epidemiology and Economic Burden

Jonathan L. Slaughter, MD, MPH[a,b,c],*

KEYWORDS

- Aerodigestive disorders • Aspiration • Cost • Dysphasia • Epidemiology
- Esophageal atresia • Gastroesophageal reflux disease • Neonate

KEY POINTS

- Disorders of the upper and lower airway and the upper gastrointestinal tract are related developmentally and functionally, since successful swallowing and respiration requires precise coordination.
- The epidemiology of many neonatal aerodigestive disorders, including their prevalence and the effectiveness and cost-effectiveness of potential treatments, is not fully characterized.
- Epidemiology and comparative effectiveness research, including pragmatic clinical trials, is important to drive health care policy and improve outcomes for infants with aerodigestive disorders.

INTRODUCTION
Prevalence and Epidemiology of Neonatal Aerodigestive Disorders

The airway and upper gastrointestinal tract are intimately connected, not only during fetal development but also during postnatal coordination of function.[1,2] Disorders of either the airway or the upper digestive tract often impact both feeding and breathing, since successful swallowing requires coordination between the two. Given limited evidence on the prevalence of aerodigestive disorders, this review focuses on the most common anomalies and functional disorders seen in neonates. Rare anomalies (≤2 in 100,000 infants) (eg, laryngeal clefts, subglottic hemangiomas, tracheal agenesis, congenital esophageal stricture) are excluded.

[a] Center for Perinatal Research, Abigail Wexner Research Institute at Nationwide Children's Hospital, Columbus, OH, USA; [b] Division of Neonatology, Department of Pediatrics, College of Medicine, The Ohio State University, Columbus, OH, USA; [c] Division of Epidemiology, College of Public Health, The Ohio State University, Columbus, OH, USA
* Nationwide Children's Hospital, Center for Perinatal Research, Research 3 Building, 5th floor, 575 Children's Crossroad, Columbus, OH 43215.
E-mail address: jonathan.slaughter@nationwidechildrens.org
Twitter: @JonathanLSlaug1 (J.L.S.)

Clin Perinatol 47 (2020) 211–222
https://doi.org/10.1016/j.clp.2020.02.003
0095-5108/20/© 2020 Elsevier Inc. All rights reserved.

perinatology.theclinics.com

Overall Economic Impact

The ability of a hospitalized infant to feed by mouth at discharge without dependence on a surgically placed gastrostomy tube is an important marker of neurodevelopmental prognosis.[3] Not only do aerodigestive disorders have treatment costs, including surgery and/or rehabilitation, but also an impact on costs related to hospital length of stay and lifelong morbidities. Cost data are important to payers and for policymakers as they determine the best means to distribute resources with a goal of improving the outcomes and well-being of infants afflicted with aerodigestive disorders. Although studies are not available on the economic impacts of many neonatal aerodigestive disorders, we include published cost estimates when able.

NASOPHARYNX AND OROPHARYNX
Choanal Atresia

The prevalence of choanal atresia, a congenital blockage of the back of the nasal passages, has been estimated at 0.82/10,000 and varies slightly between geographic locations,[4] with equal sex and race distributions.[4] There is also an equal distribution between unilateral and bilateral instances of choanal atresia.[5] When unilateral, the occlusion occurs equally in the left and right nares.[4,5] Associated malformations are present in approximately one-half of infants with choanal atresia, of which CHARGE (coloboma, heart defect, atresia choanae, retarded growth, genitourinary abnormalities, and ear anomalies) syndrome is the most common (~26%).[4,5] However, when choanal atresia is bilateral, 98% of cases are associated with specific disorders or multiple congenital anomalies. Although the full cost of choanal atresia is difficult to estimate, the 2013 weighted, median inpatient hospitalization costs were estimated at $15,000 to $20,000.[6]

Orofacial Clefts (Cleft Lip and Cleft Palate)

Cleft lips and palates occur when tissues forming the lips and palate, respectively, do not fuse properly during the first trimester. Cleft lip, with an adjusted prevalence of 10.63 (95% CI, 10.32–10.95) per 10,000 US live births, or 1 in 940 live births, was the second most common birth defect, after Trisomy 21, identified by the US Centers for Disease Control (CDC).[7] When international data were recently compiled by Tanaka and colleagues,[8] the average global prevalence of cleft lip, with or without cleft palate, was 7.94 per 10,000 live births. The CDC reported prevalence of cleft palate without cleft lip is 6.35 (95% CI, 6.11–6.60) per 10,000 US live births or 1 in 1574.[7]

The causes of orofacial clefts are not fully known. These lesions are most commonly nonsyndromic, but their causes are considered to be multifactorial.[9] Race is the only demographic variable that has been consistently associated with cleft lip. The prevalence is higher in those of Asian descent and lower in individuals of African descent relative to Whites. These differences in prevalence have persisted after global population relocations, indicating a genetic rather than environmental cause.[9,10]

Environmental exposures associated with orofacial clefts include:

1. Maternal tobacco smoking (maternal smoking and cleft lip with or without cleft palate [relative risk = 1.34; 95% CI, 1.25–1.44]) (maternal smoking and cleft palate [relative risk = 1.22; 95% CI, 1.10–1.35]) with a modest dose-effect.[11,12]
2. Pregestational and gestational diabetes mellitus (DM) (isolated cleft lip with or without cleft palate and pregestational DM [adjusted odds ratio (aOR) = 2.92; 95% CI, 1.45–5.87]) (isolated cleft lip with or without cleft palate and gestational DM [aOR = 1.45; 95% CI, 1.03–2.04]) (isolated cleft palate and pregestational

DM [aOR = 1.80; 95% CI, 0.67–4.87]) (isolated cleft palate and gestational DM [aOR = 1.54; 95% CI, 1.01–2.37]).[13]

3. Epileptic medications, including topiramate[14,15] and valproic acid[16] during pregnancy.

Children 10 years old and younger with an orofacial cleft have an annual, estimated, incremental mean medical cost difference that is $13,405 (2004 US dollars [USD]) higher than in unaffected children.[17] Total median medical costs were approximately 8 times higher for ≤10-year-old children with an orofacial cleft.[17]

Tongue Disorders

This section focuses on 3 of the most commonly diagnosed congenital tongue disorders. Macroglossia, an abnormal enlargement of the tongue, occurs in approximately 4.63 per 100,000 births with a roughly 50:50 split between isolated cases and those that are part of a syndrome.[18] Beckwith-Wiedemann syndrome, a congenital disorder consisting of macroglossia, macrosomia, hemihypertrophy, abdominal wall defects, and hypoglycemia, is the disorder most commonly associated with macroglossia (identified in ~46% of syndromic patients).[19] Isolated, but not syndromic, macroglossia is more common in females (aOR = 1.93; 95% CI, 1.45–2.56) and in African Americans (aOR = 2.02; 95% CI, 1.41–2.88) relative to Whites.[18] Macroglossia is associated with a high likelihood of feeding and respiratory problems. Isolated macroglossia has been found to increase average length of stay by 4.07 days (95% CI, 0.42–7.72 days) at an average cost of $6207 (95% CI, $576–$11,838) (2003–2012 USD) compared with 12.02 days (95% CI, 3.63–20.4 days) and a cost of $17,205 (95% CI, $374–34,035) in syndromic patients.[18]

Glossoptosis, the posterior displacement or retraction of the tongue toward the pharynx, causes airway obstruction. Glossoptosis most commonly occurs in syndromes, including Pierre Robin sequence (described with micrognathia below) and Trisomy 21.[20,21] In a small MRI study, glossoptosis was diagnosed in 63% of children with Trisomy 21 who had persistent obstructive sleep apnea despite tonsillectomy and adenoidectomy.[20]

Ankyloglossia, commonly known as tongue-tie, is the presence of an unusually short, thick, or tight lingual frenulum that restricts tongue movement and may inhibit both feeding and speech. The reported prevalence of ankyloglossia varies widely by geographic region, ranging from 0.5% to 12% of infants and diagnosis and treatment via frenectomy has increased markedly in recent years.[22–24] The lack of firm diagnostic criteria for ankyloglossia diagnosis and treatment is thought to be a cause for this diagnostic imprecision.[22]

Micrognathia (Mandibular Hypoplasia)

Micrognathia, also referred to as mandibular hypoplasia, is an undersized jaw (mandible or maxilla).[25] Its prevalence is estimated at 1 per 1500 live births.[26] Even when presenting as an isolated diagnosis on prenatal ultrasound, additional anomalies, including orofacial clefts are found postnatally in most infants.[26] Micrognathia occurs in multiple syndromes, including, but not limited to, Pierre Robin sequence, Smith-Lemli-Opitz syndrome, Cornelia De Lange syndrome, ear-patella-short stature syndrome, Catel-Manzke syndrome, Stickler syndrome, Treacher Collins syndrome, and Ehlers-Danlos syndrome.[26]

The Pierre Robin sequence is the combination of micrognathia, glossoptosis, and airway obstruction with associated neonatal respiratory distress. Its prevalence has been reported to be between 0.71 and 3.2 per 10,000 live births.[27–29] Prevalence varies regionally and is roughly twice as common in Whites relative to persons of African descent.[27] Within the United States, the estimated birth prevalence of isolated Pierre Robin sequence is 1.8 per 10,000 live births and the prevalence of syndrome-associated Pierre Robin sequence is 1.4 per 10,000 live births.[27]

SUPRAGLOTTIC/GLOTTIC/SUBGLOTTIC
Dysphagia (Swallowing Problems)

The exact, overall prevalence of neonatal dysphagia is unknown.[2,30] However, various estimates from various neonatal populations demonstrate that dysphagia is an important problem.[1] In a population-wide, self-completed questionnaire, parents of 14,138 live born children reported that 18% of their infants had a weak suck, 55% had experienced choking, and 1% had great feeding difficulties at 4 weeks postnatal.[31] Preterm birth is a major cause of neonatal dysphagia, in addition to congenital anomalies and infection.[32] In the same population-wide survey, parents reported that 17.9% of infants who had persistent feeding problems at age 15 months were born before 37 weeks gestation.[31] Neurodevelopmental delays, including cerebral palsy, increase with decreasing birth gestation. As more extremely preterm infants (born as early as 22–23 weeks gestation) continue to survive, both neurodevelopmental delays and associated dysphagia are increasing.[30,33] Although most infants of less than 28-week gestation achieve oral feeding skills by 36 to 38 weeks postmenstrual age, onset of oral feeding is significantly delayed, prolonging hospitalization and increasing associated costs.[33]

Aspiration of Feeds

Aspiration is the abnormal entry of feeds, secretions, or others substances into the airway. Although most term infants with aspiration have cerebral palsy (reported in 71% of aspirating term infants at 1 major academic children's hospital)[34] or other neurologic or structural causes,[35] aspiration leading to respiratory symptoms can occur in neurologically and structurally normal term infants (11%–13% of infants referred for video swallow evaluation).[34,36] Similar to many other aerodigestive disorders, preterm birth is a leading cause of aspiration, and a swallowing disorder and/or aspiration was identified in 28% of infants referred for fluoroscopic swallow evaluation at 1 pediatric academic center.[2,34,35]

Laryngomalacia

Laryngomalacia, a congenital anomaly in which the larynx is floppy and deviates into and partially obstructs the airway during inspiration due to a decrease in extrathoracic pressure, is reported in the pediatric otorhinolaryngology literature as the most common congenital laryngeal disorder (35%–75%)[37–39] and the most common cause of stridor in neonates,[40] although its exact prevalence in the overall neonatal population is not well documented. Within large, case series investigations, pediatric patients with laryngomalacia commonly presented with stridor (64%)[41] and swallowing dysfunction (11% in 1 study[41] and 50% in another[42]). These 2 presentations predominated in young infants (stridor as presenting symptom: mean age of diagnosis, 3.5 months; standard deviation [SD], 2.8) (swallowing dysfunction as presenting symptom: mean age, 4.8 months; SD, 4.6).[41] In most patients, laryngomalacia will improve by age 18 to 24 months.[38,43,44] Surgical treatment is only necessary in less than 10% of patients.[38]

Vocal Cord Paralysis

Paralysis of the vocal cords, usually bilateral (44%),[45] is the second most common congenital laryngeal anomaly (~30%)[39] and the second most common cause of neonatal stridor.[37,40] Bilateral vocal cord is usually idiopathic but can be associated with central nervous system disorders, including Arnold-Chiari malformation, cerebral palsy, hydrocephalus, myelomeningocele, spina bifida, and after an hypoxic-ischemic event.[37] Acquired vocal cord paralysis can occur after birth trauma,[45] but is usually left-sided (71%)[46] and discovered postoperatively after damage to the left recurrent laryngeal nerve during congenital heart surgeries involving the aortic arch (21%–27% vs 1%–4% when the aortic arch is not involved)[47,48] or patent ductus arteriosus ligation (9%–17% overall;[49,50] 40% in extremely low-birth-weight [<1000 g birth weight] infants),[51] or during esophageal surgeries, including esophageal atresia and tracheoesophageal fistula repair (3%).[40,52]

Subglottic Stenosis

The prevalence of congenital subglottic stenosis is not well reported, although it was reported to be responsible for 30.9% of congenital laryngeal anomalies at a single center[39] and has also been described as the third most common laryngeal disorder.[37] It is most commonly associated with syndromes, including Trisomy 21, CHARGE, and 22q11 deletion.[53,54] Acquired subglottic stenosis is the most common form of subglottic stenosis and has been reported to be the most common acquired laryngeal disorder.[53] Intubation is the most common cause, with 1 center reporting an intubation history in 90% of cases.[55] Two single-center studies in the 1990s[56,57] and a recent case-control study[58] have reported a <1% incidence of acquired subglottic stenosis in intubated neonates. Extreme prematurity is thought to increase acquired subglottic stenosis risk, although this has not been firmly established.[58,59] A small case-control study conducted between 2006 and 2014 found that a Sherman ratio (endotracheal tube internal diameter [millimeters]/gestational age)[60] greater than 0.1 (aOR = 6.40; 95% CI, 1.65–24.77), more than 5 previous intubations (aOR = 3.74; 95% CI, 1.15–12.19), and traumatic intubation (aOR = 3.37; 95% CI, 1.01–11.26), were risk factors for severe acquired subglottic stenosis requiring surgical intervention.[58]

TRACHEAL
Tracheal Stenosis

Tracheal stenosis is a narrowing of the tracheal lumen. The population-based incidence of congenital tracheal stenosis was estimated to be 1 per 64,500 live births at 1 major Canadian academic hospital between 1964 and 2006.[61] Congenital tracheal stenosis is usually associated with other anomalies. The isolated form, without any associated malformations, only presents in 10% to 25% of infants.[61,62] Associated cardiovascular anomalies, including vascular slings or rings (vascular encirclement of the trachea and/or esophagus by aberrant or anomalous vessels) that compress the airway are common and reported to occur in up to 50% of patients.[63] Additional reported anomalies include cardiovascular (left pulmonary artery sling, patent ductus arteriosus, ventricular septal defects, double aortic arch, aberrant subclavian artery), respiratory (pulmonary agenesis or hypoplasia, tracheal bronchus), and those involving the gastrointestinal, renal, skeletal systems.[61]

Congenital Lower Airway Malacia (Tracheomalacia, Tracheobronchomalacia, and Bronchomalacia)

Malacia of the trachea and bronchi is a softening due to cartilage abnormalities. Collapse of the trachea and/or bronchi occurs during expiration as intrathoracic pressure is increased. Tracheomalacia is isolated to the trachea, bronchomalacia to the bronchi (may be bilateral or unilateral),[64] and tracheobronchomalacia is the term when both the trachea and bronchi are involved.[65] Malacia of the trachea and bronchi is seen frequently and congenital tracheomalacia is the most common congenital tracheal abnormality.[66] Within a 7-year period, at least a 1 in 2100 incidence of congenital (primary) airway malacia was estimated by 1 major children's hospital within the Netherlands, when they extrapolated their findings from children with symptoms severe enough to be referred for bronchoscopy to the general regional population.[64] The same study reported tracheomalacia in 46%, tracheobronchomalacia in 36%, and bronchomalacia in 18%.[64] Lower airway malacia may be isolated, but is commonly associated with congenital cartilage abnormalities, tracheoesophageal fistula, congenital syndromes, including CHARGE and VACTERL (vertebral defects, anal atresia, cardiac, tracheoesophageal fistula, renal, and limb defects), prolonged intubation, or compression from external lesions (vascular ring, pectus excavatum, teratoma, hemangioma, or bronchogenic cysts).[64,65] Acquired (secondary) tracheomalacia, ~15% of cases,[67] occurs after a traumatic insult to a normally developed trachea.[66] Some potential causes include tracheotomy, external compression, infection, and inflammation.[66] Preterm birth-associated chronic lung disease is also associated with tracheobronchomalacia development. A cohort study inclusive of referral neonatal intensive care units within many major children's hospitals in the United States found that 36% of infants with bronchopulmonary dysplasia had tracheobronchomalacia.[67]

TRACHEOESOPHAGEAL
Tracheoesophageal Fistula and Esophageal Atresia

Tracheoesophageal fistula, an abnormal communication between the trachea and the esophagus, and esophageal atresia, in which a portion of the esophagus ends in a blind pouch, frequently occur together[68] (72.2% of esophageal atresia cases have an associated tracheoesophageal fistula).[69] Esophageal atresia and tracheoesophageal fistula are the most common major structural birth defects affecting the esophagus and the trachea with an estimated birth prevalence ranging from 2.1 to 2.8 per 10,000 births.[70,71] By far, the most common type is esophageal atresia with a distal tracheoesophageal fistula (fistula between the lower pouch of the esophagus and the trachea), which occurs in 86% to 89% of patients with esophageal atresia.[72,73] Esophageal atresia and tracheoesophageal fistula have remained stable over time, although the exact prevalence may vary slightly between regions.[69,72,74–76] They are associated with additional malformations in ~50% of cases, the most common of which is VACTERL Association (10%),[69] and they are associated specifically with chromosomal disorders in ~10% of affected infants.[73] A large cohort investigation estimated the median hospital cost per esophageal atresia/tracheoesophageal fistula case to be $106,673 (2015 USD), although the cost was found to vary widely between children's hospitals.[77]

ESOPHAGEAL
Gastroesophageal Reflux Disease

Gastroesophageal reflux (GER), the retrograde passage of gastric contents into the esophagus, is a normal physiologic event in neonates and occurs in all infants.[78,79] The primary mechanism of neonatal gastroesophageal reflux is transient lower esophageal sphincter relaxation.[78] GER disease (GERD) occurs when the reflux is pathologic and causes clinical symptoms.[78] However, the exact prevalence of neonatal GERD is difficult to determine because many symptoms of pathologic GER-related disease are nonspecific. These include gastrointestinal symptoms (regurgitation/spitting up milk/emesis, abdominal distension), swallowing problems, feeding problems, choking spells, bradycardia/apnea spells, and increased irritability (back arching, crying, grimacing).[80] Nonetheless, neonatal clinicians frequently make a subjective clinical diagnosis of GERD (presumed GERD) without physiologic testing.[81,82] A cohort investigation using billing records from preterm infants ($\leq$36 weeks gestation) at 33 freestanding children's hospital neonatal intensive care units within the United States found that 10% were diagnosed with GERD. However, a 13-fold variation (2%–26%) in GERD diagnosis between institutions provided evidence of diagnostic subjectivity and imprecision.[83]

Recently, pH-impedance probe testing of infants with presumed GERD, based on subjective clinical symptoms alone, demonstrated that acid reflux index (ARI) severity grade was unrelated to reported clinical symptoms (ARI < 3 [normal], 18%; ARI 3–7 [intermediate GER], 17%; ARI >7, 16% [severe acid-GERD]; P = 1.0).[84] In addition, the same research team found that air boluses[85] and refluxate volume[84] can be linked to GERD-attributable clinical symptoms. To ultimately determine the true prevalence of GERD within preterm infants and the neonatal population at large, researchers will need to first document, via pH-impedance testing within the subset of the overall population presenting with the nonspecific symptoms attributed to GERD, the proportion of infants with true pathologic GERD.

Preterm infants diagnosed with GERD have a 1-month average increase in postnatal hospitalization and an estimated care cost increase of $70,000 (2010 USD).[83] Because most hospitalized neonates diagnosed and treated for GERD continue to be treated at discharge (75% of those ever treated with a proton pump inhibitor [PPI] remained on the PPI at discharge) (52% ever treated with an histamine-2 receptor antagonist [H2RA] remained on an H2RA at discharge)[82] overall costs of GERD treatment likely continue to accumulate after discharge. Given the imprecision of current clinical GERD diagnoses, as noted above, the potential to reduce future GERD-related treatment costs through more precise, physiologic diagnosis of GERD via pH-impedance probe testing, is strong. Identifying the small subset of patients in whom ARI and clinical symptoms correlate would reduce misdiagnosis of acid-mediated GERD in the vast majority of infants who are currently treated based on subjective, nonspecific clinical symptoms alone. Thus, unnecessary and potentially harmful acid-suppressive treatment would be avoided.[78,82] Identification of, via randomized trials, the effectiveness of acid-suppressive treatment in the small subset of infants whose acid reflux is correlated with their clinical symptoms, is a worthy research goal.

SUMMARY

The epidemiology of many neonatal aerodigestive disorders, including their prevalence, is not fully characterized. Therefore, there is a clear need for studies that identify the prevalence of various aerodigestive disorders (both anomalies requiring surgical repair and functional symptoms requiring therapy and rehabilitation) in the current era of neonatal intensive care, in which the survival of extremely preterm infants and those with severe genetic and neurologic impairments is increasing.

The conduits of milk from the oropharynx to the stomach, and of air from the nasopharynx and oropharynx to the lungs, are interrelated; disorders of any of these pathways may have a negative effect on swallowing, feeding, and respiration (avoidance of aspiration). Future research to determine the exact prevalence of neonatal aerodigestive disorders, and the effectiveness and cost-effectiveness of potential treatments, is important to drive health care policy and improve the outcomes of infants with these disorders.

DISCLOSURE

The author has no commercial or financial conflicts of interest to disclose. The author is funded by the National Heart, Lung, and Blood Institute of the US National Institutes of Health (R03HL140272) (R01HL145032). However, that funding is unrelated to the topic of this article and did not contribute to this work product.

Best Practices

What is the current practice for aerodigestive disorders?

Treatment of aerodigestive disorders varies depending on the specific disorder. Surgical repair of congenital anomalies is frequently needed. Personalized diagnostic, therapeutic, and rehabilitative treatments exist to treat functional disorders, including dysphagia, aspiration, and gastroesophageal reflux disease (GERD).

What changes in current practice are likely to improve outcomes?

Major Recommendations:
1. Improved characterization of the prevalence of various aerodigestive disorders (both anomalies requiring surgical repair and functional symptoms requiring personalized therapy and rehabilitation)
2. Physiologic diagnosis of GERD via pH-impedance probe testing rather than subjective diagnoses based on nonspecific clinical symptoms
3. Research to evaluate the comparative effectiveness and cost-effectiveness of treatments for aerodigestive disorders
4. Pragmatic trials to establish whether targeted treatment of the small subsets infants with true GERD, as physiologically diagnosed by pH-impedance probe testing, is effective

Rating for the Strength of the Evidence

Weak. There is a great need for evidence to establish the effectiveness and cost-effectiveness of treatments for aerodigestive disorders

Bibliographic Source(s): *Data from* Refs.[1–3,84,85]

REFERENCES

1. Jadcherla SR. Challenges to eating, swallowing, and aerodigestive functions in infants: a burning platform that needs attention! J Pediatr 2019;211:7–9.
2. Jadcherla SR. Advances with neonatal aerodigestive science in the pursuit of safe swallowing in infants: invited review. Dysphagia 2017;32(1):15–26.
3. Jadcherla SR, Khot T, Moore R, et al. Feeding methods at discharge predict long-term feeding and neurodevelopmental outcomes in preterm infants referred for gastrostomy evaluation. J Pediatr 2017;181:125–30.e1.
4. Harris J, Robert E, Källén B. Epidemiology of choanal atresia with special reference to the CHARGE association. Pediatrics 1997;99(3):363–7.
5. Burrow TA, Saal HM, de Alarcon A, et al. Characterization of congenital anomalies in individuals with choanal atresia. Arch Otolaryngol Head Neck Surg 2009; 135(6):543–7.
6. Arth AC, Tinker SC, Simeone RM, et al. Inpatient hospitalization costs associated with birth defects among persons of all ages - United States, 2013. MMWR Morb Mortal Wkly Rep 2017;66(2):41–6.
7. Parker SE, Mai CT, Canfield MA, et al. Updated national birth prevalence estimates for selected birth defects in the United States, 2004-2006. Birth Defects Res A Clin Mol Teratol 2010;88(12):1008–16.

8. Tanaka SA, Mahabir RC, Jupiter DC, et al. Updating the epidemiology of cleft lip with or without cleft palate. Plast Reconstr Surg 2012;129(3):511e–8e.
9. Mitchell LE. Genetic epidemiology of birth defects: nonsyndromic cleft lip and neural tube defects. Epidemiol Rev 1997;19(1):61–8.
10. Leck I. The geographical distribution of neural tube defects and oral clefts. Br Med Bull 1984;40(4):390–5.
11. Little J, Cardy A, Munger RG. Tobacco smoking and oral clefts: a meta-analysis. Bull World Health Organ 2004;82(3):213–8.
12. Honein MA, Rasmussen SA, Reefhuis J, et al. Maternal smoking and environmental tobacco smoke exposure and the risk of orofacial clefts. Epidemiology 2007;18(2):226–33.
13. Correa A, Gilboa SM, Besser LM, et al. Diabetes mellitus and birth defects. Am J Obstet Gynecol 2008;199(3):237.e1-9.
14. Margulis AV, Mitchell AA, Gilboa SM, et al. Use of topiramate in pregnancy and risk of oral clefts. Am J Obstet Gynecol 2012;207(5):405.e1-7.
15. Hernandez-Diaz S, Huybrechts KF, Desai RJ, et al. Topiramate use early in pregnancy and the risk of oral clefts: a pregnancy cohort study. Neurology 2018;90(4): e342–51.
16. Werler MM, Ahrens KA, Bosco JL, et al. Use of antiepileptic medications in pregnancy in relation to risks of birth defects. Ann Epidemiol 2011;21(11):842–50.
17. Boulet SL, Grosse SD, Honein MA, et al. Children with orofacial clefts: health-care use and costs among a privately insured population. Public Health Rep 2009; 124(3):447–53.
18. Simmonds JC, Patel AK, Mildenhall NR, et al. Neonatal macroglossia: demographics, cost of care, and associated comorbidities. Cleft Palate Craniofac J 2018;55(8):1122–9.
19. Prada CE, Zarate YA, Hopkin RJ. Genetic causes of macroglossia: diagnostic approach. Pediatrics 2012;129(2):e431–7.
20. Donnelly LF, Shott SR, LaRose CR, et al. Causes of persistent obstructive sleep apnea despite previous tonsillectomy and adenoidectomy in children with down syndrome as depicted on static and dynamic cine MRI. AJR Am J Roentgenol 2004;183(1):175–81.
21. Schweiger C, Manica D, Kuhl G. Glossoptosis. Semin Pediatr Surg 2016;25(3): 123–7.
22. Segal LM, Stephenson R, Dawes M, et al. Prevalence, diagnosis, and treatment of ankyloglossia: methodologic review. Can Fam Physician 2007;53(6):1027–33.
23. Joseph KS, Kinniburgh B, Metcalfe A, et al. Temporal trends in ankyloglossia and frenotomy in British Columbia, Canada, 2004-2013: a population-based study. CMAJ Open 2016;4(1):E33–40.
24. Walsh J, Links A, Boss E, et al. Ankyloglossia and lingual frenotomy: national trends in inpatient diagnosis and management in the United States, 1997-2012. Otolaryngol Head Neck Surg 2017;156(4):735–40.
25. Joshi N, Hamdan AM, Fakhouri WD. Skeletal malocclusion: a developmental disorder with a life-long morbidity. J Clin Med Res 2014;6(6):399–408.
26. Vettraino IM, Lee W, Bronsteen RA, et al. Clinical outcome of fetuses with sonographic diagnosis of isolated micrognathia. Obstet Gynecol 2003;102(4):801–5.
27. Scott AR, Mader NS. Regional variations in the presentation and surgical management of Pierre Robin sequence. Laryngoscope 2014;124(12):2818–25.
28. Maas C, Poets CF. Initial treatment and early weight gain of children with Robin Sequence in Germany: a prospective epidemiological study. Arch Dis Child Fetal Neonatal Ed 2014;99(6):F491–4.

29. Printzlau A, Andersen M. Pierre Robin sequence in Denmark: a retrospective population-based epidemiological study. Cleft Palate Craniofac J 2004;41(1): 47–52.

30. Jadcherla S. Dysphagia in the high-risk infant: potential factors and mechanisms. Am J Clin Nutr 2016;103(2):622s–8s.

31. Motion S, Northstone K, Emond A, et al. Persistent early feeding difficulties and subsequent growth and developmental outcomes. Ambul Child Health 2001; 7(3-4):231–7.

32. Roden DF, Altman KW. Causes of dysphagia among different age groups: a systematic review of the literature. Otolaryngol Clin North Am 2013;46(6):965–87.

33. Jadcherla SR, Wang M, Vijayapal AS, et al. Impact of prematurity and co-morbidities on feeding milestones in neonates: a retrospective study. J Perinatol 2010;30(3):201–8.

34. Sheikh S, Allen E, Shell R, et al. Chronic aspiration without gastroesophageal reflux as a cause of chronic respiratory symptoms in neurologically normal infants. Chest 2001;120(4):1190–5.

35. de Benedictis FM, Carnielli VP, de Benedictis D. Aspiration lung disease. Pediatr Clin North Am 2009;56(1):173–90, xi.

36. Mercado-Deane MG, Burton EM, Harlow SA, et al. Swallowing dysfunction in infants less than 1 year of age. Pediatr Radiol 2001;31(6):423–8.

37. Daniel SJ. The upper airway: congenital malformations. Paediatr Respir Rev 2006;7(Suppl 1):S260–3.

38. Thompson DM. Laryngomalacia: factors that influence disease severity and outcomes of management. Curr Opin Otolaryngol Head Neck Surg 2010;18(6): 564–70.

39. Sakakura K, Chikamatsu K, Toyoda M, et al. Congenital laryngeal anomalies presenting as chronic stridor: a retrospective study of 55 patients. Auris Nasus Larynx 2008;35(4):527–33.

40. Rutter MJ. Evaluation and management of upper airway disorders in children. Semin Pediatr Surg 2006;15(2):116–23.

41. Cooper T, Benoit M, Erickson B, et al. Primary presentations of laryngomalacia. JAMA Otolaryngol Head Neck Surg 2014;140(6):521–6.

42. Simons JP, Greenberg LL, Mehta DK, et al. Laryngomalacia and swallowing function in children. Laryngoscope 2016;126(2):478–84.

43. Wright CT, Goudy SL. Congenital laryngomalacia: symptom duration and need for surgical intervention. Ann Otol Rhinol Laryngol 2012;121(1):57–60.

44. Isaac A, Zhang H, Soon SR, et al. A systematic review of the evidence on spontaneous resolution of laryngomalacia and its symptoms. Int J Pediatr Otorhinolaryngol 2016;83:78–83.

45. Emery PJ, Fearon B. Vocal cord palsy in pediatric practice: a review of 71 cases. Int J Pediatr Otorhinolaryngol 1984;8(2):147–54.

46. Alfares FA, Hynes CF, Ansari G, et al. Outcomes of recurrent laryngeal nerve injury following congenital heart surgery: a contemporary experience. J Saudi Heart Assoc 2016;28(1):1–6.

47. Dewan K, Cephus C, Owczarzak V, et al. Incidence and implication of vocal fold paresis following neonatal cardiac surgery. Laryngoscope 2012;122(12):2781–5.

48. Ohta N, Kuratani T, Hagihira S, et al. Vocal cord paralysis after aortic arch surgery: predictors and clinical outcome. J Vasc Surg 2006;43(4):721–8.

49. Rukholm G, Farrokhyar F, Reid D. Vocal cord paralysis post patent ductus arteriosus ligation surgery: risks and co-morbidities. Int J Pediatr Otorhinolaryngol 2012; 76(11):1637–41.

50. Zbar RI, Chen AH, Behrendt DM, et al. Incidence of vocal fold paralysis in infants undergoing ligation of patent ductus arteriosus. Ann Thorac Surg 1996;61(3): 814–6.

51. Benjamin JR, Smith PB, Cotten CM, et al. Long-term morbidities associated with vocal cord paralysis after surgical closure of a patent ductus arteriosus in extremely low birth weight infants. J Perinatol 2010;30(6):408–13.

52. Mortellaro VE, Pettiford JN, St Peter SD, et al. Incidence, diagnosis, and outcomes of vocal fold immobility after esophageal atresia (EA) and/or tracheoesophageal fistula (TEF) repair. Eur J Pediatr Surg 2011;21(6):386–8.

53. Marston AP, White DR. Subglottic stenosis. Clin Perinatol 2018;45(4):787–804.

54. Jefferson ND, Cohen AP, Rutter MJ. Subglottic stenosis. Semin Pediatr Surg 2016;25(3):138–43.

55. Rodriguez H, Cuestas G, Botto H, et al. Post-intubation subglottic stenosis in children. Diagnosis, treatment and prevention of moderate and severe stenosis. Acta Otorrinolaringol Esp 2013;64(5):339–44.

56. Choi SS, Zalzal GH. Changing trends in neonatal subglottic stenosis. Otolaryngol Head Neck Surg 2000;122(1):61–3.

57. Walner DL, Loewen MS, Kimura RE. Neonatal subglottic stenosis–incidence and trends. Laryngoscope 2001;111(1):48–51.

58. Thomas RE, Rao SC, Minutillo C, et al. Severe acquired subglottic stenosis in neonatal intensive care graduates: a case-control study. Arch Dis Child Fetal Neonatal Ed 2018;103(4):F349–54.

59. Dankle SK, Schuller DE, McClead RE. Risk factors for neonatal acquired subglottic stenosis. Ann Otol Rhinol Laryngol 1986;95(6 Pt 1):626–30.

60. Sherman JM, Lowitt S, Stephenson C, et al. Factors influencing acquired subgottic stenosis in infants. J Pediatr 1986;109(2):322–7.

61. Herrera P, Caldarone C, Forte V, et al. The current state of congenital tracheal stenosis. Pediatr Surg Int 2007;23(11):1033–44.

62. Anton-Pacheco JL, Cano I, Comas J, et al. Management of congenital tracheal stenosis in infancy. Eur J Cardiothorac Surg 2006;29(6):991–6.

63. Loeff DS, Filler RM, Vinograd I, et al. Congenital tracheal stenosis: a review of 22 patients from 1965 to 1987. J Pediatr Surg 1988;23(8):744–8.

64. Boogaard R, Huijsmans SH, Pijnenburg MW, et al. Tracheomalacia and bronchomalacia in children: incidence and patient characteristics. Chest 2005;128(5): 3391–7.

65. Patwari PP, Sharma GD. Common pediatric airway disorders. Pediatr Ann 2019; 48(4):e162–8.

66. Snijders D, Barbato A. An update on diagnosis of tracheomalacia in children. Eur J Pediatr Surg 2015;25(4):333–5.

67. Hysinger EB, Friedman NL, Padula MA, et al. Tracheobronchomalacia is associated with increased morbidity in bronchopulmonary dysplasia. Ann Am Thorac Soc 2017;14(9). https://doi.org/10.1513/AnnalsATS.201702-178OC.

68. Forrester MB, Merz RD. Epidemiology of oesophageal atresia and tracheoosophageal fistula in Hawaii, 1986-2000. Public Health 2005;119(6):483–8.

69. Pedersen RN, Calzolari E, Husby S, et al. Oesophageal atresia: prevalence, prenatal diagnosis and associated anomalies in 23 European regions. Arch Dis Child 2012;97(3):227–32.

70. Harris J, Kallen B, Robert E. Descriptive epidemiology of alimentary tract atresia. Teratology 1995;52(1):15–29.

71. Torfs CP, Curry CJ, Bateson TF. Population-based study of tracheoesophageal fistula and esophageal atresia. Teratology 1995;52(4):220–32.

72. Pini Prato A, Carlucci M, Bagolan P, et al. A cross-sectional nationwide survey on esophageal atresia and tracheoesophageal fistula. J Pediatr Surg 2015;50(9): 1441–56.
73. Shaw-Smith C. Oesophageal atresia, tracheo-oesophageal fistula, and the VAC-TERL association: review of genetics and epidemiology. J Med Genet 2006;43(7): 545–54.
74. Nassar N, Leoncini E, Amar E, et al. Prevalence of esophageal atresia among 18 international birth defects surveillance programs. Birth Defects Res A Clin Mol Teratol 2012;94(11):893–9.
75. Cassina M, Ruol M, Pertile R, et al. Prevalence, characteristics, and survival of children with esophageal atresia: a 32-year population-based study including 1,417,724 consecutive newborns. Birth Defects Res A Clin Mol Teratol 2016; 106(7):542–8.
76. Lupo PJ, Isenburg JL, Salemi JL, et al. Population-based birth defects data in the United States, 2010-2014: a focus on gastrointestinal defects. Birth Defects Res 2017;109(18):1504–14.
77. Cameron DB, Graham DA, Milliren CE, et al. Quantifying the burden of interhospital cost variation in pediatric surgery: implications for the prioritization of comparative effectiveness research. JAMA Pediatr 2017;171(2):e163926.
78. Eichenwald EC. Diagnosis and management of gastroesophageal reflux in preterm infants. Pediatrics 2018;142(1) [pii:e20181061].
79. Rosen R, Vandenplas Y, Singendonk M, et al. Pediatric gastroesophageal reflux clinical practice guidelines: joint recommendations of the North American Society for Pediatric Gastroenterology, Hepatology, and Nutrition and the European Society for Pediatric Gastroenterology, Hepatology, and Nutrition. J Pediatr Gastroenterol Nutr 2018;66(3):516–54.
80. Gulati IK, Jadcherla SR. Gastroesophageal reflux disease in the neonatal intensive care unit infant: who needs to be treated and what approach is beneficial? Pediatr Clin North Am 2019;66(2):461–73.
81. Slaughter JL, Stenger MR, Reagan PB. Variation in the use of diuretic therapy for infants with bronchopulmonary dysplasia. Pediatrics 2013;131(4):716–23.
82. Slaughter JL, Stenger MR, Reagan PB, et al. Neonatal histamine-2 receptor antagonist and proton pump inhibitor treatment at United States Children's Hospitals. J Pediatr 2016;174:63–70.e63.
83. Jadcherla SR, Slaughter JL, Stenger MR, et al. Practice variance, prevalence, and economic burden of premature infants diagnosed with GERD. Hosp Pediatr 2013;3(4):335.
84. Collins CR, Hasenstab KA, Nawaz S, et al. Mechanisms of aerodigestive symptoms in infants with varying acid reflux index determined by esophageal manometry. J Pediatr 2019;206:240–7.
85. Woodley FW, Ciciora SL, Vaz K, et al. Novel use of impedance technology shows that esophageal air events can be temporally associated with GERD-like symptoms. J Pediatr Gastroenterol Nutr 2019. https://doi.org/10.1097/MPG.0000000000002514.

Feeding and Swallowing Difficulties in Neonates
Developmental Physiology and Pathophysiology

Sreekanth Viswanathan, MD, MS[a],*, Sudarshan Jadcherla, MD[b,c]

KEYWORDS

- Suck-swallow-breath • Oral feeding • Preterm infants • Dysphagia

KEY POINTS

- Development of enteral and oral feeding milestones in infants is intricately linked to physiologic maturation of the gastrointestinal tract.
- Development of enteral and oral feeding milestones in infants is also linked to the complex interplay of the gastrointestinal tract with cardiorespiratory and central nervous system control and coordination.
- Assessment of an infant's developmental skills and maturation can guide us with targeted management approaches and prediction of feeding outcomes.

The good physician treats the disease; the great physician treats the patient who has the disease.

—*Sir William Osler*

INTRODUCTION

Independent oral feeding is one of the criteria recommended by the American Academy of Pediatrics for hospital discharge of high-risk infants.[1] Due to improved survival associated with advances in perinatal and neonatal care over the past decade, the prevalence of oral feeding difficulties in infants has increased over the past decade.[2,3] Delay in achieving timely oral feeding skills in premature infants is associated with poor postnatal growth, prolonged hospitalization, increased gastrostomy needs, and

[a] Division of Neonatology, Department of Pediatrics, Nemours Children's Hospital, University of Central Florida College of Medicine, 13535 Nemours Parkway, Orlando, FL 32827, USA; [b] Division of Neonatology, Department of Pediatrics, Nationwide Children's Hospital, The Ohio State University College of Medicine, Columbus, OH, USA; [c] Neonatal and Infant Feeding Disorders Research Program, Center for Perinatal Research, The Research Institute at Nationwide Children's Hospital, Columbus, OH, USA
* Corresponding author.
E-mail address: sreekanth.viswanathan@nemours.org

Clin Perinatol 47 (2020) 223–241
https://doi.org/10.1016/j.clp.2020.02.005
0095-5108/20/© 2020 Elsevier Inc. All rights reserved.

adverse neurodevelopmental outcomes, all with an increase in health care costs.[4–7] In this article, we review and summarize the normal physiology and maturation of oral feeding developmental process and describe the pathophysiological changes of oral feeding difficulties associated with some of the common comorbidities in infants.

EMBRYOLOGIC AND ANATOMIC CONSIDERATIONS

Embryologically, primitive foregut gives rise to pharynx, esophagus, and stomach, as well as airways, lungs, and diaphragm, and these organs share similar sensory-motor control systems. Sucking and swallowing are important early neurodevelopmental milestones. The cellular components needed for coordinated neural and muscular activity develop in the early fetal period, followed by isolated functions of sucking, swallowing, and respiration. However, maturation and integration of these neuromuscular functions occurs during mid and late gestation. The fetus starts swallowing the amniotic fluid by 11 to 12 weeks of gestation, and by 18 to 20 weeks, sucking movements appear, and by full-term gestation, the fetus can swallow and circulate nearly 500 mL of amniotic fluid.[8] During normal pregnancy, swallowing functions develop through experiences of swallowing amniotic fluid in the intrauterine environment until full-term birth. This critical developmental process of acquisition of oral feeding skills is interrupted by preterm birth, and subsequent functional maturation of these processes are affected and often delayed by the extrauterine environment in preterm infants.[9,10]

Fig. 1 illustrates the difference in anatomy of the head and neck of infants compared with adults.[11] In infants, the oral cavity is small, the hard palate is flatter, and the tongue is relatively large. The pharynx in the adult has 3 anatomic segments, that is, nasopharynx, oropharynx, and hypopharynx. However, in newborns and infants, the oropharynx is underdeveloped. The larynx and hyoid bone are higher in the neck, and the epiglottis touches the back of the soft palate, so that the larynx is open to

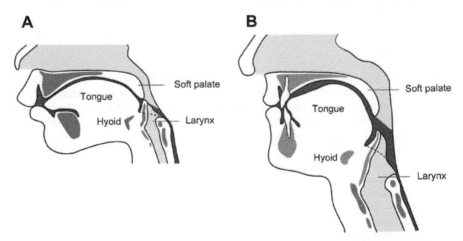

Fig. 1. Sagittal section of the head and neck in (A) infant and (B) adult. The foodway and the airway are shaded in dark and light gray, respectively. (A) In infants, the oral cavity is small, the palate is flatter, and the tongue is large. The epiglottis is touching the soft palate. The airway and foodway are separated except when swallowing. (B) In adults, the larynx is lower in the neck, and the foodway and airway cross in the pharynx (oropharynx). (*From* Matsuo K, Palmer JB. Anatomy and physiology of feeding and swallowing: normal and abnormal. Phys Med Rehabil Clin N Am. 2008; 19(4):691-707; with permission.)

the nasopharynx. The breathing and eating pathways are separated except when swallowing; the reason why infants are considered preferential nasal breathers. Infant anatomy changes with growth and development; the neck gets longer, and the pharynx gets elongated to develop the 3 distinct pharyngeal segments including oropharynx. The larynx descends to a position lower in the neck, the epiglottis loses it contact with soft palate, and the airway is now open into the hypopharynx. With this change in anatomy, the pharynx, specifically the oropharynx, becomes part of both the breathing and eating pathways.

DEVELOPMENTAL MATURATION OF ORAL FEEDING IN INFANTS

The process of swallowing (deglutition) in infants refers to the whole process of propulsion of the milk bolus from the mouth into the stomach and involves a complex coordination of rhythmic sequences of sucking, swallowing, and breathing, followed by well-timed relaxations of the upper and lower esophageal sphincter (UES and LES, respectively) and sequential esophageal contractions.[12] The normal deglutition process in infants can be divided into 3 phases based on the location of the bolus: (1) *oral phase* implicated in formation of bolus by sucking, (2) *pharyngeal phase* implicated in safe and efficient transport of the bolus into the esophagus by eliciting pharyngeal swallow reflex in coordination with UES opening while ensuring airway protection, and (3) *esophageal phase* implicated in the aboral transport of bolus toward the stomach by sequential peristaltic activity. Infants undergo a process of developmental maturation and coordination of sucking, swallowing, respiration, and esophageal motility with the goal of safe, efficient, and independent swallowing skills. In early infancy, the processes of suck, swallow, and breathing are primarily regulated by brainstem central pattern generators (CPG) that are capable of producing rapid, rhythmic motor patterns without cortical or sensory input. The CPGs for sucking/swallowing/breathing develop in parallel in early gestation, and learn to interact and coordinate with each other with advancing gestation; modulated by peripheral sensory/motor input from multimodal experiences (cortical input) from a variety of stimuli, including tactile, taste, temperature, and vision, at this critical period of development. Developmental maturation of the individual components of oral feeding (sucking, pharyngeal swallowing, respiratory coordination, and esophageal motility) in infants is summarized in the following 4 sections.

Development of Sucking

The oral phase of swallowing in early infancy is primarily a brainstem-mediated reflex (sucking reflex) with the goal of compressing the nipple and expressing its contents. The bolus is then squeezed back into the pharynx by the anterior to posterior movement of the tongue along the hard palate. Sucking can be divided into non-nutritive sucking (NNS; when the infant sucks on a pacifier, finger, or emptied breast with no milk transfer) and nutritive suck (involves milk transfer).

NNS is an oromotor rhythmic movement that appears between 28 to 33 weeks postmenstrual age (PMA) in preterm infants.[13] The NNS pattern is organized into alternating epochs of burst and pause periods. A mature NNS burst consists of 6 to 12 suck cycles followed by pause periods to accommodate respiration.[14] NNS occurs at a pace of 2 suck cycles per second. NNS involves minimal swallowing, thereby allowing sucking and respiration to function independently from one another at a more rapid pace. Each suck cycle is composed of 2 components: suction and expression. Suction corresponds to the negative intraoral pressure generated with closure of the nasal passages by the soft palate, lips tightening around breast or bottle nipple, and the lowering of the lower jaw, whereas expression corresponds to the compression of the breast or bottle nipple by the tongue against the hard palate.[15,16] *Nutritive sucking (NS),* which implies the ingestion of milk, occurs at a slower pace of 1 suck cycle per second. This lower sucking pace during NS allows the pharyngeal swallows to have the time needed to coordinate with breathing for airway safety. **Fig. 2** shows a descriptive scale of infant sucking patterns, their respective rhythmicity, and the eventual attainment of a mature rhythmic alternation of suction and expression.[15] Both NNS and NS follow a developmental pathway of increasing regularity of the suck wave (both suction and expression), increasing the length of sucking bursts and increasing consistency in the intervals between sucks within a burst with maturation, thereby improving the efficiency of sucking[15,17–19] (**Fig. 3**). It has been speculated that NS efficiency is better with bottle feeding than direct breast feeding during initial

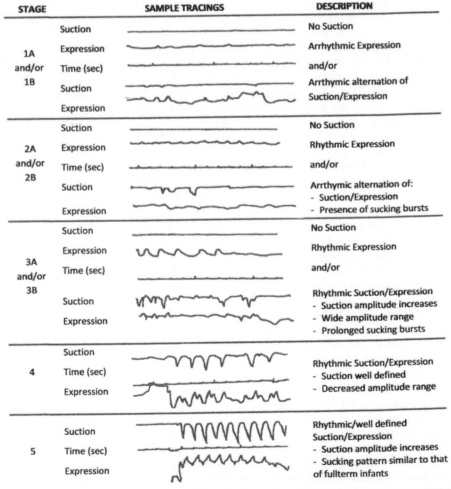

STAGE	SAMPLE TRACINGS	DESCRIPTION
1A and/or 1B	Suction	No Suction
	Expression	Arrhythmic Expression
	Time (sec)	and/or
	Suction	Arrthymic alternation of Suction/Expression
	Expression	
2A and/or 2B	Suction	No Suction
	Expression	Rhythmic Expression
	Time (sec)	and/or
	Suction	Arrthymic alternation of: - Suction/Expression - Presence of sucking bursts
	Expression	
3A and/or 3B	Suction	No Suction
	Expression	Rhythmic Expression
	Time (sec)	and/or
	Suction	Rhythmic Suction/Expression - Suction amplitude increases - Wide amplitude range - Prolonged sucking bursts
	Expression	
4	Suction	Rhythmic Suction/Expression - Suction well defined - Decreased amplitude range
	Time (sec)	
	Expression	
5	Suction	Rhythmic/well defined Suction/Expression - Suction amplitude increases - Sucking pattern similar to that of fullterm infants
	Time (sec)	
	Expression	

Fig. 2. A 5-stage descriptive scale of the development of nutritive sucking in preterm infants defined by the sequential presence and absence of the suction and expression and their respective rhythmicity. (*From* Lau C. Development of infant oral feeding skills: what do we know? Am J Clin Nutr.2016; 103(2):616S-621S; with permission.)

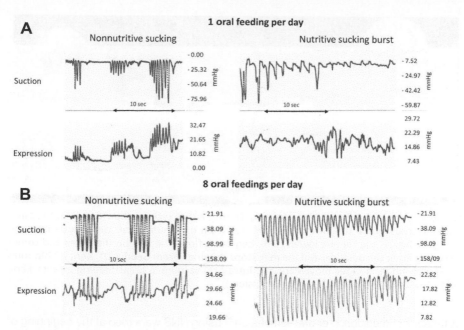

Fig. 3. Tracings of NNS (*A*) and NS (*B*) monitored 3 minutes apart during the same feeding sessions of an infant born at 33 weeks gestational age, introduced to oral feeding at 34 weeks PMA, and attaining 8 oral feedings per day at 36 weeks PMA. (*From* Lau C. Development of infant oral feeding skills: what do we know? Am J Clin Nutr. 2016; 103(2):616S-621S; with permission.)

attempts to oral feeding in preterm infants. Physiologically, the expression component of sucking matures earlier than suction. The need to generate adequate suction pressure for latching onto the breast may be the reason for initial struggles with direct breast feeding in preterm infants, which can be improved by using a nipple shield (**Fig. 4**).[17,20] With consistent and regular oromotor experiences from NNS and NS, sucking progresses from a primarily brainstem-mediated reflex in the newborn period to a volitional and purposeful activity during the later stages of infancy.

To accelerate the development of sucking and oral feeding skills in preterm infants, early prefeeding oromotor stimulation at critical time periods (between 28 and 33 weeks PMA) by various methods have been explored, and includes the use of dry pacifier, pacifier dips, orofacial stimulation, and other sensory integration modalities like kangaroo care or auditory stimulation.[21,22] These interventions are offered for short periods and stopped at any sign of adverse events, such as unstable vitals, choking, fatigue, and disorganization. These prefeeding oromotor interventions were found to be associated with reduced gavage feeding days, and decreased hospital length of stay.[23,24] Providing such oromotor stimulation also provides better parent-infant interaction, parent satisfaction, improving breastfeeding rates, infant state control, developmental maturity, and reduced stress levels.[25]

Preterm infants with more mature NNS skills (total number of sucks, suck bursts, the average number of sucks per burst, suck amplitude, burst duration, and organization), at beginning of oral feeds, are reported to have a shorter duration to reach full oral feeds, suggesting a quantitative relationship between NNS skills and feeding milestones.[26–28] Based on this observation, interventions such as rhythmic oro-

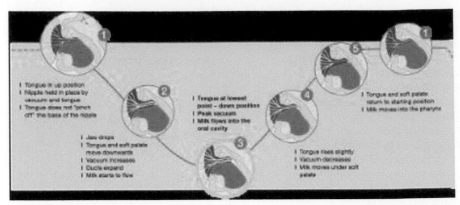

Fig. 4. Infant sucking during breastfeeding. During a suck cycle, vacuum begins at the baseline, increases as the tongue lowers, and reaches a maximum when the tongue is at the lowest point. As the tongue lowers, milk begins to flow. The tongue then rises and comes to rest again at the baseline, and the milk stops flowing. (*From* Geddes DT, Kent JC, Mitoulas LR, Hartmann PE. Tongue movement and intra-oral vacuum in breastfeeding infants. Early Hum Dev. 2008;84(7):471-477; with permission.)

cutaneous stimulation,[26] or oral stimulation[29] using NNS were tried at the beginning of oral feeds (~32–33 weeks PMA) with the assumption that improving NNS skills will facilitate the development of NS through strengthening of the muscles or neurologic stimulation. These interventions delivered at the beginning of oral feeds, although have improved the NNS skill metrics, did not show robust improvement in time to achieve full oral feeds,[25,26,30] whereas interventions to stimulate NS at the beginning of oral feeding was associated with earlier attainment of full oral feeding milestone.[31] This suggests that NNS skills alone may not be predictive of the coordination among sucking, pharyngeal swallow, and breathing that are essential for NS.[25,32] Once infants have reached a PMA of 32 to 34 weeks, it is likely that oromotor experience from NS is more likely to be effective than focusing on NNS stimulation for earlier transition from gavage feeding to independent oral feeding. Quality improvement initiatives that focus on prevention of oral feeding difficulties in preterm infants, such as SIMPLE (simplified, individualized, milestone-targeted, pragmatic, longitudinal and educational) feeding program initiatives integrate and unite many of these multiple approaches to optimize the oral feeding outcomes.[33]

Development of Pharyngeal Swallowing

In the pharyngeal stage, the soft palate elevates to close off the nasopharynx, thereby preventing bolus regurgitation into the nasopharynx. The vocal folds close to seal the glottis, the larynx moves upward and forward by the suprahyoid muscles (hyolaryngeal elevation), and the epiglottis tilts backward. The hyolaryngeal elevation results in active opening of UES. Pharyngeal constrictor muscles contract sequentially from the top to the bottom, squeezing the bolus downward via the open UES into the esophagus.

Suck-pharyngeal coordination

To trigger adequate pharyngeal swallow reflex, proper bolus formation and presentation to the pharynx is necessary. There is a tightly linked, anti-phase relationship between sucking and swallowing, where the generation and release of positive pharyngeal pressure is tightly coupled with the generation and release of negative intraoral suction (**Fig. 5**).[34] Sucking that is coupled with a pharyngeal swallow generated significantly higher milk ejection pressures than sucks that occurred in isolation. If the timing of pharyngeal swallow reflex is delayed or not efficient, that will lead to pharyngeal pooling of milk, which increases the risk for penetration and/or aspiration into the larynx.[35]

For safe and efficient swallowing, preterm infants need to attain functional maturation, control, and coordination of the processes involved in feeding.[16] Studies have shown that preterm infants have a mature 1:1 suck:pharyngeal swallow ratio and interval similar to the full-term infants when oral feedings are introduced by 33 to 34 weeks PMA.[36] Suck:pharyngeal swallow ratio can increase to 2 to 3:1 over time, as well as over the course of the feeding. However, piecemeal deglutition or multiple swallowing, defined as swallowing of 1 single bolus in 2 or more portions to empty the oral cavity, is also a common feature of infant swallowing.[37,38]

Pharyngeal–upper esophageal sphincter coordination

There is increasing interest in the use of high-resolution manometry (HRM) to understand the pathophysiology of oropharyngeal dysphagia in the infant population. Rommel and colleagues[39] performed serial high-resolution pharyngoesophageal manometry in stable preterm infants during the oral feeding development period to study the development of pharyngeal motility, UES function, and their coordination during NS. They observed that preterm infants have delayed and protracted pharyngeal phase, and poor pharyngeal pressures at the laryngeal inlet coupled with poor coordination of pharyngeal propulsion with UES relaxation (**Fig. 6**). UES metrics, including UES pressure at onset of the UES relaxation, UES nadir relaxation pressure, and duration of the UES relaxation, are similar from 31 weeks PMA onward; whereas *UES relaxation response time* (time from UES relaxation onset to complete UES relaxation) decreased with increasing PMA (a potential biomarker of pharyngeal-UES coordination maturation). In preterm infants of earlier PMA, UES

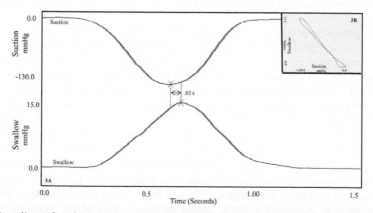

Fig. 5. Coupling of sucking and swallowing. Generation of intraoral suction demonstrating an antiphase relationship with the generation of positive pharyngeal pressure during the swallow. Upper right corner box: X-Y plot showing the relationship between increasing and decreasing negative intraoral pressure and increasing and decreasing positive pharyngeal pressure. (*From* McGrattan KE, Sivalingam M, Hasenstab KA, Wei L, Jadcherla SR. The physiologic coupling of sucking and swallowing coordination provides a unique process for neonatal survival. Acta Paediatr. 2016;105(7):790-797; with permission.)

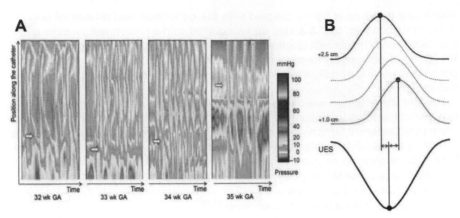

Fig. 6. (*A*) Gradual increase in peak pharyngeal pressures at 1 cm above the UES (*white arrow*) in healthy preterm infants with advancing gestational age (GA). (*B*) Averaged time differences and variability between the peak pharyngeal pressures and the UES nadir according to age and different pharyngeal segments (1.0 cm and 2.5 cm proximal to the UES). In early preterms infants, the peak pharyngeal contraction occurs before the UES nadir, whereas the pharyngeal peak tends to occur after the UES nadir with advanced GA. (*From* Rommel N, van Wijk M, Boets B, et al. Development of pharyngo-esophageal physiology during swallowing in the preterm infant. Neurogastroenterol Motil. 2011; 23(10): e401-408; with permission.)

took longer to fully relax and their peak pharyngeal contraction (responsible for pharyngeal bolus flow) occurred before the UES nadir pressure, compared with older infants. This pharyngo-UES discoordination in preterm infants potentially increases the resistance to bolus flow across the UES during each swallow, thus interrupting the suck, swallow, and breathing coordination needed for efficient nutritive swallowing, increasing the risk for aspiration and cardiorespiratory symptoms from bolus retention in the hypopharynx, and predisposing them to poor feeding endurance from fatigue.

Robust pharyngeal contractility is essential to trigger pharyngoesophageal peristalsis, and pharyngeal dysfunctions can manifest as oral feeding difficulties, inability to handle oral secretions, or supra-esophageal reflux events, and/or airway compromise. Jadcherla and colleagues[40] used HRM studies to characterize the pharyngeal motor activity and their regulatory characteristics during NS in full-term and preterm infants. Total pharyngeal contraction magnitude or vigor is assessed by pharyngeal contractile integral (PhCl), a 3-dimensional measure of pharyngeal contractile pressure, length, and duration of contraction (**Fig. 7**). They observed that PhCl is distinct in the proximal and distal part of the pharynx, and PhCl was lower when UES nadir pressures were low. Preterm infants at term PMA, compared with full-term infants, have lower pharyngeal contraction frequency, but higher PhCl per individual contraction associated with lower milk intake.[41] This is likely from the immaturity of PhCl and UES coordination in preterm infants, similar to the findings of the study by Rommel and colleagues[39] mentioned previously. These data suggest that postnatal maturation of UES to relax rapidly and fully is a major determinant of the full oral feeding milestone in preterm infants.

Emerging technologies like pharyngeal high-resolution impedance manometry with pressure flow analysis, which provides a visual depiction of pressure flow of bolus during pharyngeal deglutition, is a promising bedside tool.[42] Research is ongoing to

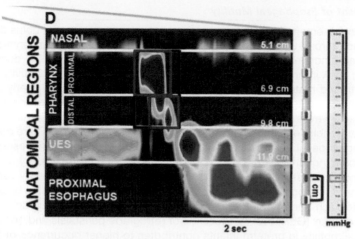

Fig. 7. Pharyngeal vigor measured by PhCI (*red space-time box*) is distinct in proximal and distal pharyngeal regions. (*From* Jadcherla SR, Prabhakar V, Hasenstab KA, et al. Defining pharyngeal contractile integral during high-resolution manometry in neonates: a neuromotor marker of pharyngeal vigor. Pediatr Res. 2018; 84(3):341-347; with permission.)

standardize the objective swallow metrics derived from this biomechanically based approach, and its validation in the infant population.

Development of Respiratory Coordination with Swallowing

The adult pattern of swallowing, which appears only after infancy, is "exhale-swallow-exhale" (exhalation surrounds the swallows) where the swallows occur when airflow is minimal and the positive airflow with post-swallow exhalation helps to provide airway clearance. Preterm infants swallow at all phases of respiration. While transitioning to oral feeding during the developmental window of 32 to 36 weeks, the most common pattern observed is apneic pauses in breathing (deglutition apnea [DA]) associated with pharyngeal swallows ("DA-swallow-DA").[36,43,44] If swallowing mechanism is not swift and efficient, that duration of DA increases. Such disruption to respiration (reduced tidal volume and minute ventilation) if prolonged can result in desaturations and bradycardia attributed to oral feeding.[43,45–47] With maturation, the pharyngeal swallows gradually get integrated within the respiratory cycle, the DA events are superseded by a pattern of attenuated respiration with swallows, and ultimately progress to a safer "inhale-swallow-exhale" pattern, as seen in healthy term infants.[36,48,49] The pattern of "DA-swallow-DA" disappears at approximately 9 months of age,[50,51] likely coinciding with the anatomic development of laryngeal descent, lengthening of pharynx, and the epiglottis loosing contact with the velum. Studies in full-term infants have shown that post-swallow exhalation becomes the predominant pattern during second half of infancy. For exhalation to follow a swallow, there must be sufficient air within the lungs, and the pattern of "inhale-swallow-exhale" ensures this during infancy.[48,49] Inhalation before a swallow decreases the pressure in the esophagus in preparation for bolus entry when the UES opens at the end of the pharyngeal phase. When exhalation occurs after a swallow, the esophageal pressure will gradually increase, thereby facilitating downstream bolus transit.[48] Monitoring respiratory signals during NNS and NS helps to determine the swallow-breathing coordination and to identify neonates with an increased risk of aspiration.

Development of Esophageal Motility

Once the bolus enters the esophagus, a peristalsis wave carries the bolus down into the stomach through the LES. Jadcherla and colleagues[52] have demonstrated that longitudinal functional maturation of pharyngoesophageal motility occurs with advancing PMA in preterm infants. Resting UES and LES tone and activity increase with growth and maturation. Also, esophageal lengthening occurs linearly in infants with growth. Esophageal motility comprises peristaltic and nonperistaltic waveforms. The peristaltic waves can be anterograde or retrograde in nature, whereas the nonperistaltic waves include synchronous and incomplete wave patterns. There are 2 types of esophageal peristalsis: esophageal deglutition reflex (a peristaltic response triggered by pharyngeal swallow reflex often accompanied by a respiratory pause [DA]) and secondary peristalsis (swallow-independent peristalsis triggered by esophageal provocation).[53,54] Together, these peristaltic mechanisms propagate the bolus distally into the stomach during swallowing and also to clear the esophagus during gastroesophageal reflux (GER) events. Presence of retrograde peristalsis and nonperistaltic esophageal motility in preterm infants contributes to higher occurrence of GER and poor clearance of refluxed material. However, with maturation, the occurrence of nonperistaltic waves and retrograde peristalsis decreases, whereas that of anterograde peristaltic waves increases (especially develops more frequent and robust secondary peristalsis), leading to better and faster clearance of esophagus with reduction in GER severity.

Infant with feeding difficulties: underlying physiologic alterations and its clinical relevance

As previously described, the different components that are essential for safe and efficient oral feeding mature at different times and rates in neonates, and unsafe and inefficient oral feeding may be caused by delay in functional maturation or coordination at any level. In addition to the physiologic immaturity, development of oral feeding skills and endurance in preterm infants is further impacted by the multiple comorbidities that they develop during the extrauterine life.[55] Factors affecting the postnatal maturation of these processes are often heterogeneous, and thus a targeted PMA (eg, full-term PMA) alone may not be a good indicator for the acquisition of functional swallowing skills. It is important to understand the functional maturity level and the pathophysiological mechanisms behind the oral feeding difficulty in each individual patient to provide personalized management strategies to optimize the feeding outcomes. A brief summary of various clinical tools available with their advantages and limitations to understand the structural and functional pathophysiology of oral difficulty in infants is given in **Table 1**. Further, we are describing the physiologic alterations associated with conditions that are commonly associated with oral feeding difficulties in infants. We have excluded the anatomic/structural defects of the upper aerodigestive tract in the discussion, as it is beyond the scope of this article.

Chronic lung disease of prematurity

In preterm infants with chronic lung disease of prematurity (CLD), the need for prolonged respiratory support often deprives them of the sensory and oromotor feeding experience at critical developmental periods. The oral feeding difficulties in infants with CLD have multifactorial etiology.

- Infants with severe CLD have lower sucking pressure, sucking frequency, shorter sucking burst duration, and lower frequency of swallows compared with infants without CLD, thus affecting the oral feeding endurance and efficiency.[26,56] The

Table 1
Clinical tools to evaluate oral feeding difficulties in infants: advantages and limitations

Test	Advantages	Limitations
Upper gastrointestinal fluoroscopy study	Evaluation of gastrointestinal anatomy	Not sensitive or specific for either dysphagia or GER Significant radiation exposure
Video fluoroscopic swallow study (VFSS)	Structural and functional study of swallowing Swallowing safety: quantify the risk for airway penetration and aspiration Swallowing efficiency: recommendation to compensate for the structural and functional dysfunction	Time limited (average time 2–3 minutes/study) Uncommon feeding positions and situation (potentially impair adaptive aerodigestive reflexes) Barium products may not mimic infant formula VFSS metrics based on qualitative interpretation of image data are not correlating with feeding outcomes Significant radiation exposure
Fiberoptic endoscopic evaluation of swallowing (FEES)	Direct visualization of upper aerodigestive structures Dynamic view of the oral-pharyngeal transfer Natural feeding position No barium products Bedside procedure Not time-limited No radiation exposure	Only indirect evidence of pharyngoesophageal transfer May overestimate the amount of pharyngeal residue Data in infant population are limited Qualitative interpretation of image data
Multichannel intraluminal impedance (MII)-pH monitoring	Detect acid and nonacid gastroesophageal reflux (GER) Differentiate between liquid, gas, and mixed GER Quantify the GER events and symptom association Basal impedance to assess esophageal mucosal inflammation	Lack of validated normative standards to diagnose infant gastroesophageal reflux disease Analysis and symptom association depends on the symptom diary Value of symptom association indices to predict outcomes is not proven Analysis is semiautomated, and labor intensive

(continued on next page)

Table 1
(continued)

Test	Advantages	Limitations
Pharyngoesophageal manometry High-resolution impedance manometry	Assess esophageal body pressures, peristalsis and upper/lower esophageal sphincter responses to swallow and GER events at baseline and secondary to provocative stimulation Impedance metrics capture bolus flow Swallowing skills can be tested in infants with minimal oral feeding Natural feeding position No barium products Bedside procedure Not time-limited No radiation exposure	Require highly skilled personnel to perform, analysis and interpretation Not readily available Need standardization of procedure, validation of metrics in infants Limited data on manometric metrics to predict feeding outcomes, determine therapeutic targets, and as a tool to evaluate different feeding interventions

lower frequency of sucking and swallowing is likely to compensate for their poor coordination of suck-swallow-breath.

- The suck-swallow-breath coordination maturation is often delayed or does not follow the predicted maturation pattern.[57]
- The DA or attenuated respiration associated with swallowing may not be well tolerated or sustainable for entire feeds, resulting in feeding-related cardiorespiratory compromise that prolongs the transition time from gavage to oral feeding.[45,56]
- Repeated exposure to noxious sensory stimulation (tubes, cannulas, and tapes placed on the infant's face) results in orosensory aversion, which presents a challenge when introducing oral feeding interventions.
- Supplemental oxygen during feeding may help to reduce the desaturations and improve feeding endurance, especially in infants with underlying severe anemia of prematurity.[58–60]
- Infants with CLD often have clinical symptoms suggestive of GER; however, studies have shown that rather than higher impedance-positive GER, impaired esophageal motility and heightened vagal reflex responses to esophageal provocation from underlying inflammatory state may be contributing to the symptom generation.[61,62] Infants who are continuous positive airway pressure (CPAP) dependent were observed to have a reduced number of GER events, as CPAP may help to inhibit GER events by passive increase in LES basal pressure and direct mechanical compression of the esophagus.[62–64]
- Infants with severe CLD often have growth failure and will need a gastrostomy tube to support long-term growth and development while gradually progressing toward independent oral feeding.

Gastroesophageal reflux disease

Gastroesophageal reflux disease (GERD) is a commonly attributed cause of feeding problems in infants. The best available objective test to diagnose GERD in infants is a 24-hour esophageal pH-impedance study, which helps to quantify acid and nonacid GER events; differentiates among liquid, gas, and mixed GER; and performs symptom association.

- The esophagus clears the refluxed material from the lumen back into the stomach either by a swallow-dependent peristalsis originating in the pharynx or by a more mature, swallow-independent secondary peristalsis originating within the esophageal body, which usually occurs concurrently with an increase in UES pressure that increases the pressure barrier against the entry of refluxate into the pharynx. With maturation, the peristaltic response becomes faster and more efficient with greater intraluminal esophageal pressure and faster esophageal clearance, especially with more frequent and robust secondary peristaltic activity.[54] Esophageal dysmotility can affect the clearance mechanism of GER. Some pH-impedance study metrics, like acid clearance time, and bolus clearance time, basal mucosal impedance (marker of mucosal inflammation) will give an indication of underlying esophageal dysmotility.
- GER is often implicated as a possible culprit of apparent life threatening events (ALTE) and brief resolved unexplained events (BRUE) in infants and empirical acid-suppressive medication use for presumed acid-GERD is common. However, the temporal or causal relationship of these events with GER is not proven.[65] Pharyngoesophageal manometry studies have shown that the impairments in swallowing and respiratory interaction, lower esophageal contractile pressure, and incomplete propagation of esophageal peristalsis resulting in inefficient

pharyngeal and esophageal clearance are the plausible mechanisms underlying such events rather than the reflux burden or ascent of GER.[66] Data also suggest that such events are more common in the immediate postprandial period, which are more likely to be nonacid GER, whereas acid-GER usually happens later during feeding, suggesting that acid-suppressant medications are unlikely to be helpful in these scenarios. Similarly, feeding-related spells (apnea, bradycardia, and desaturations) in preterm infants are found to be more likely the result of aberrant pharyngoesophageal motility and respiratory dysregulation that resulted in repetitive swallowing, prolonged respiratory rhythm disturbance, and immature esophageal motility than GER.[44]

Hypoxic ischemic encephalopathy

Poor feeding is a sensitive indicator of central nervous system disease.[67] Infants with hypoxic ischemic encephalopathy (HIE) have feeding difficulties manifesting as oropharyngeal inertia, pooling of secretions, inadequate airway protection, and GER. Pharyngoesophageal manometry studies have shown that infants with HIE have increased UES basal tone, increased frequency of pharyngeal waveforms per stimulus, decreased proximal esophageal contractile amplitude, prolonged proximal esophageal contractile duration, and decreased frequency of LES relaxation.[68] Increased skeletal muscle hypertonicity at UES and proximal esophagus and dysregulation at LES may explain the pathophysiological basis for pooling of secretions, improper bolus clearance, and aspiration risk in infants with HIE. Maturation with increasing PMA modifies some of these responses with reduced UES basal tone, decreased pharyngeal contractions, and reduced latency to terminal swallow at pharynx.[69]

Infants of diabetic mothers

Feeding difficulties are a major problem in infants of diabetic mothers (IDMs) and are a key reason for prolonged hospital stay and parent-infant separation.[70,71] Pharyngoesophageal manometry studies in IDMs with severe oral feeding difficulties have demonstrated longer response latency to esophageal peristalsis onset and prolonged LES nadir duration, likely from the neurologic dampening secondary to prolonged hyperglycemia exposure in utero, which may improve with maturation postnatally.[72] Also, body composition studies have shown that IDMs have a greater percentage of body fat compared with non-IDMs.[73,74] IDMs were found to have higher umbilical cord–leptin concentration at birth, the major satiety hormone secreted by adipocytes in proportion to the fat mass.[75,76] The presence of higher body fat and leptin level may be associated with early satiety and reduced interest in oral feeding.

SUMMARY

- Prevalence of dysphagia in infants is increasing, especially with the improved survival of high-risk preterm infants.
- Management of oral feeding difficulties in infants should be tailored around the functional maturity level rather than be based on their corrected gestation.
- Standardized/protocolized management of oral feeding difficulties in infants is problematic due to the heterogeneity of feeding problems and underlying comorbidities.
- Timely initiation of oromotor therapies for central and enteric nervous system interactions at critical developmental periods may provide opportunities for improved progression of feeding skills, as well as improvement in neurodevelopmental outcomes.

- Personalized management based on objective multidisciplinary assessment of pathophysiological basis of troublesome symptoms during oral feeding across the phases of the swallow is likely to be more effective to improve the outcomes.

DISCLOSURE

A. Guarantor of the article: S. Viswanathan.
  B. Any potential competing conflicts of interests: None.
  Statement of financial support: None.

Best Practices

What is the current practice related to Feeding and Swallowing Difficulties in Neonates?

Empiric and non–evidence-based diagnosis feeding modification strategies are common. Many centers do not have feeding and nutrition guidelines that are guided by physiologic principles. Our objectives in this article were to clarify and expand on the following:

- NNS and NS are often introduced based on gestational maturity (targeted PMA) rather than functional maturity. This may delay the acquisition and integration of sucking, swallowing, and breathing at critical developmental periods.
- GER is often implicated in feeding-related spells (apnea, bradycardia, and desaturation), and ALTE/BRUE episodes in infants. The use of empirical acid-suppressive medication for presumed acid-GERD is very prevalent.
- Assessment of infants with oral feeding difficulties is often based on subjective clinical assessment of symptoms and qualitative testing. A standardized approach, when applied to a complex, heterogeneous problem brings out better outcomes.

What changes in the current practice are likely to improve outcomes?

- Management of oral feeding difficulties in infants should be tailored around the functional maturity level rather than be based on their corrected gestation. Inefficient oral skill may be caused by delay in functional maturation or coordination at any level: upstream or downstream.

- To accelerate the development of sucking and oral feeding skills in preterm infants, introduction of timely oromotor stimulation and swallowing experiences at critical periods is important.

- The deglutition apnea or attenuated respiration associated with swallowing is common in preterm infants and may cause feeding-related spells and delays the transition from gavage to oral feeding. Supplemental oxygen during feeding may help to reduce the severity of desaturations and improve feeding endurance, especially in infants with underlying severe anemia of prematurity.

- GER is not the main cause of oral feeding-related spells, and they are more likely the result of inefficient reflux clearance mechanisms from inefficient pharyngoesophageal motility and respiratory dysregulation. The use of acid-suppressive medication should be limited to objectively proven acid-GERD in infants.

- It is important to understand the functional maturity level and the pathophysiological mechanisms behind the oral feeding difficulty in each individual patient to provide personalized management strategies to optimize the feeding outcomes.

Summary statement

Prevalence of dysphagia in infants is increasing, and caregivers should be cognizant of underlying physiologic alterations in sucking, swallowing, esophageal peristalsis, sphincteric functions, and airway protective mechanisms to optimize clinical outcomes.

REFERENCES

1. Newborn AAoPCoFa. Hospital discharge of the high-risk neonate. Pediatrics 2008;122(5):1119–26.

2. Stoll BJ, Hansen NI, Bell EF, et al. Trends in care practices, morbidity, and mortality of extremely preterm neonates, 1993-2012. JAMA 2015;314(10):1039–51.

3. Horton J, Atwood C, Gnagi S, et al. Temporal trends of pediatric dysphagia in hospitalized patients. Dysphagia 2018;33(5):655–61.

4. Jadcherla SR, Khot T, Moore R, et al. Feeding methods at discharge predict long-term feeding and neurodevelopmental outcomes in preterm infants referred for gastrostomy evaluation. J Pediatr 2017;181:125–30.e1.

5. Lainwala S, Kosyakova N, Power K, et al. Delayed achievement of oral feedings is associated with adverse neurodevelopmental outcomes at 18 to 26 months follow-up in preterm infants. Am J Perinatol 2019. https://doi.org/10.1055/s-0039-1681059.

6. Walsh MC, Bell EF, Kandefer S, et al. Neonatal outcomes of moderately preterm infants compared to extremely preterm infants. Pediatr Res 2017;82(2):297–304.

7. Hatch LD, Scott TA, Walsh WF, et al. National and regional trends in gastrostomy in very low birth weight infants in the USA: 2000-2012. J Perinatol 2018;38(9):1270–6.

8. Bosma JF. Development and impairments of feeding in infancy and childhood. In: Groher ME, editor. Dysphagia: diagnosis and management. 3rd edition. Boston: Butterworth-Heinemann; 1997. p. 131–67.

9. Illingworth RS, Lister J. The critical or sensitive period, with special reference to certain feeding problems in infants and children. J Pediatr 1964;65:839–48.

10. Jadcherla S. Dysphagia in the high-risk infant: potential factors and mechanisms. Am J Clin Nutr 2016;103(2):622S–8S.

11. Matsuo K, Palmer JB. Anatomy and physiology of feeding and swallowing: normal and abnormal. Phys Med Rehabil Clin N Am 2008;19(4):691–707, vii.

12. Singendonk MM, Rommel N, Omari TI, et al. Upper gastrointestinal motility: prenatal development and problems in infancy. Nat Rev Gastroenterol Hepatol 2014; 11(9):545–55.

13. Hack M, Estabrook MM, Robertson SS. Development of sucking rhythm in preterm infants. Early Hum Dev 1985;11(2):133–40.

14. Barlow SM, Finan DS, Lee J, et al. Synthetic orocutaneous stimulation entrains preterm infants with feeding difficulties to suck. J Perinatol 2008;28(8):541–8.

15. Lau C. Development of infant oral feeding skills: what do we know? Am J Clin Nutr 2016;103(2):616S–21S.

16. Lau C, Alagugurusamy R, Schanler RJ, et al. Characterization of the developmental stages of sucking in preterm infants during bottle feeding. Acta Paediatr 2000;89(7):846–52.

17. Lau C, Sheena HR, Shulman RJ, et al. Oral feeding in low birth weight infants. J Pediatr 1997;130(4):561–9.

18. Capilouto GJ, Cunningham TJ. Objective assessment of a preterm infant's nutritive sucking from initiation of feeding through hospitalization and discharge. Neonatal Intensive Care 2016;29(1):40–5.

19. Capilouto GJ, Cunningham TJ, Giannone PJ, et al. A comparison of the nutritive sucking performance of full term and preterm neonates at hospital discharge: a prospective study. Early Hum Dev 2019;134:26–30.

20. Geddes DT, Kent JC, Mitoulas LR, et al. Tongue movement and intra-oral vacuum in breastfeeding infants. Early Hum Dev 2008;84(7):471–7.

21. Pickler RH, Wetzel PA, Meinzen-Derr J, et al. Patterned feeding experience for preterm infants: study protocol for a randomized controlled trial. Trials 2015; 16:255.

22. Song D, Jegatheesan P, Nafday S, et al. Patterned frequency-modulated oral stimulation in preterm infants: a multicenter randomized controlled trial. PLoS One 2019;14(2):e0212675.

23. Say B, Simsek GK, Canpolat FE, et al. Effects of pacifier use on transition time from gavage to breastfeeding in preterm infants: a randomized controlled trial. Breastfeed Med 2018;13(6):433–7.

24. Arora K, Goel S, Manerkar S, et al. Prefeeding oromotor stimulation program for improving oromotor function in preterm infants - a randomized controlled trial. Indian Pediatr 2018;55(8):675–8.

25. Harding C, Frank L, Van Someren V, et al. How does non-nutritive sucking support infant feeding? Infant Behav Dev 2014;37(4):457–64.

26. Barlow SM, Lee J, Wang J, et al. Frequency-modulated orocutaneous stimulation promotes non-nutritive suck development in preterm infants with respiratory distress syndrome or chronic lung disease. J Perinatol 2014;34(2):136–42.

27. Bingham PM, Ashikaga T, Abbasi S. Prospective study of non-nutritive sucking and feeding skills in premature infants. Arch Dis Child Fetal Neonatal Ed 2010; 95(3):F194–200.

28. Grassi A, Sgherri G, Chorna O, et al. Early intervention to improve sucking in pre-term newborns: a systematic review of quantitative studies. Adv Neonatal Care 2019;19(2):97–109.

29. Fucile S, Gisel EG, McFarland DH, et al. Oral and non-oral sensorimotor interventions enhance oral feeding performance in preterm infants. Dev Med Child Neurol 2011;53(9):829–35.

30. Bache M, Pizon E, Jacobs J, et al. Effects of pre-feeding oral stimulation on oral feeding in preterm infants: a randomized clinical trial. Early Hum Dev 2014;90(3): 125–9.

31. Lau C, Smith EO. Interventions to improve the oral feeding performance of pre-term infants. Acta Paediatr 2012;101(7):e269–74.

32. Harding C, Frank L, Dungu C, et al. The use of nonnutritive sucking to facilitate oral feeding in a term infant: a single case study. J Pediatr Nurs 2012;27(6): 700–6.

33. Jadcherla SR, Dail J, Malkar MB, et al. Impact of process optimization and quality improvement measures on neonatal feeding outcomes at an all-referral neonatal intensive care unit. JPEN J Parenter Enteral Nutr 2016;40(5):646–55.

34. McGrattan KE, Sivalingam M, Hasenstab KA, et al. The physiologic coupling of sucking and swallowing coordination provides a unique process for neonatal survival. Acta Paediatr 2016;105(7):790–7.

35. Goldfield EC, Richardson MJ, Lee KG, et al. Coordination of sucking, swallowing, and breathing and oxygen saturation during early infant breast-feeding and bottle-feeding. Pediatr Res 2006;60(4):450–5.

36. Lau C, Smith EO, Schanler RJ. Coordination of suck-swallow and swallow respiration in preterm infants. Acta Paediatr 2003;92(6):721–7.

37. Pouderoux P, Logemann JA, Kahrilas PJ. Pharyngeal swallowing elicited by fluid infusion: role of volition and vallecular containment. Am J Physiol 1996;270(2 Pt 1):G347–54.

38. Ferris L, King S, McCall L, et al. Piecemeal deglutition and the implications for pressure impedance dysphagia assessment in pediatrics. J Pediatr Gastroenterol Nutr 2018;67(6):713–9.

39. Rommel N, van Wijk M, Boets B, et al. Development of pharyngo-esophageal physiology during swallowing in the preterm infant. Neurogastroenterol Motil 2011;23(10):e401–8.

40. Jadcherla SR, Prabhakar V, Hasenstab KA, et al. Defining pharyngeal contractile integral during high-resolution manometry in neonates: a neuromotor marker of pharyngeal vigor. Pediatr Res 2018;84(3):341–7.

41. Prabhakar V, Hasenstab KA, Osborn E, et al. Pharyngeal contractile and regulatory characteristics are distinct during nutritive oral stimulus in preterm-born infants: implications for clinical and research applications. Neurogastroenterol Motil 2019;31(8):e13650.

42. Omari TI, Ciucci M, Gozdzikowska K, et al. High-resolution pharyngeal manometry and impedance: protocols and metrics-recommendations of a high-resolution pharyngeal manometry International Working Group. Dysphagia 2019. https://doi.org/10.1007/s00455-019-10023-y.

43. Thoyre SM, Carlson J. Occurrence of oxygen desaturation events during preterm infant bottle feeding near discharge. Early Hum Dev 2003;72(1):25–36.

44. Thoyre SM. Challenges mothers identify in bottle feeding their preterm infants. Neonatal Netw 2001;20(1):41–50.

45. Hasenstab KA, Nawaz S, Lang IM, et al. Pharyngoesophageal and cardiorespiratory interactions: potential implications for premature infants at risk of clinically significant cardiorespiratory events. Am J Physiol Gastrointest Liver Physiol 2019; 316(2):G304–12.

46. Mathew OP, Clark ML, Pronske ML, et al. Breathing pattern and ventilation during oral feeding in term newborn infants. J Pediatr 1985;106(5):810–3.

47. Miller MJ, DiFiore JM. A comparison of swallowing during apnea and periodic breathing in premature infants. Pediatr Res 1995;37(6):796–9.

48. Gross RD, Trapani-Hanasewych M. Breathing and swallowing: the next frontier. Semin Speech Lang 2017;38(2):87–95.

49. Reynolds EW, Grider D, Caldwell R, et al. Swallow-breath interaction and phase of respiration with swallow during nonnutritive suck among low-risk preterm infants. Am J Perinatol 2010;27(10):831–40.

50. Weber F, Woolridge MW, Baum JD. An ultrasonographic study of the organisation of sucking and swallowing by newborn infants. Dev Med Child Neurol 1986;28(1): 19–24.

51. Kelly BN, Huckabee ML, Jones RD, et al. The first year of human life: coordinating respiration and nutritive swallowing. Dysphagia 2007;22(1):37–43.

52. Jadcherla SR, Shubert TR, Gulati IK, et al. Upper and lower esophageal sphincter kinetics are modified during maturation: effect of pharyngeal stimulus in premature infants. Pediatr Res 2015;77(1–1):99–106.

53. Gupta A, Gulati P, Kim W, et al. Effect of postnatal maturation on the mechanisms of esophageal propulsion in preterm human neonates: primary and secondary peristalsis. Am J Gastroenterol 2009;104(2):411–9.

54. Viswanathan S, Jadcherla SR. Development of gastrointestinal motility reflexes. In: Neu J, editor. Gastroenterology and nutrition: neonatology questions and controversies. 3rd edition. Philadelphia: Elsevier; 2019. p. 15–28.

55. Jadcherla SR, Wang M, Vijayapal AS, et al. Impact of prematurity and co-morbidities on feeding milestones in neonates: a retrospective study. J Perinatol 2010;30(3):201–8.

56. Mizuno K, Nishida Y, Taki M, et al. Infants with bronchopulmonary dysplasia suckle with weak pressures to maintain breathing during feeding. Pediatrics 2007;120(4):e1035–42.

57. Gewolb IH, Bosma JF, Taciak VL, et al. Abnormal developmental patterns of suck and swallow rhythms during feeding in preterm infants with bronchopulmonary dysplasia. Dev Med Child Neurol 2001;43(7):454–9.

58. Duan J, Kong X, Li Q, et al. Association between anemia and bronchopulmonary dysplasia in preterm infants. Sci Rep 2016;6:22717.
59. Bromiker R, Kasinetz Y, Kaplan M, et al. Sucking improvement following blood transfusion for anemia of prematurity. Arch Pediatr Adolesc Med 2012;166(10):897–901.
60. Viswanathan S, Jadcherla SR. Impact of anemia of prematurity on oral feeding milestones in premature infants. Am J Perinatol 2019.
61. Nobile S, Noviello C, Cobellis G, et al. Are infants with bronchopulmonary dysplasia prone to gastroesophageal reflux? A prospective observational study with esophageal pH-impedance monitoring. J Pediatr 2015;167(2):279–85.e1.
62. Jadcherla SR, Hasenstab KA, Sitaram S, et al. Effect of nasal noninvasive respiratory support methods on pharyngeal provocation-induced aerodigestive reflexes in infants. Am J Physiol Gastrointest Liver Physiol 2016;310(11):G1006–14.
63. Djeddi D, Cantin D, Samson N, et al. Nasal continuous positive airway pressure inhibits gastroesophageal reflux in newborn lambs. PLoS One 2014;9(9):e107736.
64. Fournier MR, Kerr PD, Shoenut JP, et al. Effect of nasal continuous positive airway pressure on esophageal function. J Otolaryngol 1999;28(3):142–4.
65. Rossor T, Andradi G, Ali K, et al. Gastro-oesophageal reflux and apnoea: is there a temporal relationship? Neonatology 2018;113(3):206–11.
66. Hasenstab KA, Jadcherla SR. Respiratory events in infants presenting with apparent life threatening events: is there an explanation from esophageal motility? J Pediatr 2014;165(2):250–5.e1.
67. Volpe JJ, Hill H. Disorders of sucking and swallowing in the newborn infant: clinicopathological correlations. In: Korofiken R, Guilleminault C, editors. Progress in perinatal neurology, vol. 1. Baltimore (MD): Williams & Wilkins; 1981. p. 157–81.
68. Gulati IK, Shubert TR, Sitaram S, et al. Effects of birth asphyxia on the modulation of pharyngeal provocation-induced adaptive reflexes. Am J Physiol Gastrointest Liver Physiol 2015;309(8):G662–9.
69. Jensen PS, Gulati IK, Shubert TR, et al. Pharyngeal stimulus-induced reflexes are impaired in infants with perinatal asphyxia: does maturation modify? Neurogastroenterol Motil 2017;29(7). https://doi.org/10.1111/nmo.13039.
70. Kitzmiller JL, Cloherty JP, Younger MD, et al. Diabetic pregnancy and perinatal morbidity. Am J Obstet Gynecol 1978;131(5):560–80.
71. Tolosa JN, Calhoun DA. Maternal and neonatal demographics of macrosomic infants admitted to the neonatal intensive care unit. J Perinatol 2017;37(12):1292–6.
72. Malkar MB, Viswanathan SK, Jadcherla SR. Pilot study of pharyngoesophageal dysmotility mechanisms in dysphagic infants of diabetic mothers. Am J Perinatol 2019;36(12):1237–42.
73. Logan KM, Gale C, Hyde MJ, et al. Diabetes in pregnancy and infant adiposity: systematic review and meta-analysis. Arch Dis Child Fetal Neonatal Ed 2017;102(1):F65–72.
74. Kara M, Orbak Z, Döneray H, et al. The relationship between skinfold thickness and leptin, ghrelin, adiponectin, and resistin levels in infants of diabetic mothers. Fetal Pediatr Pathol 2017;36(1):1–7.
75. Lausten-Thomsen U, Christiansen M, Hedley PL, et al. Adipokines in umbilical cord blood from children born large for gestational age. J Pediatr Endocrinol Metab 2016;29(1):33–7.
76. Tapanainen P, Leinonen E, Ruokonen A, et al. Leptin concentrations are elevated in newborn infants of diabetic mothers. Horm Res 2001;55(4):185–90.

Gastroesophageal Reflux Disease in the Neonatal Intensive Care Unit Neonate

Controversies, Current Understanding, and Future Directions

Kathryn A. Hasenstab, BS, BME[a],
Sudarshan R. Jadcherla, MD, FRCPI, DCH[a,b,c,d],*

KEYWORDS

- Infant • Gastroesophageal reflux disease • Mechanisms
- Aerodigestive pathophysiology

KEY POINTS

- Distinguishing gastroesophageal reflux (GER) and GER disease (GERD) remains a conundrum in infants. Clinically based diagnosis remains unclear as symptoms are largely heterogeneous.
- GERD-type symptoms are often managed with changes in diet, feeding methods, and acid-suppressive therapy; all these empiric therapies lack objectivity and practice variation is wide.
- Complications due to true GERD are likely multifaceted and involve aerodigestive systems. Better diagnostic strategies involving evaluation for anomalies, pH-impedance testing, symptom correlation with acid and nonacid events, column extent, and nutritive and feeding assessment are needed to inform better therapeutic options and anticipatory guidance.

[a] Innovative Infant Feeding Disorders Research Program, Nationwide Children's Hospital, Center for Perinatal Research, Abigail Wexner Research Institute, 575 Children's Crossroads, Columbus, OH 43215, USA; [b] Division of Neonatology, Nationwide Children's Hospital, Columbus, OH, USA; [c] Division Pediatric Gastroenterology, Hepatology and Nutrition, Department of Pediatrics, Nationwide Children's Hospital, Columbus, OH, USA; [d] Department of Pediatrics, College of Medicine, The Ohio State University College of Medicine, Columbus, OH, USA
* Corresponding author. Innovative Infant Feeding Disorders Research Program, Nationwide Children's Hospital, Center for Perinatal Research, Abigail Wexner Research Institute, 575 Children's Crossroads, Columbus, OH 43215.
E-mail address: Sudarshan.Jadcherla@nationwidechildrens.org

Clin Perinatol 47 (2020) 243–263
https://doi.org/10.1016/j.clp.2020.02.004
0095-5108/20/© 2020 Elsevier Inc. All rights reserved.

INTRODUCTION

Accurate diagnosis and management of gastroesophageal reflux disease (GERD) in neonatal intensive care units (NICUs) remains problematic owing to heterogeneity of infants' maturational status, constantly changing physiology and pathophysiology of evolving diseases, nonspecific nature of aerodigestive and cardiorespiratory symptoms, and variability in approaches among multidisciplinary providers. The consequences of empiric therapies in this fragile infant population can be detrimental. We aim to clarify the current controversies, explain the potential role of GERD in causing symptoms and complications from a physiologic and pathophysiologic perspective, and highlight current advances in the field.

DEFINITIONS FOR GASTROESOPHAGEAL REFLUX DISEASE IN THE NEONATAL INTENSIVE CARE UNIT INFANT SETTING

Gastroesophageal reflux (GER) involves movement of gastric contents into the esophagus, and is a common physiologic process in infants, often resolving with growth and maturation.[1,2] Regurgitation is a common presentation (occurring daily in 70% of healthy infants, and resolving with maturation by 12–14 months of age) and is considered troublesome if accompanied by other symptoms, such as failure to thrive or hematemesis.[3–6] GERD definitions have changed marginally over the last 2 decades (**Box 1**).

PREVALENCE AND BURDEN

True prevalence and economic burden of GERD in NICU infants is unknown because of unclear diagnostic definitions, lack of gold standard testing, and frequent empiric treatment strategies.[1,7–11] In preterm infants, the GERD diagnosis rates across US NICUs average 10% to 22%, varying widely from 2% to 88%, and costs approximately $70K per admission averaging an extra 30 days of hospitalization.[10,11] Prescriptions are often off-label and average 24% to 37% of infants' receiving them, with treatment durations lasting approximately 10 months, which are much longer than GERD guideline recommendations of 4 to 8 weeks.[7,12,13] As GER medications have been associated with adverse events and side effects,[1,2,7,14–18] the true impact of prolonged GERD therapy on economic burden and long-term consequences in NICU survivors remains unknown.

DEVELOPMENTAL NEUROPHYSIOLOGY OF AERODIGESTIVE SYSTEMS

Understanding the links between the neural circuitry assist in understanding the multiple systems involved in GER physiology, GERD pathophysiology, and heterogeneity

---

Box 1
Common definitions associated with gastroesophageal reflux

- Regurgitation[4–6]: Visualization of gastric contents, does not require medical intervention, and does not have negative long-term consequences.
- GER[2,7–9]: The passage of gastric contents into the esophagus with or without regurgitation and vomiting, a common physiologic process
- GER disease (GERD)[7–9]:GER leading to troublesome symptoms that affect daily functioning
- Refractory GERD[7]: No response to medical therapy

with symptom occurrences. Knowledge of aerodigestive system development, structure, and function is important to assist providers in clarifying normal from abnormal.[19] The developing neural tube forming the central nervous system, and the neural crest cells forming the peripheral nervous system play an important role for afferent (sensory) and efferent (motor) neurotransmission within and between brain-airway-foregut.[20] Embryonic development of the aerodigestive tract occurs approximately between 3 and 4 weeks to form the foregut and respiratory diverticulum.[20] The diaphragm develops from pleuroperitoneal folds, with the crural portion surrounding the lower esophageal sphincter (LES) of the esophagus to form the gastroesophageal junction (GEJ).[21–23] Developmental abnormalities of aerodigestive systems may include tracheal stenosis, tracheal agenesis, tracheaesophageal fistula, craniofacial abnormalities, congenital diaphragmatic hernia, hiatal hernia, esophageal atresia, pyloric stenosis, and malrotation; these conditions increase susceptibility to reflux pathophysiologies.[7]

The glossopharyngeal nerve (IX) provides sensory connections to the tongue and pharynx, and the vagus nerve (X) provides sensory and motor connections to the respiratory system, pharynx, esophagus, stomach, and heart.[24] The vagus nerve plays a vital role in influencing cross-system effects via the pharyngeal branch (pharyngoesophageal nerve), superior laryngeal nerve, inferior laryngeal nerve, recurrent laryngeal nerve, cervical and thoracic cardiac branches, pulmonary branches, esophageal branches, and gastric branches.[24] An image of the aerodigestive tract, its nerves, functions, and potential responses to GER is shown (**Fig. 1**).

APPLIED PHYSIOLOGY AND POTENTIAL THERAPEUTIC TARGETS

An understanding of GERD mechanisms and their potential role in symptom causation is discussed along with therapeutic targets. The stomach accommodates saliva, ingested food, mucus, and gastric juices, and rhythmic migratory gastric contractions empty the contents periodically into the duodenum. Sling fibers (smooth muscle) around the greater curvature of the stomach contributes to the GEJ integrity[25] by acting as a flap valve in preventing reflux during fundal distention.[26] GER events may occur when intra-abdominal pressure overcomes the barrier role of LES and this mechanism is most commonly observed immediately after feeds.[27,28] Gastric accommodation and transient LES relaxation (TLESR) have a negative correlation, suggesting that treatments targeting impaired accommodation may be beneficial.[27,29] Currently there is poor evidence for delayed gastric emptying as a physiologic mechanism for GER;[28,30] however, this has been a therapeutic target. Secretion of gastric acid by neuronal and hormonal influence helps with digestion while protecting against infection. Exposure of gastric acid into esophagus increases until approximately 9 months and then declines.[31] However, inappropriate and chronic exposure along with poor clearance and protective mechanisms can result in esophageal tissue damage and inflammation.

The LES in conjunction with the diaphragmatic crural sling fibers forms the GEJ and maintains its integrity.[22,23] As measured with pharyngoesophageal manometry,[32–36] basal LES tone can be low (hypotonic) or high (hypertonic), and appropriately relax (with swallowing, peristalsis) or inappropriately relax for prolonged periods. In neonates, LES lengths ranges from 0.8 to 1 cm between 33 and 36 weeks postmenstrual age,[37] and continues to strengthen with growth and maturation, particularly the intra-abdominal part of the LES.[37,38] Although LES hypotonicity is a risk factor for GER, relaxation is the main mechanism in infants, primarily due to spontaneous TLESR, or swallow-induced LES relaxation (SLESR)[28,39,40] (**Fig. 2**). In preterm infants, LES

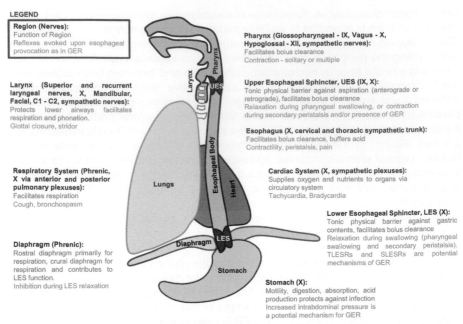

Fig. 1. Neuroanatomic relations and neurophysiologic functions within the aerodigestive tract: implications for causal and ameliorating mechanisms of gastroesophageal reflux. Each anatomic region with corresponding nerves are listed in black bold text, region function in green text, and potential response to refluxate in blue text. Note that responses to esophageal provocation can manifest as symptoms, and these can be from the direct effects of the stimulus (Reflux Theory) regionally, or from the sensory-motor effects (Reflex Theory).

relaxation improves with maturation.[38] TLESRs are common in healthy infants but increased in those with GERD, and are affected by body position with lateral left side-lying position being favorable to decreased TLESR frequency.[41,42] Regarding SLESRs, average relaxation duration during esophageal provocation-induced swallowing is 4.5 seconds at 35 weeks postmenstrual age,[38] and is terminated by esophageal peristalsis.[23,28,32–36,38,39] Thus, the potential for GER events occurs when LES relaxation duration is prolonged and/or in the presence of peristaltic failure. Therefore, rapid activation of peristaltic reflexes, bolus clearance mechanisms, prevention of proximal ascent, protection of airway, and rapid restoration of LES integrity, are all potential therapeutic targets. These complex functions of LES are mediated by excitatory (cholinergic) and inhibitory (nitric oxide or vasoactive intestinal polypeptide) transmission at the GEJ. Stimulation of $GABA_B$ pathways inhibit TLESRs, and therefore decrease the propensity to GER.[23]

The esophagus facilitates bolus transit and comprises striated muscle proximally, and smooth muscle distally, with the transition zone in between.[43] Infant esophageal length averages 6.5 cm and is correlated with somatic growth and postnatal maturation.[37] Esophageal reflexes are activated during GER to safely clear the refluxate.[44] Poor and ineffective clearance may be due to peristaltic failure or delays, and increased LES resistance, and therefore can result in symptoms. Acid exposure to the esophagus can trigger symptoms by altering sensory perception of the esophagus.[45,46] Esophageal provocation activates pharyngoesophageal reflexes, during which multisystemic responses may occur (**Fig. 3**) with or without symptoms.[32–34,47,48]

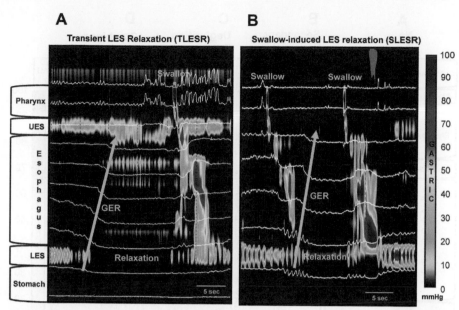

Fig. 2. Important causal and protective mechanisms for GER in infants. UES and LES are the upper and lower esophageal sphincter, respectively. Depicted is high-resolution impedance manometry with white lines representing impedance (a measurement method to detect bolus direction) and colored plots representing esophago-pressure topography (a measurement method to detect swallowing activity with low pressures in *blue* and high pressures in *purple*). Common mechanisms of GER events in infants include: (*A*) TLESR, the primary mechanism of GER is characterized by spontaneous prolonged LES relaxation (>10 seconds) with retrograde bolus (GER) detected by impedance drop. The GER may trigger peristaltic reflexes (swallowing) to facilitate clearance, and/or symptoms. (*B*) SLESR is characterized by LES relaxation with pharyngeal activity and often poor esophageal propagation. Note the second peristaltic sequence with complete esophageal propagation facilitates bolus clearance (return to impedance baseline).

For example, mechanosensitivity, osmosensitivity, or chemosensitivity can modify afferent and efferent responses, thus contributing to sensory-motor effects. These vagus nerve-mediated esophageal reflexes are modified by gestational and postnatal maturation, sleep, and disease states.[32–34,49–55]

Another critical function of the esophagus is mucosal tissue resistance, which provides protection via preepithelial defense, acid buffering, and decreasing intercellular spaces.[44] Esophageal mucosal inflammation has been associated with esophagitis, increased acid exposure, frequency of GER events, delayed clearance, and greater prevalence of aerodigestive symptoms.[56–62] In preterm and term infants, esophageal inflammation is decreased with chronologic age or proton pump inhibitor treatment.[62,63] However, although distal esophageal inflammation may be correlated to vomiting, acid-suppressive treatment may not improve acute symptoms as there is low correlation with overall symptom score, coughing, crying, and other aerodigestive symptoms.[62,63]

The upper esophageal sphincter(UES) forms a physical dynamic barrier between the pharynx and esophagus that is comprises the cervical esophagus, cricopharyngeous, and inferior constrictor muscles.[64] Because of its proximity to the airway introitus, this proximal sphincter has a vital role and includes agility and time-determined

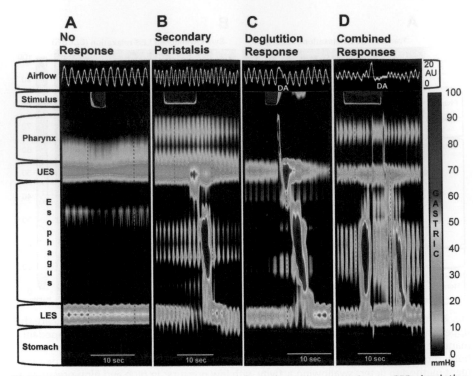

Fig. 3. Clearance mechanisms in the event of esophageal provocation: a GER simulation model. UES and LES are the upper and lower esophageal sphincter, respectively. Midesophageal infusion (stimulus) simulates GER. Media include air (gas), water (nonacid liquid), or apple juice (acid liquid). As depicted using high-resolution manometry and nasal airflow thermistor methods, potential responses may include: (A) no response characterized by absence of pharyngoesophageal activity, (B) secondary peristalsis characterized by UES contraction, esophageal body contraction, LES relaxation, and no respiratory change, (C) deglutition characterized by pharyngeal contraction, UES relaxation, esophageal body contraction, LES relaxation, and pause in breathing, or deglutition apnea (DA), or (D) combination of multiple peristaltic responses. Symptoms may occur in any of these scenarios. Responses are affected by subject maturation, stimulus media, and stimulus volume. It is currently unknown how infants with proven GERD respond to midesophageal stimuli.

response sensitivity in relation to respiratory phases, sleep, swallowing, ascending reflux events, coughing, and pharyngeal clearance. In addition, by maintaining a tonic state, the UES prevents air insufflation into the gut with inspiration.[64] UES basal tone averages 17 mm Hg in preterm infants and 26 mm Hg in full-term infants.[34] Therefore, the UES barrier function can be of increased importance in the chronic esophageal exposure to refluxate. In adult and animal models, sleep decreases UES tone,[65,66] and acid exposure decreases sensitivity of UES contraction.[67]

The oropharynx communicates with the oral cavity, nasopharynx, larynx, hypopharynx, and esophagus. The superior, middle, and inferior pharyngeal constrictor muscles maintain pharyngeal functions.[68] Pharyngeal stimuli frequently trigger pharyngeal reflexive swallowing along with deglutition apnea (a biomarker of glottal closure)[55,69–73] (Fig. 4). During multiple pharyngeal swallows, respiratory changes are prolonged; however, duration and efficiency of swallowing improves with maturation.[69] GER events reaching the pharynx (known as supraesophageal reflux,

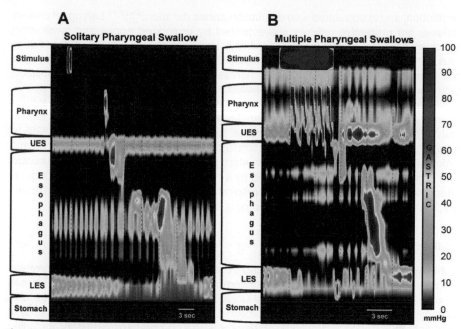

Fig. 4. Clearance mechanisms in the event of pharyngeal provocation: a proximal GER-simulation model. UES and LES are the upper and lower esophageal sphincter, respectively. As depicted in high-resolution manometry, the most common responses to pharyngeal stimulus (sterile water) are: (*A*) solitary pharyngeal reflexive swallow characterized by pharyngeal contraction, UES relaxation, esophageal peristalsis, and LES relaxation, or (*B*) multiple pharyngeal reflexive swallowing characterized by multiple pharyngeal contractions, esophageal peristalsis, and LES relaxation. Responses are dependent on stimulus volume and subject maturation. It is currently unknown how pharyngeal swallowing differs in infants with proven GERD.

extraesophageal reflux, or laryngopharyngeal reflux) may also trigger these reflexes and is believed to contribute to chronic cough, aspiration, failure to thrive, and throat clearing in the pediatric population.[74,75] In adult supraesophageal reflux disease, UES and esophageal responses to simulated liquid reflux are impaired.[76] Thus, supraesophageal reflux may be problematic in infants with dysphagia and/or sensory issues (as is common in neurologic NICU infants) presenting with inability to clear secretions, weak pharyngeal contractility, or dysfunctional swallowing. The role of acid-suppressive therapy or surgical therapies among those infants who are susceptible to supraesophageal acid injury in infants remains to be clarified.[74,75]

The main function of the diaphragm is to facilitate inspiration; however, it is also involved in other nonventilatory behaviors, such as coughing, sneezing, and emesis.[20,21] The costal diaphragm facilitates respiratory mechanics, whereas the crural diaphragm is important for both respiration and augmenting LES tone during inspiration when the risk from reflux can be greater. Hiatal hernia occurs when there is separation between the LES and the diaphragm, in which the upper part of the stomach slides into the thoracic cavity, and can be detected radiographically or via esophageal high-resolution manometry.[77] Hiatal hernia is an increased risk factor for GERD.[78]

The larynx protects the airway and facilitates respiration and phonation. Glottal (vocal cord) closure reflex during pharyngeal and esophageal stimuli augments airway protection, and is correlated with deglutition apnea duration.[35,72,79] Laryngeal chemoreflexes are protective reflexes characterized by prolonged apnea and swallowing, which are sensitive to acid (chemosensitivity), low chloride (osmosensitivity), and stimulus volume, and improves with maturation.[80–84] Exaggeration or lack of laryngeal chemoreflexes have the potential for increased risks in the neurogenic population, with the concern of aspiration during swallowing and or reflux events.[85]

Numerous studies have conflicting results whether or not cardiorespiratory system events are linked to GER,[86–91] and acid-suppressive therapy may not be beneficial.[92–95] In preterm infants, HR decrease is prevalent with approximately 32% of pharyngeal stimuli and dependent on stimulus characteristics and maturation.[55] Maturation of vagal functions in healthy premature infants, particularly in relation to control and regulation of breathing is achieved by 44 weeks postmenstrual age. Inadequate integration of aerodigestive and cardiorespiratory reflexes can result in delayed recovery,[55] and therefore troublesome symptoms that include dysphagia.

CURRENT DIAGNOSTIC STRATEGIES

Controversies exist in the diagnosis and treatment of GERD in infants. A differential diagnosis is a first step to distinguish uncomplicated versus complicated GER based on clinical presentation and behavioral signs, symptom scores, and/or a short trial of therapy.[1,2,7–11,13,96,97] NASPGHAN guidelines for infants aged 0 to 12 month with frequent regurgitation and/or vomiting recommend a comprehensive history, including age of symptom onset, feeding history, pattern of regurgitation, family medical history, physical examination, environmental triggers, patient growth, and any pharmacologic or diet changes.[7] Clinical presentation and complications thought to be due to GERD are shown in **Box 2**. Additional differential diagnoses may include malrotation, autonomic dysfunction, achalasia, gastroparesis, sepsis/meningitis/intracranial illness,

---

Box 2
Signs/symptoms/complications thought due to gastroesophageal reflux disease in neonatal intensive care unit infants

Signs/Symptoms
- GERD related: Distressed behavior (excessive crying/irritability/posturing)
- Dysphagia related: Poor oral feeds or refusal, failure to thrive/poor growth
- Respiratory related: Chronic cough, stridor, apnea, recurrent lower respiratory tract infections
- Cardiopulmonary related: Apnea/bradycardia/desaturation
- Other: Nasal congestion, sinusitis, recurrent otitis media, anemia

Complications
- Reflux esophagitis
- Strictures
- Recurrent aspiration pneumonia
- Nasopharyngeal and laryngeal symptoms, recurrent otitis media

Red flags suggesting potential conditions other than GERD requiring further investigation
- Vomiting: Pyloric stenosis, urinary tract infection, intracranial pathologies
- Fever: Infection
- Bile-stained vomit: Intestinal obstruction is a strong consideration
- Hematemesis: Gastrointestinal bleeding
- Bloody stools: Milk protein allergy, bacteria, acute surgical condition
- Abdominal distension: Intestinal obstruction, dysmotility, anatomic abnormalities
- Chronic diarrhea: Milk protein allergy

and urinary tract-related pathologies (especially for vomiting and poor feeding).[7] Infant GER symptom scores have recently been developed taking into account clinical presentation and parent/provider perception.[96,97] However, controversy remains as to whether these metrics are true metrics of GERD as they did not use evidence-based GERD diagnosis, and differences between inpatient and outpatient populations exist.[97] Empiric proton pump inhibitor therapy for GERD diagnosis is not currently supported in infants, due to poor evidence in decreasing symptoms.[7]

Advantages and disadvantages of testing methods are shown (**Table 1**). Although no gold standard currently exists for the diagnosis of GERD in high-risk infants, pH-impedance is currently the preferred method over pH-metry alone as pH-impedance is able to measure additional GER bolus characteristics (anterograde/retrograde, gas/liquid/mixed, height, clearance times) (**Fig. 5**) and symptom correlation via symptom indices.[1,98–103] Proposed thresholds: (a) esophageal acid exposure utilizing acid reflux index are greater than 7% or greater than 10%,[9,104] (b) GER frequency (acid or nonacid) greater than 70 events/per day (>18 for acid, >51 for weakly acid, >1 for weakly alkaline). However, even in the event of crossing thresholds, it does not necessarily mean there is a symptom correlation. As GERD is multifactorial, it is likely that a combination of clinical and evidence-based metrics (acid exposure, inflammation, symptom correlation) may assist in true diagnosis and effective treatment strategies.[101]

CURRENT TREATMENT STRATEGIES

Guidelines for management of infant GERD[2,7] using stepwise approaches are summarized in **Box 3**. Evidence and controversies of potential interventions are discussed below.

i. Nonpharmacologic (conservative) therapies[1,2,7] include body positioning and feeding modifications. Body positioning goes against current American Academy of Pediatrics guidelines of positioning infants in supine position for the prevention of sudden infant death syndrome.[105,106] Therefore, position management for GER is not recommended in sleeping infants.[1,2,7] Furthermore, caution should be exercised for infants with anomalies and airway vulnerability. Anticipatory guidance must be provided to parents about airway safety and safe swallowing. Feeding modifications include feeding changes, such as increasing duration, decreasing volume, decreasing milk flow rate, thickening formula, and elimination of cow's milk protein. If thickening with rice or oatmeal, extreme caution is needed as such methods can quickly cross safe osmolality thresholds[107] and has numerous potential adverse events with minimal benefit in preterm infants.[18,107–111]

ii. Pharmacologic therapies include antacids, acid-suppressive strategies, mucosal protectants, prokinetics, alginates, and drugs targeting TLESRs. Antacids may include aluminum or magnesium hydroxides or phosphates, magnesium trisilicate, or carbonate and bicarbonate salts but are not recommended in infants.[18] NICE guidelines do not recommend acid-suppressive therapies to treat overt regurgitation as an isolated symptom, and the American Academy of Pediatrics supports avoidance of routine empiric antireflux medications for reflux-type of symptoms or apnea and desaturation events in preterm infants.[1,2,14] If at all used based on objective evidence, treatment should be short term (4–8 weeks)[2,7] due to risks of prolonged use.[7,15–17] Testing via pH-impedance with symptom correlation and baseline impedance is needed to determine acid as the true cause of symptoms, or esophageal inflammation respectively.[62,101] Further placebo-controlled clinical trials are needed in objectively defined GERD.[2,7] Mucosal protectants, such as

Table 1
Current diagnostic testing modalities for gastroesophageal reflux disease and its potential advantages and disadvantages in infants

Testing Modality	Advantages	Disadvantages
Upper GI	• Targets foregut anatomic considerations (hiatal hernia, malrotation, pyloric stenosis, intestinal stricture, achalasia, and tracheo-esophageal fistula) • Useful for those undergoing Gastrostomy or antireflux surgery and evaluation of extraesophageal symptoms	• Not supported to diagnose GERD • Radiation exposure
Ultrasonography	• Targets foregut anatomic considerations (pyloric stenosis or gastric dysmotility, other diagnoses triggering vomiting, such as non-GI causes—renal or liver origins)	• Limited value with GERD evaluation
Esophago-gastro-duodenoscopy	• Can be performed with/without biopsy, targets esophagitis (erosive, microscopic, eosinophilic), GERD complications or conditions mimicking GERD	• Normal endoscopy does not rule out GERD • Not supported to diagnose GERD in infants
Biomarkers	• Uses salivary pepsin to determine cause of extraesophageal symptoms	• Lack of normal values, insufficient to diagnose extraesophageal reflux disease • Unknown if it correlates with severity of symptoms
Scintigraphy	• Targets gastric emptying and GERD, can detect possible aspiration of refluxate	• Lack of standardization, not supported for diagnosis of GERD in infants
Pharyngoesophageal manometry	• Targets GI motility (dysmotility) and/or LES function (outlet obstruction, hiatal hernia, TLESRs, hypotonicity) and assesses mechanisms • Detailed evaluation of aerodigestive protection (peristalsis, UES, LES, airway responses) in response to simulated reflux and cause of aerodigestive and cardiorespiratory symptoms, such as cough and pathologic apnea • Personalized approaches using concurrent technologies (impedance, cardiorespiratory monitoring, video-fluoroscopy, ultrasonography • Fundoplication and postsurgery LES evaluations	• Not supported to diagnose GERD in infants • Requires specialized equipment and expertise • Labor intensive

	Advantages	Limitations
pH-metry	• Determines pathologic esophageal acid exposure (acid-GERD) • Acute symptom correlation with acid reflux episodes • Can evaluate acid-suppressive therapy efficacy	• Lack of healthy control data • Not sensitive to nonacid or ascending reflux, and not preferred over pH-MII
pH-impedance (pH-MII)	• Determines pathologic esophageal acid exposure, and can detects nonacid refluxate and height of refluxate • Distinguishes physical (gas, liquid, mixed) and chemical (acid, weakly acid, weakly alkaline) characteristics of refluxate • Acute symptom correlation with reflux events • Baseline impedance as a surrogate for esophageal inflammation • Determine acid-suppressive therapy efficacy	• Limited availability • Lack of control data • Reflux episodes may be underestimated • Time consuming and needs expertise to interpret • Reliance on bedside caregivers dedicated to symptom documentation

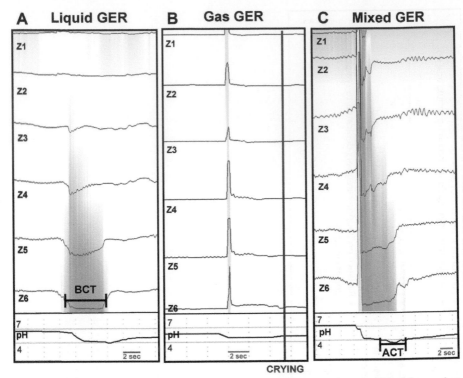

Fig. 5. Characterization of GER events during pH-impedance. 24-hour pH-impedance characterizes physico-chemical (liquid/gas/mixed, acid/nonacid) and spatio-temporal (height, clearance times) GER characteristics and symptom correlation. Potential examples are: (*A*) liquid acid characterized by retrograde drop in impedance and pH drop below 4. Note this is not full-column GER (does not reach Z1). Bolus clearance time (BCT) determines bolus contact and clearance efficiency. (*B*) Gas nonacid characterized by rapid rise in impedance reaching the most proximal impedance channel (Z1) and pH > 4. Crying is associated with this GER event. (*C*) Mixed acid characterized by liquid and gas components with pH < 4. Acid clearance time (ACT) measures esophageal acid contact time. As numerous iterations are possible, it is important to discern the true cause of symptoms for effective diagnosis and therapies.

sucralfate, may be beneficial to promote healing but is contraindicated in preterm infants and has been associated with bezoars.[112] Prokinetics generally are not recommended in NICU infants; if used, specialized advice is recommended.[1,2,7,16,17] Although alginates may be beneficial, apnea frequency is not altered[113] and chronic use is not recommended due to risk of adverse events.[7,18] Drugs targeting TLESRs: Medications that inhibit TLESR include atropine, baclofen, cannabinoid receptor agonists, cholecystokinin A receptor antagonists, metabotropic glutamate receptor antagonists, morphine, and nitric oxide.[23] The safety and efficacy of these drugs in NICU infants is unknown.

iii. Surgical therapies include fundoplication and enteral tube feeding strategies. Fundoplication is a surgical procedure for refractory GERD. LES tone, GEJ anatomy, presence of swallowing and aerodigestive protective reflexes should be considered in the decision-making. Fundoplication can strengthen the barrier function at the GEJ, but infant's inability to swallow and belch, and lack of emetic reflex

---

Box 3
Stepwise infant gastroesophageal reflux disease management approaches according to current guidelines

NASPGHAN Guidelines[7]
- History and physical exam
- Alarm sign/red flags → testing and referral
- Feeding modifications (avoid overfeeding by reducing volume with more frequent feeds, thicken feeds, continue breastfeeding) management if improved
- 2–4 wk protein hydrolysate or amino acid-based formula, or elimination of cow's milk in mother's diet if breastfed
- Pediatric gastrointestinal (GI) referral, if referral not possible consider 4–8 wk trial of acid-suppressive therapy and wean if symptoms improve (if no improvement then revisit differential al diagnosis, testing, and short-term medication trial)

NICE Guidelines[2]
- Parental education/reassurance
- Determine complicated vs uncomplicated GER, red flags/complications → testing/clinical judgment/referral
- Frequent regurgitation
  Formula fed: feeding history → reduce feeding volume if excessive
  → smaller more frequent feeds
  → thickened formula → 1–2-wk alginate therapy
  Breast fed: breastfeeding assessment → 1–2-wk alginate trial
- 4-wk acid-suppressive therapy trial in (1) overt regurgitation + unexplained feeding difficulties, distressed behavior, or poor growth, (2) endoscopy-proven esophagitis
- Enteral tube feeding for poor growth with overt regurgitation, Jejunal feeds in those with intragastric intolerance or concern for reflux-related pulmonary aspiration

---

can result in new symptoms.[7] Enteral tube feeding strategies include gastrostomy or transpyloric feeding and may be recommended for poor growth when associated with dysphagia. Transpyloric feeding is not supported by best evidence at this time.

OTHER CONTROVERSIES TO CONSIDER IN THE COMPLEX NEONATAL INTENSIVE CARE UNIT INFANT

i. Specific risk factors: Coexisting morbidities with maturation occurring ex utero may increase risk of GERD and include congenital anomalies, bronchopulmonary dysplasia, or neuropathology.[114,115] On another note, the use of caffeine and bronchodilators can worsen GERD due to increasing gastric acid secretions and decreasing LES tone.[116,117]

ii. Symptoms-based treatment trials: The basis of symptoms needs to be determined in the context of reflux events, and may be related to heightened esophageal sensitivity, acid neutralization delays, poor clearance mechanism, dysmotility, or inflammation. True causality of symptoms should be determined, particularly for airway symptoms such as coughing and stridor, and cannot be attributed to GERD unless tested.[118] Reflux as the cause of prolonged cardiorespiratory events is extremely rare, and is more likely caused by dysfunctional swallowing mechanisms,[94] which can only be recognized when tested. Thus, symptom-based treatment trials are obsolete as the causal and ameliorating mechanisms are multifactorial.

SUMMARY AND FUTURE DIRECTIONS

We clarified the current controversies (**Box 4**), explained the potential role of GERD in causing symptoms and complications from physiologic and pathophysiologic perspectives, and highlighted current advances in the field. Evidence basis for the

---

Box 4
Current gastroesophageal reflux disease controversies that remain to be resolved in neonatal intensive care unit infants

True GERD definitions, prevalence, and identification of troublesome symptoms/complications

By anatomic region
- Pharynx: Diagnosis, prevalence, and burden of supraesophageal GERD
- UES: Impact of acid exposure on UES protection
- Esophagus: Impact of GERD on esophageal reflexes
- LES: Identifying TLESR thresholds, and safe therapies targeting TLESRs
- Stomach: Long-term effects of modifying gastric acid
- Larynx: GER as true cause of apnea/bradycardia/desaturation events
- Maturation vs maladaptation vs malfunction

Development of diagnostic criteria to define true GERD in nonverbal infants
- Identification of true cause of symptoms

Development of effective GERD therapies
- Conservative therapies
- Thickening is controversial and should be monitored
- Use of acid-suppressive therapies and duration
- Role of surgical therapies (fundoplication, tracheostomy, gastrostomy) and transpyloric feeds
- Timing, duration, and definition of therapeutic success

---

diagnostic strategies were discussed, and involve evaluation for anomalies, pH-impedance testing to evaluate symptom correlation with GER events (acid and nonacid) and its column extent and feeding assessment. Distinguishing physiologic from pathophysiological basis of symptoms attributed to GERD is needed before dietary modification, pharmacotherapies, or surgical procedures. Because of the heterogeneity and multifactorial nature of symptom generation, better diagnostic strategies and treatment algorithms are needed as consequences of therapies can be a concern. Well-controlled clinical trials are needed to answer these questions regarding GERD in NICU neonates.

ACKNOWLEDGMENTS

The authors thank Roseanna Helmick, BS, BME, for assistance with figures.

DISCLOSURE

The authors have nothing to disclose.

Best Practices

Neonatal Gastroesophageal Reflux Disease (GERD)

What is the current practice?
- Symptoms-based empiric pharmacologic therapies and feeding modifications of uncertain duration
- Practice variation is wide

Best Practice/Guideline/Care Path Objective(s)
- Determine physiologic vs pathophysiologic GER
- History and physical exam, parental education, and reassurance

What changes in current practice are likely to improve outcomes?
- Symptoms are nonspecific and heterogeneous. Avoid empiric therapies
- Proper identification for the basis of symptoms and consideration of maturation vs maladaptation vs malfunction

Major Recommendations
- Evidence-based diagnosis using pH-impedance and symptom correlation testing for appropriate management
- Short-term therapies if utilized

Summary Statement
History, physical exam, and parental education are important in determining suspicion of GERD. If suspicion is high, objective evidence-based diagnosis is essential to manage true GERD.

Bibliographic Source(s): *Data from* Refs.[1,2,7]

REFERENCES

1. Eichenwald E, Committee on Fetus and Newborn. Diagnosis and management of gastroesophageal reflux in preterm infants. Pediatrics 2018;142(1). https://doi.org/10.1542/peds.2018-1061.

2. National Collaborating Centre for Women's and Children's Health (UK). Gastro-oesophageal reflux disease: recognition, diagnosis and management in children and young people. London: National Institute for Health and Care Excellence (UK); 2015.

3. Vandenplas Y, Hauser B, Devreker T, et al. Infant regurgitation and pediatric gastroesophageal reflux disease. New York: Humana Press; 2013.

4. Hegar B, Dewanti NR, Kadim M, et al. Natural evolution of regurgitation in healthy infants. Acta Paediatr 2009;98(7):1189–93.

5. Nelson SP, Chen EH, Syniar GM, et al. Prevalence of symptoms of gastroesophageal reflux during infancy. A pediatric practice-based survey. Pediatric Practice Research Group. Arch Pediatr Adolesc Med 1997;151(6):569–72.

6. Zeevenhooven J, Koppen IJ, Benninga MA. The New Rome IV criteria for functional gastrointestinal disorders in infants and toddlers. Pediatr Gastroenterol Hepatol Nutr 2017;20(1):1–13.

7. Rosen R, Vandenplas Y, Singendonk M, et al. Pediatric gastroesophageal reflux clinical practice guidelines: joint recommendations of the North American Society for Pediatric Gastroenterology, Hepatology, and Nutrition and the European Society for Pediatric Gastroenterology, Hepatology, and Nutrition. J Pediatr Gastroenterol Nutr 2018;66(3):516–54.

8. Rudolph CD, Mazur LJ, Liptak GS, et al. Guidelines for evaluation and treatment of gastroesophageal reflux in infants and children: recommendations of the North American Society for Pediatric Gastroenterology and Nutrition. J Pediatr Gastroenterol Nutr 2001;32(Suppl 2):S1–31.

9. Vandenplas Y, Rudolph CD, Di Lorenzo C, et al. Pediatric gastroesophageal reflux clinical practice guidelines: joint recommendations of the North American Society for Pediatric Gastroenterology, Hepatology, and Nutrition (NASPGHAN) and the European Society for Pediatric Gastroenterology, Hepatology, and Nutrition (ESPGHAN). J Pediatr Gastroenterol Nutr 2009;49(4):498–547.

10. Jadcherla SR, Slaughter JL, Stenger MR, et al. Practice variance, prevalence, and economic burden of premature infants diagnosed with GERD. Hosp Pediatr 2013;3(4):335–41.

11. Dhillon AS, Ewer AK. Diagnosis and management of gastro-oesophageal reflux in preterm infants in neonatal intensive care units. Acta Paediatr 2004;93(1): 88–93.

12. D'Agostino JA, Passarella M, Martin AE, et al. Use of gastroesophageal reflux medications in premature infants after NICU discharge. Pediatrics 2016;138(6).

13. Slaughter JL, Stenger MR, Reagan PB, et al. Neonatal histamine-2 receptor antagonist and proton pump inhibitor treatment at United States Children's Hospitals. J Pediatr 2016;174:63–70.e63.

14. Ho T, Dukhovny D, Zupancic JA, et al. Choosing wisely in newborn medicine: five opportunities to increase value. Pediatrics 2015;136(2):e482–9.

15. Trikha A, Baillargeon JG, Kuo YF, et al. Development of food allergies in patients with gastroesophageal reflux disease treated with gastric acid suppressive medications. Pediatr Allergy Immunol 2013;24(6):582–8.

16. Safe M, Chan WH, Leach ST, et al. Widespread use of gastric acid inhibitors in infants: are they needed? Are they safe? World J Gastrointest Pharmacol Ther 2016;7(4):531–9.

17. Corvaglia L, Monari C, Martini S, et al. Pharmacological therapy of gastroesophageal reflux in preterm infants. Gastroenterol Res Pract 2013;2013:714564.

18. Vandenplas Y, Salvatore S, Hauser B. The diagnosis and management of gastro-oesophageal reflux in infants. Early Hum Dev 2005;81(12):1011–24.

19. Mansfield LE. Embryonic origins of the relation of gastroesophageal reflux disease and airway disease. Am J Med 2001;111(Suppl 8A):3S–7S.

20. Bolender D, Kaplan S. Basic embryology. In: Polin R, Abman S, Rowitch D, et al, editors. Fetal and neonatal physiology, vol. 1. Philadelphia: Elsevier; 2017. p. 23–9.

21. Mantilla C, Fahim M, JE B, et al. Functional development of respiratory muscles. In: Polin R, Abman S, Rowitch D, et al, editors. Fetal and neonatal physiology, vol. 1. Philadelphia: Elsevier; 2017. p. 692–705.

22. Mittal RK, Balaban DH. The esophagogastric junction. N Engl J Med 1997; 336(13):924–32.

23. Mittal RK, Goyal RK. Sphincter mechanisms at the lower end of the esophagus. GI Motility Online 2006. https://doi.org/10.1038/gimo14.

24. Gray H. The nervous system. In: Pickering Pick T, Howden R, editors. Gray's anatomy. New York: Fall River Press; 2012. p. 727–33.

25. Liebermann-Meffert D, Allgower M, Schmid P, et al. Muscular equivalent of the lower esophageal sphincter. Gastroenterology 1979;76(1):31–8.

26. Goyal RK, Rattan S. Nature of the vagal inhibitory innervation to the lower esophageal sphincter. J Clin Invest 1975;55(5):1119–26.

27. Hunt RH, Camilleri M, Crowe SE, et al. The stomach in health and disease. Gut 2015;64(10):1650–68.

28. Omari TI, Barnett C, Snel A, et al. Mechanisms of gastroesophageal reflux in healthy premature infants. J Pediatr 1998;133(5):650–4.

29. Pauwels A, Altan E, Tack J. The gastric accommodation response to meal intake determines the occurrence of transient lower esophageal sphincter relaxations and reflux events in patients with gastro-esophageal reflux disease. Neurogastroenterol Motil 2014;26(4):581–8.

30. Ewer AK, Durbin GM, Morgan ME, et al. Gastric emptying and gastro-oesophageal reflux in preterm infants. Arch Dis Child Fetal Neonatal Ed 1996; 75(2):F117–21.

31. Vandenplas Y, Sacre-Smits L. Continuous 24-hour esophageal pH monitoring in 285 asymptomatic infants 0-15 months old. J Pediatr Gastroenterol Nutr 1987; 6(2):220–4.

32. Gupta A, Gulati P, Kim W, et al. Effect of postnatal maturation on the mechanisms of esophageal propulsion in preterm human neonates: primary and secondary peristalsis. Am J Gastroenterol 2009;104(2):411–9.

33. Jadcherla SR, Duong HQ, Hoffmann RG, et al. Esophageal body and upper esophageal sphincter motor responses to esophageal provocation during maturation in preterm newborns. J Pediatr 2003;143(1):31–8.

34. Jadcherla SR, Duong HQ, Hofmann C, et al. Characteristics of upper oesophageal sphincter and oesophageal body during maturation in healthy human neonates compared with adults. Neurogastroenterol Motil 2005;17(5):663–70.

35. Jadcherla SR, Gupta A, Coley BD, et al. Esophago-glottal closure reflex in human infants: a novel reflex elicited with concurrent manometry and ultrasonography. Am J Gastroenterol 2007;102(10):2286–93.

36. Jadcherla SR, Shaker R. Esophageal and upper esophageal sphincter motor function in babies. Am J Med 2001;111(Suppl 8A):64S–8S.

37. Gupta A, Jadcherla SR. The relationship between somatic growth and in vivo esophageal segmental and sphincteric growth in human neonates. J Pediatr Gastroenterol Nutr 2006;43(1):35–41.

38. Pena EM, Parks VN, Peng J, et al. Lower esophageal sphincter relaxation reflex kinetics: effects of peristaltic reflexes and maturation in human premature neonates. Am J Physiol Gastrointest Liver Physiol 2010;299(6):G1386–95.

39. Omari TI, Benninga MA, Barnett CP, et al. Characterization of esophageal body and lower esophageal sphincter motor function in the very premature neonate. J Pediatr 1999;135(4):517–21.

40. Omari TI, Miki K, Davidson G, et al. Characterisation of relaxation of the lower oesophageal sphincter in healthy premature infants. Gut 1997;40(3):370–5.

41. van Wijk MP, Benninga MA, Dent J, et al. Effect of body position changes on postprandial gastroesophageal reflux and gastric emptying in the healthy premature neonate. J Pediatr 2007;151(6):585–90, 590.e1-2.

42. Loots C, Smits M, Omari T, et al. Effect of lateral positioning on gastroesophageal reflux (GER) and underlying mechanisms in GER disease (GERD) patients and healthy controls. Neurogastroenterol Motil 2013;25(3):222–229,e1-2.

43. Ghosh SK, Janiak P, Schwizer W, et al. Physiology of the esophageal pressure transition zone: separate contraction waves above and below. Am J Physiol Gastrointest Liver Physiol 2006;290(3):G568–76.

44. Orlando R. Esophageal mucosal defense mechanisms. GI Motility Online 2006. https://doi.org/10.1038/gimo15.

45. Sarkar S, Hobson AR, Furlong PL, et al. Central neural mechanisms mediating human visceral hypersensitivity. Am J Physiol Gastrointest Liver Physiol 2001; 281(5):G1196–202.

46. Sarkar S, Thompson DG, Woolf CJ, et al. Patients with chest pain and occult gastroesophageal reflux demonstrate visceral pain hypersensitivity which may be partially responsive to acid suppression. Am J Gastroenterol 2004;99(10): 1998–2006.

47. Jadcherla SR. Manometric evaluation of esophageal-protective reflexes in infants and children. Am J Med 2003;115(Suppl 3A):157S–60S.

48. Jadcherla SR, Hoffmann RG, Shaker R. Effect of maturation of the magnitude of mechanosensitive and chemosensitive reflexes in the premature human esophagus. J Pediatr 2006;149(1):77–82.

49. Jadcherla SR, Stoner E, Gupta A, et al. Evaluation and management of neonatal dysphagia: impact of pharyngoesophageal motility studies and multidisciplinary feeding strategy. J Pediatr Gastroenterol Nutr 2009;48(2):186–92.

50. Jadcherla SR, Parks VN, Peng J, et al. Esophageal sensation in premature human neonates: temporal relationships and implications of aerodigestive reflexes and electrocortical arousals. Am J Physiol Gastrointest Liver Physiol 2012; 302(1):G134–44.

51. Hill CD, Jadcherla SR. Esophageal mechanosensitive mechanisms are impaired in neonates with hypoxic-ischemic encephalopathy. J Pediatr 2013;162(5): 976–82.

52. Jadcherla SR, Chan CY, Fernandez S, et al. Maturation of upstream and downstream esophageal reflexes in human premature neonates: the role of sleep and awake states. Am J Physiol Gastrointest Liver Physiol 2013;305(9):G649–58.

53. Malkar MB, Jadcherla S. Neuromotor mechanisms of pharyngoesophageal motility in dysphagic infants with congenital heart disease. Pediatr Res 2014; 76(2):190–6.

54. Collins CR, Hasenstab KA, Nawaz S, et al. Mechanisms of aerodigestive symptoms in infants with varying acid reflux index determined by esophageal manometry. J Pediatr 2019;206:240–7.

55. Hasenstab KA, Nawaz S, Lang IM, et al. Pharyngoesophageal and cardiorespiratory interactions: potential implications for premature infants at risk of clinically significant cardiorespiratory events. Am J Physiol Gastrointest Liver Physiol 2019;316(2):G304–12.

56. Cohen Sabban J, Bertoldi GD, Ussher F, et al. Low-impedance baseline values predict severe esophagitis. J Pediatr Gastroenterol Nutr 2017;65(3):278–80.

57. Borrelli O, Salvatore S, Mancini V, et al. Relationship between baseline impedance levels and esophageal mucosal integrity in children with erosive and non-erosive reflux disease. Neurogastroenterol Motil 2012;24(9). 828-e394.

58. Zhong C, Duan L, Wang K, et al. Esophageal intraluminal baseline impedance is associated with severity of acid reflux and epithelial structural abnormalities in patients with gastroesophageal reflux disease. J Gastroenterol 2013;48(5): 601–10.

59. Salvatore S, Salvatoni A, Van Steen K, et al. Behind the (impedance) baseline in children. Dis Esophagus 2014;27(8):726–31.

60. Salvatore S, Salvatoni A, Van Berkel M, et al. Esophageal impedance baseline is age dependent. J Pediatr Gastroenterol Nutr 2013;57(4):506–13.

61. Kessing BF, Bredenoord AJ, Weijenborg PW, et al. Esophageal acid exposure decreases intraluminal baseline impedance levels. Am J Gastroenterol 2011; 106(12):2093–7.

62. Jadcherla SR, Hanandeh N, Hasenstab KA, et al. Differentiation of esophageal pH-impedance characteristics classified by the mucosal integrity marker in human neonates. Pediatr Res 2019;85(3):355–60.

63. Loots CM, Wijnakker R, van Wijk MP, et al. Esophageal impedance baselines in infants before and after placebo and proton pump inhibitor therapy. Neurogastroenterol Motil 2012;24(8):758–762,e1-2.

64. Lang I. Upper esophageal sphincter. GI Motility Online 2006. https://doi.org/10. 1038/gimo12.

65. Eastwood PR, Katagiri S, Shepherd KL, et al. Modulation of upper and lower esophageal sphincter tone during sleep. Sleep Med 2007;8(2):135–43.

66. Bajaj JS, Bajaj S, Dua KS, et al. Influence of sleep stages on esophago-upper esophageal sphincter contractile reflex and secondary esophageal peristalsis. Gastroenterology 2006;130(1):17–25.

67. Lang IM, Medda BK, Shaker R. Effects of esophageal acidification on esophageal reflexes controlling the upper esophageal sphincter. Am J Physiol Gastrointest Liver Physiol 2019;316(1):G45–54.

68. German R. Anatomy and development of oral cavity and pharynx. GI Motility Online 2006. https://doi.org/10.1038/gimo5.

69. Hasenstab KA, Sitaram S, Lang IM, et al. Maturation modulates pharyngeal-stimulus provoked pharyngeal and respiratory rhythms in human infants. Dysphagia 2018;33(1):63–75.

70. Jadcherla SR, Shubert TR, Gulati IK, et al. Upper and lower esophageal sphincter kinetics are modified during maturation: effect of pharyngeal stimulus in premature infants. Pediatr Res 2015;77(1–1):99–106.

71. Jadcherla SR, Gupta A, Stoner E, et al. Pharyngeal swallowing: defining pharyngeal and upper esophageal sphincter relationships in human neonates. J Pediatr 2007;151(6):597–603.

72. Jadcherla SR, Gupta A, Wang M, et al. Definition and implications of novel pharyngo-glottal reflex in human infants using concurrent manometry ultrasonography. Am J Gastroenterol 2009;104(10):2572–82.

73. Jadcherla SR, Prabhakar V, Hasenstab KA, et al. Defining pharyngeal contractile integral during high-resolution manometry in neonates: a neuromotor marker of pharyngeal vigor. Pediatr Res 2018;84(3):341–7.

74. Yilmaz T, Bajin MD, Gunaydin RO, et al. Laryngopharyngeal reflux and *Helicobacter pylori*. World J Gastroenterol 2014;20(27):8964–70.

75. Postma G, Halum S. Laryngeal and pharyngeal complications of gastroesophageal reflux disease. GI Motility Online 2006. https://doi.org/10.1038/gimo46.

76. Babaei A, Venu M, Naini SR, et al. Impaired upper esophageal sphincter reflexes in patients with supraesophageal reflux disease. Gastroenterology 2015;149(6):1381–91.

77. Weijenborg PW, van Hoeij FB, Smout AJ, et al. Accuracy of hiatal hernia detection with esophageal high-resolution manometry. Neurogastroenterol Motil 2015; 27(2):293–9.

78. Kahrilas PJ, Pandolfino JE. Hiatus hernia. GI Motility Online 2006. https://doi.org/10.1038/gimo48.

79. Jadcherla SR, Gupta A, Stoner E, et al. Correlation of glottal closure using concurrent ultrasonography and nasolaryngoscopy in children: a novel approach to evaluate glottal status. Dysphagia 2006;21(1):75–81.

80. Thach BT. The role of the upper airway in SIDS and sudden unexpected infant deaths and the importance of external airway-protective behaviors. In: Duncan JR, Byard RW, editors. SIDS sudden infant and early childhood death: the past, the present and the future. Adelaide: University of Adelaide Press; 2018.

81. Pickens DL, Schefft G, Thach BT. Prolonged apnea associated with upper airway protective reflexes in apnea of prematurity. Am Rev Respir Dis 1988; 137(1):113–8.

82. Davies AM, Koenig JS, Thach BT. Characteristics of upper airway chemoreflex prolonged apnea in human infants. Am Rev Respir Dis 1989;139(3):668–73.

83. Davies AM, Koenig JS, Thach BT. Upper airway chemoreflex responses to saline and water in preterm infants. J Appl Physiol (1985) 1988;64(4):1412–20.

84. Pickens DL, Schefft GL, Thach BT. Pharyngeal fluid clearance and aspiration preventive mechanisms in sleeping infants. J Appl Physiol (1985) 1989;66(3): 1164–71.

85. Sasaki CT, Hundal JS, Kim YH. Protective glottic closure: biomechanical effects of selective laryngeal denervation. Ann Otol Rhinol Laryngol 2005;114(4):271–5.

86. Funderburk A, Nawab U, Abraham S, et al. Temporal association between reflux-like behaviors and gastroesophageal reflux in preterm and term infants. J Pediatr Gastroenterol Nutr 2016;62(4):556–61.

87. Kenigsberg K, Griswold PG, Buckley BJ, et al. Cardiac effects of esophageal stimulation: possible relationship between gastroesophageal reflux (GER) and sudden infant death syndrome (SIDS). J Pediatr Surg 1983;18(5):542–5.

88. Rossor T, Andradi G, Ali K, et al. Gastro-oesophageal reflux and apnoea: is there a temporal relationship? Neonatology 2018;113(3):206–11.

89. Di Fiore J, Arko M, Herynk B, et al. Characterization of cardiorespiratory events following gastroesophageal reflux in preterm infants. J Perinatol 2010;30(10): 683–7.

90. Corvaglia L, Zama D, Spizzichino M, et al. The frequency of apneas in very pre-term infants is increased after non-acid gastro-esophageal reflux. Neurogastroenterol Motil 2011;23(4):303–307,e2.

91. Corvaglia L, Zama D, Gualdi S, et al. Gastro-oesophageal reflux increases the number of apnoeas in very preterm infants. Arch Dis Child Fetal Neonatal Ed 2009;94(3):F188–92.

92. Nobile S, Marchionni P, Noviello C, et al. Correlation between cardiorespiratory events and gastro-esophageal reflux in preterm and term infants: analysis of predisposing factors. Early Hum Dev 2019;134:14–8.

93. Cresi F, Martinelli D, Maggiora E, et al. Cardiorespiratory events in infants with gastroesophageal reflux symptoms: is there any association? Neurogastroenterol Motil 2018;30(5):e13278.

94. Hasenstab KA, Jadcherla SR. Respiratory events in infants presenting with apparent life threatening events: is there an explanation from esophageal motility? J Pediatr 2014;165(2):250–5.e1.

95. Wheatley E, Kennedy KA. Cross-over trial of treatment for bradycardia attributed to gastroesophageal reflux in preterm infants. J Pediatr 2009;155(4):516–21.

96. Kleinman L, Rothman M, Strauss R, et al. The infant gastroesophageal reflux questionnaire revised: development and validation as an evaluative instrument. Clin Gastroenterol Hepatol 2006;4(5):588–96.

97. Singendonk MMJ, Rexwinkel R, Steutel NF, et al. Development of a core outcome set for infant gastroesophageal reflux disease. J Pediatr Gastroenterol Nutr 2018. https://doi.org/10.1097/MPG.0000000000002245.

98. Breumelhof R, Smout AJ. The symptom sensitivity index: a valuable additional parameter in 24-hour esophageal pH recording. Am J Gastroenterol 1991; 86(2):160–4.

99. Ward BW, Wu WC, Richter JE, et al. Ambulatory 24-hour esophageal pH monitoring. Technology searching for a clinical application. J Clin Gastroenterol 1986;8(Suppl 1):59–67.

100. Weusten BL, Roelofs JM, Akkermans LM, et al. The symptom-association probability: an improved method for symptom analysis of 24-hour esophageal pH data. Gastroenterology 1994;107(6):1741–5.

101. Sivalingam M, Sitaram S, Hasenstab KA, et al. Effects of esophageal acidification on troublesome symptoms: an approach to characterize true acid GERD in dysphagic neonates. Dysphagia 2017;32(4):509–19.

102. Jadcherla SR, Peng J, Chan CY, et al. Significance of gastroesophageal refluxate in relation to physical, chemical, and spatiotemporal characteristics in symptomatic intensive care unit neonates. Pediatr Res 2011;70(2):192–8.

103. Jadcherla SR, Gupta A, Fernandez S, et al. Spatiotemporal characteristics of acid refluxate and relationship to symptoms in premature and term infants with chronic lung disease. Am J Gastroenterol 2008;103(3):720–8.

104. Vandenplas Y, Goyvaerts H, Helven R, et al. Gastroesophageal reflux, as measured by 24-hour pH monitoring, in 509 healthy infants screened for risk of sudden infant death syndrome. Pediatrics 1991;88(4):834–40.

105. Task Force On Sudden Infant Death Syndrome. SIDS and other sleep-related infant deaths: updated 2016 recommendations for a safe infant sleeping environment. Pediatrics 2016;138(5). https://doi.org/10.1542/peds.2016-2938.

106. Moon RY, Task Force On Sudden Infant Death Syndrome. SIDS and other sleep-related infant deaths: evidence base for 2016 updated recommendations for a safe infant sleeping environment. Pediatrics 2016;138(5). https://doi.org/10.1542/peds.2016-2940.

107. Levy DS, Osborn E, Hasenstab KA, et al. The effect of additives for reflux or dysphagia management on osmolality in ready-to-feed preterm formula: practice implications. JPEN J Parenter Enteral Nutr 2019;43(2):290–7.

108. Corvaglia L, Ferlini M, Rotatori R, et al. Starch thickening of human milk is ineffective in reducing the gastroesophageal reflux in preterm infants: a crossover study using intraluminal impedance. J Pediatr 2006;148(2):265–8.

109. Corvaglia L, Aceti A, Mariani E, et al. Lack of efficacy of a starch-thickened preterm formula on gastro-oesophageal reflux in preterm infants: a pilot study. J Matern Fetal Neonatal Med 2012;25(12):2735–8.

110. Bosscher D, Van Caillie-Bertrand M, Van Cauwenbergh R, et al. Availabilities of calcium, iron, and zinc from dairy infant formulas is affected by soluble dietary fibers and modified starch fractions. Nutrition 2003;19(7–8):641–5.

111. Beal J, Silverman B, Bellant J, et al. Late onset necrotizing enterocolitis in infants following use of a xanthan gum-containing thickening agent. J Pediatr 2012; 161(2):354–6.

112. Guy C, Ollagnier M. [Sucralfate and bezoars: data from the system of pharmacologic vigilance and review of the literature]. Therapie 1999;54(1):55–8.

113. Corvaglia L, Spizzichino M, Zama D, et al. Sodium Alginate (Gaviscon(R)) does not reduce apnoeas related to gastro-oesophageal reflux in preterm infants. Early Hum Dev 2011;87(12):775–8.

114. Gulati IK, Jadcherla SR. Gastroesophageal reflux disease in the neonatal intensive care unit infant: who needs to be treated and what approach is beneficial? Pediatr Clin North Am 2019;66(2):461–73.

115. Romano C, van Wynckel M, Hulst J, et al. European Society for Paediatric Gastroenterology, Hepatology and Nutrition guidelines for the evaluation and treatment of gastrointestinal and nutritional complications in children with neurological impairment. J Pediatr Gastroenterol Nutr 2017;65(2):242–64.

116. Foster LJ, Trudeau WL, Goldman AL. Bronchodilator effects on gastric acid secretion. JAMA 1979;241(24):2613–5.

117. Stein MR, Towner TG, Weber RW, et al. The effect of theophylline on the lower esophageal sphincter pressure. Ann Allergy 1980;45(4):238–41.

118. Jadcherla SR, Hasenstab KA, Shaker R, et al. Mechanisms of cough provocation and cough resolution in neonates with bronchopulmonary dysplasia. Pediatr Res 2015;78(4):462–9.

Approach to Feeding Difficulties in Neonates and Infants: A Comprehensive Overview

Ish K. Gulati, MD[a,b,c,d,]*, Zakia Sultana, BA[a,d],
Sudarshan R. Jadcherla, MD, FRCPI, DCH[a,b,c,d,e]

KEYWORDS

- Deglutition • Infant • Dysphagia • Feeding difficulties • Mechanisms
- Aerodigestive pathophysiology

KEY POINTS

- Deglutition disorders (DD) in neonates encompass the spectrum of feeding difficulties, swallowing disorders, aerodigestive sequelae, and pulmonary consequences; the prevalence of these entities is unacceptably high and current diagnostic and therapeutic approaches lack objectivity and practice variation is wide.
- Complications caused by DD are likely multifaceted and involve neurologic, aerodigestive, and cardiopulmonary systems, all of which impact long-term development. Better diagnostic strategies involving structural and functional assessment, and nutritive and feeding assessment are needed to inform better therapeutic options and anticipatory guidance.
- In the evaluation and management DD, maturational aspects must be first considered prior to the development of life-style changing long-term tube-feeding plans.

INTRODUCTION

Feeding difficulties or deglutition disorders (DD) in infants encompass a wide spectrum of oral feeding problems, swallowing disorders, pharyngoesophageal motility, and aerodigestive concerns, and their pulmonary consequences. The prevalence of these entities is universal and is unacceptably high. These difficulties can manifest as an inability to adequately eat and maintain hydration and nutrition while thriving normally. This is caused by ineffective suck, swallow, or poor airway-digestive

---

[a] Innovative Infant Feeding Disorders Research Program, Nationwide Children's Hospital, Columbus, OH, USA; [b] Division of Neonatology, Nationwide Children's Hospital, Columbus, OH, USA; [c] Department of Pediatrics, College of Medicine, The Ohio State University College of Medicine, Columbus, OH, USA; [d] Center for Perinatal Research, Abigail Wexner Research Institute, Nationwide Children's Hospital, 575 Children's Crossroads, Columbus, OH 43215, USA; [e] Division Pediatric Gastroenterology, Hepatology and Nutrition, Department of Pediatrics, Nationwide Children's Hospital, Columbus, OH, USA
* Corresponding author. Center for Perinatal Research, Abigail Wexner Research Institute, Nationwide Children's Hospital, 575 Children's Crossroads, Columbus, OH 43215.
E-mail address: Ish.Gulati@nationwidechildrens.org

Clin Perinatol 47 (2020) 265–276
https://doi.org/10.1016/j.clp.2020.02.006
0095-5108/20/© 2020 Elsevier Inc. All rights reserved.

transit along the upper gastrointestinal tract. Because of complex developmental physiology and pathophysiology of airway-digestive pathways and lack of specific diagnostic approaches, infants are often not oral-fed but gavage-fed, while maintaining airway with continuous positive airway pressure, high-flow nasal cannula, or other assisted ventilation strategies. All such airway-protective and maintenance approaches delay the acquisition of complicated sucking and swallowing milestones. Although airway maintenance and oral-pharyngeal swallowing go hand-in-hand, evaluation and management of such DDs at crib-side remains a major problem on a day-to-day basis; as such, feeding providers are conflicted with multiple nonevidence-based opinions, all of which further contribute to practice variation and variable outcomes. A focused clinical and objective evaluation of these DDs in infants is needed for optimal and personalized therapies. In this article, we discuss the following:

1. Feeding concerns in infants, its prevalence and economic burden
2. Prioritization and stratification of investigations for diagnoses
3. Recommendations for optimal feeding and growth in infants

PREVALENCE, ECONOMIC BURDEN, AND COMORBIDITIES OF DEGLUTITION DISORDERS

DDs are widely prevalent globally, and the exact prevalence is not known in infants with or without comorbidities (**Table 1**). Feeding difficulties encompass broad-spectrum disorders that are common among preterm and term infants, healthy and chronically sick infants, inpatients, and outpatients at birthing hospitals and all-referral hospitals. Feeding difficulties in premature infants born less than 37 weeks of gestational age is about 10.5%, which increases to about 24.5% among those born at less than 1500 g.[1] These problems are also related to the degree of birth gestation in that infants born less than 28 weeks' gestational age had significantly prolonged feeding delays and chronic hospitalization compared with those born after 28 weeks' gestational age. However, in this observational study, most infants born less than 28 weeks gestational age reached oral feeds by 38 weeks postmenstrual age but had chronic lung disease.[2] Feeding difficulties are prevalent in about 80% of preterm-born infants associated with neurodevelopmental delay and are a major reason for chronic clinic visits.[3] On the contrary, among those with chronic feeding difficulties during the neonatal intensive care unit (NICU) stay, infants discharged on oral feeding had superior neurodevelopmental outcomes at 2 years compared with those discharged on gastrostomy tube

Table 1	
Common comorbidities in preterm and term infants	
Preterm	**Term**
Pharyngoesophageal and gastrointestinal dysmotility manifested by feeding intolerance, gastroparesis, gastroesophageal reflux symptoms	Infant of mother with diabetes
	Brief resolved unexplained event
	Neonatal abstinence syndrome
Intraventricular hemorrhage	Hypothyroidism
Bronchopulmonary dysplasia	Congenital heart disease
Aspiration syndromes	Chronic lung disease
	Thoracoabdominal surgeries
	Congenital anomalies
	Chromosomal/genetic abnormalities

feeding. Bronchopulmonary dysplasia (BPD) or chronic lung disease is an invariable outcome among NICU graduates; the prevalence and severity of this condition varies. About 31% of preterm infants with BPD have feeding difficulties.[4] The spectrum of DDs has an impact on health care economics. Although exact health care costs are unclear and are variable in different settings and countries, we have noted that approximate health care costs for infants discharged on feeding tubes in the United States cost approximately $180,000 per infant up to 5 years and about $46,875 in the first year alone.[5] These costs, unadjusted for inflation and time periods, are only likely to increase the burden of DDs globally given the advancement of technologies and their applications.

Another burning problem associated with DDs is the diagnosis of gastroesophageal reflux (GER) and gastroesophageal reflux disease (GERD). Infants present with common symptoms that are not easily differentiated from those arising from airway-digestive dysfunctions and are often misunderstood to be caused by GERD. Symptoms and cues are often heterogeneous, and diagnostic precision is clinically difficult. As a result, providers resort to empirical therapy for antireflux medications; we noted a 13-fold variation in the usage of antireflux therapies in convalescing NICU infants.[6] Furthermore, increasing prematurity rates, better survival rates with increased risk of comorbidities, and changing practice to shorten hospital stay with early discharges have led to surge in gastrostomy placements from 12 to 23 per 1000 very-low-birthweight infants.[7] In addition, fundoplication rates vary from 0% to 64%, suggesting a significant variation in practice, whereas proper definition of the disease or need for procedure and focused testing is not always feasible.[8]

DD in its various forms is commonly prevalent in premature and high-risk NICU infants, and the comorbidities, such as airway and pulmonary disease, neurologic sequelae, variations of GERD entities, and congenital anomalies, are all contributory to the lack of progress with feeding milestones. Thus, variability in feeding disorders management from lack of diagnostic precision and appropriate crib-side therapies lead to dissatisfaction among parents and providers, albeit with escalating morbidities and health care costs.[9]

UNDERSTANDING THE PHYSIOLOGIC BASIS FOR DEGLUTITION DISORDERS

Symptomatic infants with feeding difficulties present with bradycardia, desaturations, apnea, coughing and choking spells, back-arching and fussiness, limited intake and endurance to complete the prescribed feeding volume, or food refusal and aversion on the extreme. Often symptoms are attributed to anterograde aspiration, such as may happen during oral, pharyngeal, or esophageal phase of swallowing.[10,11] Sometimes such conditions are also attributed to retrograde aspiration, such as may happen during GER events or esophageal dysmotility wherein esophageal transit is delayed.[12] Most providers observe for a symptom-free period of 5 to 7 days before discharge, the rationale of which is not entirely clear.[13] We have shown that these bradycardiac events in otherwise orally feeding infants have aberrant responses across respiratory, digestive, and cardiovascular system related to maladaptive maturation of parasympathetic system.[14] Data from pharyngeal-esophageal motility studies in infants reveal that acid reflux severity grade has no relationship with symptom generation and that symptoms alone should not be a diagnostic criteria for GERD diagnosis and or prescription for medical or surgical treatment strategies.[15]

Potential pharyngoesophageal swallowing mechanisms during resting state or on pharyngeal or oral stimulation in **Fig. 1** suggest that the safe swallowing involves

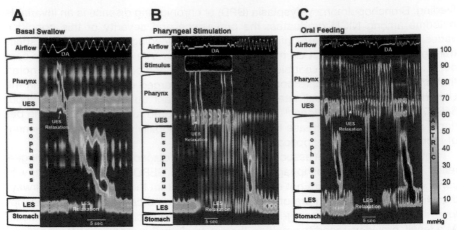

Fig. 1. Primary peristalsis. Described are anatomic regions during high-resolution manometry, which uses pressure topography plots encoded in color with pressures corresponding to the scale shown on the vertical axis (*right*) and time on the horizontal axis. (*A*) Depicted is an example of primary peristalsis during spontaneous basal swallowing. Note the upper esophageal sphincter (UES) and lower esophageal sphincter (LES) relaxation with robust peristalsis and integrity of breathing represented by a brief deglutition apnea (DA) in the airflow sensor. (*B*) Depicted is an example of pharyngeal infusion (stimulus) induced multiple pharyngeal swallows. Note the multiple pharyngeal contractions after the onset of infusion followed by a fully propagated terminal swallow characterized by UES relaxation, esophageal peristalsis, and LES relaxation. (*C*) Depicted is an example of peristaltic rhythms during oral feeding challenge. Note the presence of multiple pharyngeal contractions, DA, and respiratory regulation, followed by fully propagated swallow with UES and LES relaxation.

pharyngeal, upper esophageal sphincter, esophageal body, and lower esophageal sphincter coordination along with cross-systems interaction with airway ventilation. These reflexes are distinct in premature and full-term infants during oral nutritive challenge (**Fig. 2**) in that the efficiency of peristalsis is not completely developed in preterm-born infants at full-term equivalent age and the presence of comorbidities may be contributory. Specific abnormalities and interactions associated with DDs in infants with specific diseases are shown in **Table 2**.

The functional act of deglutition is a complex process divided into five phases: (1) preparatory, (2) oral, (3) pharyngeal, (4) esophageal, and (5) gastric phase (**Table 3**). Healthy term infants are usually capable of regulating these five phases effectively while maintaining physiologic stability manifested by airway-digestive protection and cardiorespiratory modulation during swallowing or during physiologic GER events.[14,16] However, dysfunctional patterns associated with eating and peristalsis or GER events in high-risk infants are distinct, and may result from immaturity, maladaptation, malfunction, or maldevelopment of the reflexes associated with safe eating and peristalsis.[17,18] The basis of symptoms during oral feeding is shown in **Fig. 3**.

APPROACH TO EVALUATE INFANTS WITH EATING DIFFICULTIES

A thorough history and clinical assessment must be undertaken to evaluate predisposing individualized risk factors (**Table 4**). Clinical assessment involves a detailed examination including special attention to structural and functional evaluation.

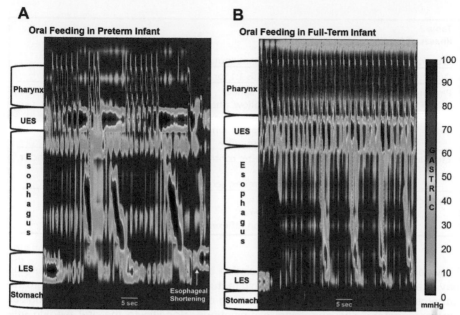

Fig. 2. Oral feeding in preterm and full-term infant. Example of oral feeding in a preterm infant (*A*) and full-term infant (*B*) during high-resolution manometry are displayed. In the preterm infant, note the lesser number of pharyngeal contractions, and presence of esophageal shortening versus the full-term infant with sustained pharyngeal contractions with appropriate lower esophageal sphincter relaxation. LES, lower esophageal sphincter; UES, upper esophageal sphincter.

Table 2	
Potential dysmotility mechanisms associated with infant feeding difficulty	
Hypoxic ischemic encephalopathy[28,29]	Aberrant upper esophageal sphincter function
	Increased upper esophageal sphincter contractility reflex
	Decreased lower esophageal sphincter basal tone
	Increased lower esophageal sphincter relaxation reflex
	Poorly coordinated esophageal peristaltic response
Bronchopulmonary dysplasia[30]	Clustered cough events caused by nonpropagating swallows or upper esophageal sphincter contractile reflex
	Primary peristalsis restores posttussive normalcy
Neonatal abstinence syndrome[31]	High basal lower esophageal sphincter pressures
	Increased duration of esophageal peristalsis
Infant of mother with diabetes[32]	Lower frequency of deglutitive apnea
	Prolonged upper esophageal sphincter relaxation
Brief resolved unexplained event[16]	Frequent primary peristalsis
	Significant propagation failure
	Decreased upper esophageal sphincter protective contractile reflex
Prematurity[33]	Esophageal propagation velocity and frequency advance with maturation
	Propagation is faster with secondary peristalsis

Table 3
Phases of feeding and characteristics

Preparatory[27]	Alert and active, rooting, nonnutritive sucking
Oral[34]	Sucking and swallowing is 1:1 for preterm and term infants
Pharyngeal[35]	Deglutition, deglutition apnea Pharyngeal reflexive swallow, pharyngeal upper esophageal sphincter contractile and relaxation reflexes Pharyngeal lower esophageal sphincter relaxation Pharyngeal glottal closure reflex
Esophageal[33]	Upper esophageal sphincter contractile reflex, upper esophageal sphincter relaxation reflex Esophageal deglutition reflex, secondary peristalsis
Gastric[36–38]	Gastric emptying Migrating motor complexes Periodic pyloric relaxation reflexes

Providers must understand the association between DDs and comorbidities and pay attention to recognizing dysmorphic features and anomalies; evaluating growth patterns and reasons for aberrance; feeding and nutrition status; and neurological, cardiorespiratory, and abdominal examinations. Specific to the oral feeding efficiency, critical components of a well-targeted examination must include assessment of oromotor activity during an oral feeding session; airway-digestive apparatus; functions of cranial nerves V, VII, IX, X, XI, and XII; and airway-

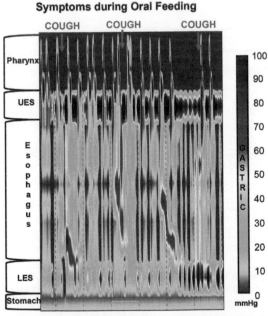

Fig. 3. Symptoms during oral feeding. Depicted are common symptoms during oral feeding that may happen during propagated swallow or nonpropagated swallow. Noted here are multiple cough events during the challenge, but the infant continues to swallow. UES, upper esophageal sphincter.

Table 4	
Pertinent history for feeding difficulty in infant	
Maternal	Thyroid dysfunction, diabetes, asthma, cardiac abnormality, neuropsychiatric illness, and drug abuse
Antenatal	Nature of pregnancy, antenatal visits, congenital anomalies, prior children with any chronic feeding problems
Birth history and postnatal history	Adverse events affecting neurologic stability, hypoxic ischemic encephalopathy, chromosomal/ genetic syndromes and metabolic disorders, postnatal neurologic injury and feeding intolerance, necrotizing enterocolitis, and stools frequency
Feeding milestones	Nonnutritive and nutritive breastfeeding, nuzzling, latching, sucking, swallowing, oral intake progression, cardiorespiratory events

breathing regulatory status. Abnormal facies or syndromic signs must be noted, because several syndromic infants have feeding difficulties and developmental delays. Abdominal examination is vital to understand abnormalities, such as congenital hypertrophic pyloric stenosis, inguinal hernia, impaired peristalsis, abdominal distention suspicious of strictures or inflammatory changes, or functional motility disorders. Importance of stool frequency and type should not be underestimated, because dysmotility of small or large bowel often manifests with abnormal stooling patterns. A neurologic examination is pertinent for truncal and peripheral tone (abnormal in infant of mothers with diabetes, hypothyroidism, perinatal asphyxia, congenital myasthenia gravis, and metabolic disorders).[19] The value of watching a complete oral feeding session cannot be overstated. Important things to consider during such observations are alertness level, latching, swallowing, body tone, respiratory effort, drooling if any, and pauses in between sucking and swallowing.

Risk factors for DDs, such as abnormalities of swallowing, GERD, or airway-digestive dysfunctions, include anatomic and developmental malformations, gut anomalies including craniofacial birth defects, pharyngeal clefts, pharyngeal achalasia, esophageal webs/atresia, tracheoesophageal fistula, hiatus hernia, diaphragmatic hernia, omphalocele, gastroschisis, duodenal stenosis/atresia/web, and intestinal malrotation. Extraluminal causes of dysphagia need to be considered if associated with stridor or suspicion of proximal obstruction. Primary vocal cord paralysis or secondary to cardiothoracic surgery, aberrant vascular arches, need to be evaluated. Other causes of DDs and GERD include milk protein allergy, sepsis and eosinophilic esophagitis, and other nonspecific systemic inflammatory states.

Instrumental and diagnostic evaluation of DD is usually overperformed at most centers, and often a thorough clinical assessment is adequate. Sucking and swallowing dysfunction need a focused anatomic and physiologic approach and sometimes therapeutic strategies also are diagnostic. More than one diagnostic study may be needed to correlate anatomic with functional aspect. Upper gastrointestinal fluoroscopy study and video fluoroscopic swallow study are the usual standard investigations performed for anatomical evaluation and bolus transit. Ideally, infants should feed contrast media by mouth instead of inserting via feeding tube.

However, these studies are of limited value in infants with oromotor inertia and tube-fed infants. The risk of radiation exposure does not permit prolonged studies, and lack of standardization of techniques and interpretation is a major concern for accurate diagnosis. Functional evaluation of oropharyngeal and pharyngoesophageal reflexes and motility include pH impedance and basal and/or provocative manometry to test for adaptive reflexes and eating efficiency skills. In observational studies, we noted that oral milk stimuli provoked a distinctively underdeveloped pharyngeal contractility in preterm infants at term age compared with term-born infants.[20]

Video fluoroscopic swallowing study is often used to assess infant dysphagia. However, its indications, testing methods, interpretations, and recommendations are not standardized for infants. Fiberoptic endoscopic evaluation of swallowing is sometime used at tertiary centers as an alternative to video fluoroscopic swallowing study.[21] However, further research is needed to compare efficacy. Aspiration and/or penetration seen on video fluoroscopic swallowing study is considered diagnostic of feeding difficulty and formulas are commonly modified to improve growth. Our group has noted that alteration of ready-to-feed preterm formulas may significantly increase osmolality. Caution and monitoring should be exercised with modification of preterm formulas.[22] Any of the evaluation techniques have advantages and disadvantages and are described in **Table 5**.

Table 5
Diagnostic procedures for dysphagia: merits and limitations

Test	Merits	Limitations
Video fluoroscopic swallow study	Evaluates anatomy of upper airway, digestive tract Bolus movement detection during swallowing Laryngeal penetration, airway aspiration detection	Radiation exposure Variability in indication, testing methods, interpretations, and recommendations
Upper gastrointestinal fluoroscopy study	Anatomic abnormalities in upper gastrointestinal tract	Radiation exposure Not diagnostic of GER
24-h pH with multichannel intraluminal impedance	Differentiate acid and nonacid GER events Detects differences in liquid, gas, and mixed GER events Detects frequency, duration, and height of refluxate in association with clinical symptoms	Labor-intensive analysis No quantitative data regarding pressure and volume mechanisms
Basal and adaptive pharyngoesophageal manometry	Mechanistic sensory motor evaluation of pharyngeal swallows and esophageal peristalsis at rest and on provocation Useful for application of personalized therapies	Less commonly available Clinical correlation needed

RECOMMENDATIONS FOR OPTIMAL FEEDING STRATEGIES IN INFANTS

Prevention of feeding disorders is the best option. Variability in feeding practices is dependent on infants' heterogeneity and on multiple interdisciplinary providers and institutional feeding protocols. Furthermore, a lack of adequate communication among parents, providers, and allied health care professionals creates more barrier in making optimal management plans. The implementation of a feeding quality program and institutional guidelines in NICU accelerates acquisition of feeding milestones and overall length of stay. We have observed that simplified, individualized, milestone-targeted, pragmatic, longitudinal, and educational (SIMPLE) feeding strategy improved feeding and outcome metrics.[23] When this approach was applied to more complicated infants with BPD, advanced maturity with early acquisition of feeding and lower length of stay were noted regardless of BPD severity, thereby lowering resource use.[24]

Despite following a rigorous feeding quality program, some infants have additional comorbidities that limit progression of their feeding milestones compared with their healthy peers. These infants require individualized feeding management strategies. Our group has previously established proof of concept for an individualized evidence-based approach to modify outcomes for infants referred for gastrostomy tube evaluation.[25] The predictive ability of this approach helps optimal resource use. The salient features of the innovative approach are as follows:

1. Manometry-based findings characterized the clinical and neuromotor motility correlations at evaluation, which differed between successful oral feeders and feeding failures. Specifically, successful oral feeders had a greater frequency of peristaltic responses to esophageal and pharyngeal infusions, a greater tendency to pass the oral feeding challenge test, and more suck-swallow-breath-esophageal swallow sequences were seen in the success group compared with failures.
2. Multidisciplinary feeding strategies in implementing early and consistent oral feeding methods. Nonnutritive sucking methods have a limited role in enhancing feeding capabilities.[26,27] Standardized cue-based feeding approaches based on feeding readiness scores show early acquisitions of oral feeding milestones. Oral feeding attempts are advanced in stepwise manner based on feeding skills and quality of feeding while observing the lack of symptoms. Symptomatic infants require consistent pacing techniques using modification of milk flow rates using slower-flow nipples. The best strategy for feeding difficulty is a cautious and consistent feeding process to avoid confusion among the providers.
3. For infants with GERD-like symptoms, objectively proven acid GERD is treated pharmacologically for short durations.[19] Nonacid GERD requires nonpharmacologic approaches, which may include feeding strategy modifications, such as optimizing osmolality, pacing, position, and trial of elemental formula. Application of consensus guidelines on GERD is helpful in such infants.[19] Fundoplication is only reserved for infants with objectively documented GERD and poor airway-protective mechanisms when abnormalities of gastroesophageal junction are noted. Transpyloric feeds may be an alternative to fundoplication. All of the previously mentioned observational and experiential strategies have not been tested in well-controlled clinical trials.

DISCLOSURE

The authors have nothing to disclose.

Best Practices

What is the current practice?

- Symptoms related to DDs are heterogeneous, and are often managed empirically with no objective testing

- Wide practice variation in identification and evaluation of DDs

Best practice/guideline/care path objectives

- Determine physiologic basis for infants with DDs

- Understand the association between DDs and other comorbidities

- Clinical assessment and personalized management plan

What changes in current practice are likely to improve outcomes?

- Timely identification of DDs in preterm and term infants

- Early diagnostic evaluation with personalized management plan leading to shorter hospital stay and more opportunities for better neurodevelopmental outcomes

Major recommendations

- Objective testing of upper and lower aerodigestive reflexes to evaluate integrity of swallowing and breathing function

- Individualized evidence-based feeding strategies

- Multidisciplinary participation and parental education are necessary to optimize management plans

Summary statement

A thorough history, clinical assessment, and other comorbidities should be considered in determining a feeding strategy. Objective evidence-based diagnosis is necessary.

Bibliographic Sources: Data from Refs.[9,22,23]

REFERENCES

1. Motion S, Northstone K, Emond A, et al. Early feeding problems in children with cerebral palsy: weight and neurodevelopmental outcomes. Dev Med Child Neurol 2002;44(1):40–3.

2. Jadcherla SR, Wang M, Vijayapal AS, et al. Impact of prematurity and comorbidities on feeding milestones in neonates: a retrospective study. J Perinatol 2010;30(3):201–8.

3. Field D, Garland M, Williams K. Correlates of specific childhood feeding problems. J Paediatr Child Health 2003;39(4):299–304.

4. Mercado-Deane MG, Burton EM, Harlow SA, et al. Swallowing dysfunction in infants less than 1 year of age. Pediatr Radiol 2001;31(6):423–8.

5. Jadcherla SR, Stoner E, Gupta A, et al. Evaluation and management of neonatal dysphagia: impact of pharyngoesophageal motility studies and multidisciplinary feeding strategy. J Pediatr Gastroenterol Nutr 2009;48(2):186–92.

6. Slaughter JL, Stenger MR, Reagan PB, et al. Neonatal histamine-2 receptor antagonist and proton pump inhibitor treatment at United States children's hospitals. J Pediatr 2016;174:63–70.e3.

7. Greene NH, Greenberg RG, O'Brien SM, et al. Variation in gastrostomy tube placement in premature infants in the United States. Am J Perinatol 2019;36(12):1243–9.

8. Stey AM, Vinocur CD, Moss RL, et al. Hospital variation in rates of concurrent fundoplication during gastrostomy enteral access procedures. Surg Endosc 2018; 32(5):2201–11.

9. Jadcherla SR, Slaughter JL, Stenger MR, et al. Practice variance, prevalence, and economic burden of premature infants diagnosed with GERD. Hosp Pediatr 2013;3(4):335–41.

10. Arvedson J, Rogers B, Buck G, et al. Silent aspiration prominent in children with dysphagia. Int J Pediatr Otorhinolaryngol 1994;28(2–3):173–81.

11. Rosenbek JC, Robbins JA, Roecker EB, et al. A penetration-aspiration scale. Dysphagia 1996;11(2):93–8.

12. Logemann JA. Swallowing physiology and pathophysiology. Otolaryngol Clin North Am 1988;21(4):613–23.

13. Quinn JM, Sparks M, Gephart SM. Discharge criteria for the late preterm infant: a review of the literature. Adv Neonatal Care 2017;17(5):362–71.

14. Hasenstab KA, Nawaz S, Lang IM, et al. Pharyngoesophageal and cardiorespiratory interactions: potential implications for premature infants at risk of clinically significant cardiorespiratory events. Am J Physiol Gastrointest Liver Physiol 2019; 316(2):G304–12.

15. Collins CR, Hasenstab KA, Nawaz S, et al. Mechanisms of aerodigestive symptoms in infants with varying acid reflux index determined by esophageal manometry. J Pediatr 2019;206:240–7.

16. Hasenstab KA, Jadcherla SR. Respiratory events in infants presenting with apparent life threatening events: is there an explanation from esophageal motility? J Pediatr 2014;165(2):250–5.e1.

17. Jadcherla S. Dysphagia in the high-risk infant: potential factors and mechanisms. Am J Clin Nutr 2016;103(2):622S–8S.

18. Jadcherla SR. Advances with neonatal aerodigestive science in the pursuit of safe swallowing in infants: invited review. Dysphagia 2017;32(1):15–26.

19. Rosen R, Vandenplas Y, Singendonk M, et al. Pediatric gastroesophageal reflux clinical practice guidelines: joint recommendations of the North American Society for Pediatric Gastroenterology, Hepatology, and Nutrition and the European Society for Pediatric Gastroenterology, Hepatology, and Nutrition. J Pediatr Gastroenterol Nutr 2018;66(3):516–54.

20. Prabhakar V, Hasenstab KA, Osborn E, et al. Pharyngeal contractile and regulatory characteristics are distinct during nutritive oral stimulus in preterm-born infants: implications for clinical and research applications. Neurogastroenterol Motil 2019;31(8):e13650.

21. Reynolds J, Carroll S, Sturdivant C. Fiberoptic endoscopic evaluation of swallowing: a multidisciplinary alternative for assessment of infants with dysphagia in the neonatal intensive care unit. Adv Neonatal Care 2016;16(1):37–43.

22. Levy DS, Osborn E, Hasenstab KA, et al. The effect of additives for reflux or dysphagia management on osmolality in ready-to-feed preterm formula: practice implications. JPEN J Parenter Enteral Nutr 2019;43(2):290–7.

23. Jadcherla SR, Dail J, Malkar MB, et al. Impact of process optimization and quality improvement measures on neonatal feeding outcomes at an all-referral neonatal intensive care unit. JPEN J Parenter Enteral Nutr 2016;40(5):646–55.

24. Bapat R, Gulati IK, Jadcherla S. Impact of SIMPLE feeding quality improvement strategies on aerodigestive milestones and feeding outcomes in BPD infants. Hosp Pediatr 2019;9(11):859–66.

25. Jadcherla SR, Peng J, Moore R, et al. Impact of personalized feeding program in 100 NICU infants: pathophysiology-based approach for better outcomes. J Pediatr Gastroenterol Nutr 2012;54(1):62–70.

26. Shubert TR, Sitaram S, Jadcherla SR. Effects of pacifier and taste on swallowing, esophageal motility, transit, and respiratory rhythm in human neonates. Neurogastroenterol Motil 2016;28(4):532–42.

27. Pinelli J, Symington A. Non-nutritive sucking for promoting physiologic stability and nutrition in preterm infants. Cochrane Database Syst Rev 2005;(4):CD001071.

28. Gulati IK, Shubert TR, Sitaram S, et al. Effects of birth asphyxia on the modulation of pharyngeal provocation-induced adaptive reflexes. Am J Physiol Gastrointest Liver Physiol 2015;309(8):G662–9.

29. Jensen PS, Gulati IK, Shubert TR, et al. Pharyngeal stimulus-induced reflexes are impaired in infants with perinatal asphyxia: does maturation modify? Neurogastroenterol Motil 2017;29(7).

30. Jadcherla SR, Hasenstab KA, Shaker R, et al. Mechanisms of cough provocation and cough resolution in neonates with bronchopulmonary dysplasia. Pediatr Res 2015;78(4):462–9.

31. Hart BJ, Viswanathan S, Jadcherla SR. Persistent feeding difficulties among infants with fetal opioid exposure: mechanisms and clinical reasoning. J Matern Fetal Neonatal Med 2019;32(21):3633–9.

32. Malkar MB, Viswanathan SK, Jadcherla SR. Pilot study of pharyngoesophageal dysmotility mechanisms in dysphagic infants of diabetic mothers. Am J Perinatol 2019;36(12):1237–42.

33. Jadcherla SR, Duong HQ, Hoffmann RG, et al. Esophageal body and upper esophageal sphincter motor responses to esophageal provocation during maturation in preterm newborns. J Pediatr 2003;143(1):31–8.

34. Lau C. Development of suck and swallow mechanisms in infants. Ann Nutr Metab 2015;66(Suppl 5):7–14.

35. Hasenstab KA, Sitaram S, Lang IM, et al. Maturation modulates pharyngeal-stimulus provoked pharyngeal and respiratory rhythms in human infants. Dysphagia 2018;33(1):63–75.

36. Berseth CL. Neonatal small intestinal motility: motor responses to feeding in term and preterm infants. J Pediatr 1990;117(5):777–82.

37. Jadcherla SR, Klee G, Berseth CL. Regulation of migrating motor complexes by motilin and pancreatic polypeptide in human infants. Pediatr Res 1997;42(3):365–9.

38. Jadcherla SR, Berseth CL. Effect of erythromycin on gastroduodenal contractile activity in developing neonates. J Pediatr Gastroenterol Nutr 2002;34(1):16–22.

Physiological Basis of Neonatal Aerodigestive Difficulties in Chronic Lung Disease

Shabih U. Hasan, MD[a],*, Abhay K. Lodha, MD[b],
Kamran Yusuf, MD[a], Stacey Dalgleish, RN, MN[c]

KEYWORDS

- Respiratory rhythmogenesis • Central swallow pattern generator
- Suck-swallow-breathe coordination • Preterm infants • Chronic lung disease
- Oromotor skills • Oral feeding • Noninvasive ventilation

KEY POINTS

- Establishment of full oral feeds, a major challenge for preterm infants, becomes magnified among those on noninvasive respiratory support and/or with chronic lung disease.
- Coordination of respiratory and swallowing central pattern generators is critical for successful integration of oral feeding and breathing to achieve full oral feeds and maintain adequate ventilation.
- Prolonged gavage feeding in preterm infants is an independent risk factor for adverse neurodevelopmental outcomes, speech impairment, and feeding difficulties during childhood.
- Feeding protocol such as Safe Individualized Nipple-Feeding Competence facilitates initiation and advancing of oral feeds.
- Interdisciplinary collaborative research efforts based on evidence-informed data are vital to treat and/or prevent aerodigestive disorders.

INTRODUCTION

Globally, 15 million infants are born preterm, defined as those born less than 37 weeks postmenstrual age (PMA). In the United States, after an initial decline, preterm birth

[a] Department of Pediatrics, Alberta Health Services, Cumming School of Medicine, Health Sciences Centre, 3330 Hospital Drive Northwest, Calgary, Alberta T2N 4N1, Canada; [b] Department of Pediatrics, Alberta Health Services, Cumming School of Medicine, Foothills Medical Centre, 1403-29th Street Northwest, Calgary, Alberta T2N 2T9, Canada; [c] Neonatal Intensive Care Unit, Alberta Health Services, Cumming School of Medicine, Alberta Children's Hospital, 28 Oki Drive Northwest, Calgary, Alberta T3B 6A8, Canada
* Corresponding author.
E-mail address: hasans@ucalgary.ca

Clin Perinatol 47 (2020) 277–299
https://doi.org/10.1016/j.clp.2020.03.001
0095-5108/20/© 2020 Elsevier Inc. All rights reserved.

rates have steadily increased for the fourth straight year since 2014 (https://www.cdc.gov/nchs/pressroom/sosmap/preterm_births/preterm.htm). Because of multisystem immaturity, preterm infants, especially those born before 33 weeks PMA, face many life-threatening challenges including (1) establishment of pulmonary gas exchange[1-6] and (2) provision of adequate nutrition, which are vital for their survival, somatic growth, and neurodevelopment.[7-9] Mechanical ventilation and supplemental oxygen can lead to upper airway and/or parenchymal lung injury, increased risk of sepsis, bronchopulmonary dysplasia (BPD),[10-13] and neurodevelopmental impairment (NDI).[14] To minimize lung injury, infants are weaned off the invasive mechanical ventilation and placed on noninvasive respiratory support, which may be required for several weeks. During the initial weeks of postnatal period, very low birth weights (VLBW) defined as less than or equal to 1500 g are almost always fed via gavage, as they are either endotracheally intubated or have not yet developed suck-swallow-breathe coordination. One of the major milestones for preterm infants is to establish full oral feeds via breast and/or bottle, as it is one of the criteria for discharge home from the neonatal intensive care unit (NICU).[15-21] The preterm infants have the ability to coordinate suck-swallow-breathing from 32 weeks PMA onwards.[20,22] However, prematurity, pulmonary insufficiency, and respiratory support restrict their ability to achieve these critical milestones and almost one-third of the preterm infants with BPD have airway and digestive issues.[18] Suboptimum oral sensory stimulation, lack of oral feeding protocols, reluctance of health care providers to feed preterm infants orally while on continuous positive airway pressure (CPAP), and chronic inflammation affecting the neural plasticity[23-28] compound the aerodigestive disorders. Prolonged gavage feeding in preterm infants is an independent risk factor for NDI, speech impairment, and feeding difficulties during childhood.[18,20,29-37] Thus, a combination of unstable/immature respiratory control, prolonged respiratory support for pulmonary insufficiency, delayed introduction of oral feeds, and cerebral dysfunction can lead to aerodigestive difficulties in preterm infants, especially those with chronic lung disease. Here, the authors provide an overview of the respiratory and swallowing pattern generators, physiology and pathophysiology of suck-swallow-breathe responses, impact of respiratory support and chronic lung disease (CLD) on achieving feeding milestones, and strategies to mitigate aerodigestive difficulties.

AN OVERVIEW OF CENTRAL RESPIRATORY AND SWALLOWING PATTERN GENERATORS
Ontogeny of Central Respiratory Rhythm and Pattern Generator During Development

To appreciate the pathophysiology of aerodigestive disorders in preterm infants, it is necessary to review the ontogeny and physiology of suck-swallow-breathe sequence.[1,15,16,22,38-43] Since 450 BC or earlier, respiratory gas exchange has been of interest to the physicians and philosophers.[44,45] Over the past 40 years, sophisticated series of in-vitro and in-vivo studies in reduced and intact rodent and chronic fetal sheep preparations have contributed to our understanding of respiratory rhythmogenesis and pattern generator. Central pattern generator refers to "a group of neurons or neuronal circuits, when activated can control a complex motor response involving several motor nuclei."[38,46] Marked changes in respiratory rhythmogenesis and breathing pattern formation occur from the embryonic period to postnatal life and adulthood. In both the mammalian and nonmammalian species, the respiratory rhythm originates and is controlled by 3 anatomically and functionally distinct oscillators, located in the medullary-pontine areas of the brain. The respiratory rhythm can be broadly divided in to (1) inspiratory, (2) postinspiratory, and (3) active expiratory phases. As removal of ventrolateral medullary pre-Bötzinger complex (preBötC) eliminated the respiratory rhythm in rodents, a group of glutamatergic excitatory neurons in the preBötC have been accepted as the *noeud vital* or pacemakers for the inspiratory phase of rhythmogenesis.[47,48] The postinspiratory rhythm originates from the postinspiratory complex (PiCo) and not from the BötC as previously thought. BötC located in the rostral ventrolateral medulla has a subgroup of inhibitory neurons, which are vital for the phase switching between inspiratory and expiratory activities. Because of the impact of postinspiratory phase in determining the inspiratory and expiratory durations, PiCo plays a critical role in the coordination of breathing and swallowing motor behaviors. The duration of postinspiratory phase depends on the interaction between the neurons of nucleus tract solitarius (NTS) and the dorsolateral pontine Kölliker-Fuse nucleus. The NTS receives afferent input from the pulmonary stretch receptors and superior laryngeal nerves (SLNs) (via X cranial nerve), which can induce swallowing or other airway protective responses. The active expiratory rhythm initiates from the lateral parafacial nucleus (pF_L) oscillators, located within the retrotrapezoid nucleus parafacial respiratory group (RTN/pFRG). A fascinating and developmentally regulated interaction has been reported between the preBötC and pF_L. Evidence suggests that although pF_L interneurons control the active expiratory rhythm, its activity precedes the inspiratory rhythm generator, preBötC.[49] During the embryonic period pF_L provides excitatory input to preBötC, and it is after the coupling of preBötC and pF_L when fetal breathing movements (FBM) are observed. During the postnatal period, the dominant preBötC provides both excitatory and inhibitory stimuli to pF_L. During adult life, preBötC can generate inspiratory rhythm without the excitatory input from pF_L (**Fig. 1**).

In the human and other mammalian fetuses, episodic, rapid, irregular, and sleep-state–dependent[26] FBM play a critical role in lung-liquid regulation, maintaining fetal

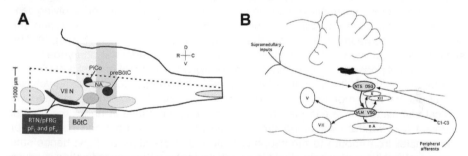

Fig. 1. Central respiratory and swallow pattern generators. (*A*) Anatomic map of oscillators in the ventral respiratory column. Schematic representation of the brainstem from a sagittal view illustrating 3 respiratory rhythm generators. PreBötC, preBötzinger complex; PiCo, postinspiratory complex; RTN/pFRG, retrotrapezoid nucleus parafacial respiratory group; PFL, parafacial nucleus; VII N, facial nucleus; NA, nucleus ambiguus.(*B*). Swallowing central pattern generator (CPG) comprising 2 main groups of neurons within the medulla oblongata including (1) dorsal swallowing group (DSG) within the nucleus tractus solitarii (NTS) and the adjacent reticular formation and (2) ventral swallowing group (VSG) located in the ventrolateral medulla (VLM) adjacent to the nucleus ambiguus (NA). The cranial nerves are represented as trigeminal nerve (V), facial nerve (VII), vagus nerve (X), and hypoglossal nerve (XII). Figure 1 A : Adapted from : Anderson TM and Ramirez JM. Respiratory rhythm generation: triple oscillator hypothesis [version 1; referees: 3approved] F1000Research 2017, 6(F1000 Faculty Rev):139 (doi: 10.12688/f1000research.10193.1). Figure 1 B: Adapted from Jean A. Brain stem control of swallowing: neuronal network and cellular mechanisms. Physiological Reviews 2001;81(2):929-69.

lungs in a distended state and fetal lung development, and have been considered entrainment or "practice for postnatal adaptation." The rate, amplitude, and duration of FBM increase with advancing gestational age.[50–54] The 5% to 10% mechanical stretch and distortion against semiclosed glottis in the developing lung lead to maintenance of transpulmonary pressures, increased DNA synthesis, pulmonary cellular proliferation and differentiation via platelet-derived growth factor B and β-receptor, and mitogen-activated protein kinase.[55–58] In humans, FBM can be observed as early as 10 weeks of PMA and increase in frequency, duration, and organization from 28 weeks PMA onwards. Similar to the postnatal period, in-utero FBM are suppressed by maternal hypoxia and stimulated by hypercarbia.[50–53] The hypoxia-mediated suppression of FBM seem to be influenced by supramedullary structures, as midcollicular sectioning disinhibits the suppression of hypoxia-mediated FBM.[59] Postnatally, vagal afferent feedback is critically important for the initiation and maintenance of regular breathing and gas exchange and neonatal survival.[60–63] Finally, although FBM play a vital role in fetal lung development, unilateral or bilateral pneumonectomy had little impact on various components of FBM or sleep state, suggesting an absence of a negative feedback loop in lung development.[64]

In summary, the central respiratory pattern generator, leading to coordinated respiratory motor activity is engendered from (1) the relative timing of the 3 excitatory rhythm generators (preBötC, PiCo, and RTN/pFRG), (2) a group of resetting glycinergic inhibitory interneurons located within the preBötC itself, (3) suprapontine input, (4) peripheral afferent feedback that includes upper airway and various pulmonary (myelinated and unmyelinated) stretch receptors, (5) chemoreceptors, and (6) metabolic demands.

Swallowing Central Pattern Generators and Pathways

Oral feeding is the most complex and highly organized multisystem sensorimotor process for newborns, especially preterm infants, as it involves multiple and evolving central respiratory and swallow pattern generators, 5 cranial nerves (V, VII, IX, X, and XII), spinal motor interneurons, and more than 2 dozen sets of muscles[41,65] (**Fig. 2**). The suck-swallow activity has been divided into (1) oral preparatory, (2) pharyngeal, and (3) esophageal phases. All three phases are controlled by distinct central pattern generators and include V (trigeminal), VII (facial), and XII (hypoglossal) cranial nerves;NA, and upper cervical motoneurons.[38] The voluntary oral phase can be initiated via cortical stimulation, whereas the involuntary pharyngeal phase is under the control of dorsal and ventral swallowing groups. The pharynx is a common passage for food transfer from mouth to the esophagus and for respiratory air flow; hence safe pharyngeal swallows play critical role in airway protection. Such coordination involves reconfiguration of central respiratory pattern generator (see **Fig. 2**) consisting of several sequential repertoires: backward roller-like tongue movements, contraction of pharyngeal and mylohyoid muscles, vocal cords adduction, tilting of the laryngeal apparatus, anterior and superior movement of the hyolaryngeal complex, laryngeal protection by epiglottis, and decreased diaphragmatic contraction (see **Fig. 2**).

The swallowing phase is controlled by the tightly synchronized swallowing central pattern generators comprising dorsal and ventral swallowing groups (DSG and VSG, respectively). Stimulation of the internal branch of the SLN can trigger swallows. Considerable evidence demonstrated that the swallowing phase is initiated in the DSG located in the NTS and reticular formation, which have neuronal interconnections with the vagal afferents and SLNs.[42] The SLN, which is a branch of the vagus nerve, arises from the middle of the nodose ganglion and also receives contributions from the superior cervical sympathetic ganglion. It divides into an internal sensory branch

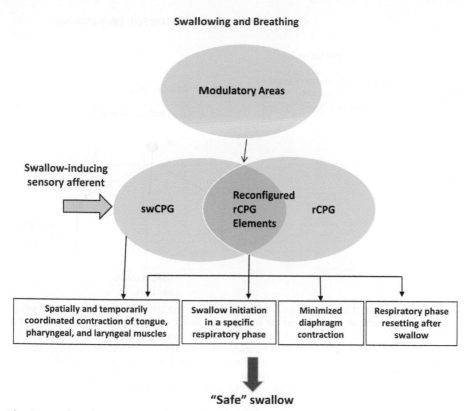

Fig. 2. A safe reflexive swallow with a reconfigured respiratory central pattern generator (rCPG). Swallow-inducing stimuli are relayed to the swallow central pattern generator (swCPG). The "traditional" definition of the swCPG produces the timing cues for the sequential contraction (or dilation) of tongue, pharyngeal, and laryngeal muscles during the pharyngeal stage of swallow. However, elements of the rCPG are reconfigured to ensure that swallows are coordinated with breathing. Other areas outside the current definitions of the swCPG and rCPG may serve to modulate the interaction between the 2 CPGs. Adapted from Bautista TG, Sun Q-J, Pilowsky PM. Chapter 13 - The generation of pharyngeal phase of swallow and its coordination with breathing: Interaction between the swallow and respiratory central pattern generators. In: Holstege G, Beers CM, Subramanian HH, editors. Progress in Brain Research, 2014, 212, 253-275.

innervating the pharynx and an external motor branch, which innervates the cricothyroid muscle. Because of its airway protection role, stimulation of SLN can induce swallowing and other airway protection responses. Furthermore, ascending sensory glossopharyngeal nerve and descending cortical pathway involved in swallowing reflex also converge on the NTS. Because pulmonary and upper airway sensory afferents and esophageal afferents also terminate in the NTS, a significant overlap occurs between the swallowing and the respiratory central pattern generators leading to inhibition of inspiration to allow for safe swallows. DSG initiates, controls the timing and shape of the rhythmic swallowing pattern, and relays it to the VSG located in the ventrolateral medulla. Compared with DSG, stimulation of VSG does not initiate well-organized swallows; however, it transmits the relayed information from the DSG to several groups of motoneurons (**Fig. 3**). Safe swallows are achieved via the

CENTRAL PATTERN GENERATOR FOR SWALLOWING

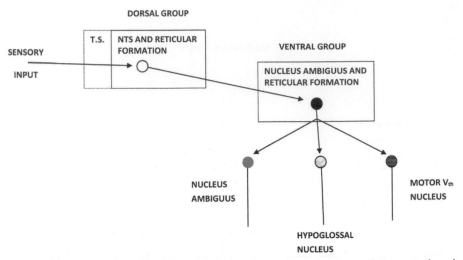

Fig. 3. Components of the central swallowing pathway: the critical core of the central swallowing pathway; dorsal area around the nucleus solitarius; and a ventral region around the nucleus ambiguus. The dorsal region receives the inputs that trigger pharyngeal and esophageal swallowing. The ventral region organizes the sequential activation of motor nuclei groups. Driving interneurons for the esophageal control may reside in both the dorsal and ventral regions. (*Adapted from* Miller AJ. The search for the central swallowing pathway: the quest for clarity. Dysphagia. 1993 ;8(3): 185-194; with permission.)

coordination of central respiratory and swallowing pattern generators, and dorsal respiratory group neurons may be the initial site for the integration of swallowing and respiratory central pattern generators. Bautista and colleagues[41] proposed nucleus reticularis gigantocellularis (NRG) as the synchronizing site for breathing and swallowing. The NRG is composed of giant neuronal cells and occupies a large portion of the brainstem reticular formation.[66,67] Although NRG is not directly involved in breathing or swallowing motor function, it is a part of the circuitry involved in their motor function, and certain tonically active nonrespiratory neurons may be specifically activated during swallowing.[41]

The esophageal phase involves relaxation of upper and lower esophageal sphincters (UES and LES, respectively) and coordination of striated and smooth and circular and longitudinal esophageal muscles in the esophagus.[16,38,46] In contrast to the pharyngeal phase, esophageal peristalsis is regulated by the enteric ganglia more than the descending central nervous system pathways. The preganglionic neural control for the striated muscles originates from the NA and for smooth muscles from the dorsal motor nucleus. The neuronal fibers from the dorsal motor nucleus innervate the myenteric plexus between the circular and longitudinal muscles, which in turn innervate the smooth muscles. The striated musculature is excitatory, whereas the postganglionic fibers for the smooth muscle release both excitatory and inhibitory neurotransmitters. The internal branch of the SLN, which facilitates airway protective responses, can elicit pharyngeal swallows and esophageal peristalsis through both striated and smooth muscles. Both the afferent and efferent pathways from the striated muscles terminate and originate, respectively from the central subnucleus of the NTS, whereas afferents from the smooth muscle terminate in the medial rather than central part of the NTS. Transport of food from the oropharynx to stomach requires the relaxation of both UES and LES and antegrade peristalsis (for review, see Jadcherla).[15]

COORDINATION OF SWALLOWING AND RESPIRATORY CENTRAL PATTERN GENERATORS
Physiologic Consideration

Coordination of swallowing sequence and timing of the respiratory cycle is critical for the maintenance of adequate gas exchange and for achieving safe swallows. The normal suck-swallow coordination begins during early embryonic life and continues during fetal and infancy periods.[68-70] During fetal life, gas exchange is accomplished via maternal-placental unit and lungs are distended with lung liquid with semiadducted vocal cords, allowing egress of lung liquid and little mixing of amniotic and pulmonary fluids. Pharyngeal swallowing, which plays an important role in the regulation of amniotic fluid volume and gastrointestinal tract development, initiates between 10 to 14 weeks PMA (similar to the onset of FBM), and consistent swallowing is observed between 22 and 24 weeks PMA.[70] True in-utero sucking begins between 18 and 24 weeks PMA as defined by the tongue movements. In-utero pharyngeal swallowing follows the sequential relaxation of the upper esophageal sphincter and primary and secondary esophageal peristalsis followed by relaxation of lower esophageal sphincter. Suckling oromotor activity is broadly divided in to nonnutritive and nutritive sucking (NNS and NS, respectively). NNS is defined when no milk or fluids are involved and the infant sucks on a pacifier (soother/dummy), whereas NS involves ingesting milk from a nipple (breast or bottle). In-utero NNS and swallowing can be observed by 15 weeks PMA and continues to mature postnatally. NNS pattern consists of burst-pause at 2 sucks per second followed by rest and subsequent return to burst-pause pattern. The number of NNS bursts per minute and peak pressures increase with advancing PMA. NS pattern comprises ~1 suck per second and 4 to 10 sucks occur per burst. The lower number of sucks per second during NS compared with those during NNS are likely due to the time needed for the completion of pharyngeal stage of swallowing and maintenance of adequate ventilation. Healthy infants can coordinate suck-swallow-breathing activity at ~32 weeks PMA and can be completely orally fed by 35 to 36 weeks PMA. For both nonnutritive and nutritive sucking, the process comprises of (1) suction and (2) expression. Suction generates negative intraoral pressure, which draws milk or liquid into mouth, and is achieved via lowering of the mandible, closure of the nasal passages by the soft palate and tight seal by the lips around the nipple. The expression phase involves the positive pressure, stripping of the breast and/or nipple by the tongue movements against the hard palate, and drawing milk or liquid into the mouth. Preterm infants can accomplish breastfeeding, albeit inefficiently, using expression primarily as the suction component needed to latch or grip the maternal nipple is weak.

Nonnutritive Sucking

It has previously been postulated that after birth, NNS does not require intricate coordination, as the risk of tracheal aspiration is minimal as long as the infants can handle their oropharyngeal secretions. However, Reynolds and colleagues[71] have demonstrated that infants born before 35 weeks PMA coordinate their NNS swallows and various expiratory phases, and such coordination matures with advancing PMA. A total of 176 swallows during 35 NNS periods were examined in 16 infants over a period of several weeks. Forty-six, twenty, and nine percent of the NNS swallows occurred during the end, beginning, or the midexpiratory phases, respectively. Seven percent occurred during midinspiration and 15% during apneas (swallow apneas). Furthermore, with advancing PMA, NNS swallows coincided more with the midexpiratory phase rather than at the end of expiratory or cusp of the expiratory-inspiratory phase. With increasing PMA, the breathing pauses changed from central and obstructive apneas to attenuated respiration; however, neither the oxygen desaturation nor bradycardiac episodes were reported. Hence the relationship of NNS to oxygen desaturation events, especially those occurring during midinspiration, is not known. Nonetheless, the data suggested improving coordination of NNS, swallows, and respiration with advancing PMA. Bingham and colleagues[72] reported the NNS to be a maturational process with increasing organization coinciding with gestational maturity (**Fig. 4**). Furthermore, a greater organized NNS pattern was associated with attaining full oral feeds. From functional perspectives, NNS has several benefits such as acceleration from gavage to oral feeds, start of oral feeds to reaching full oral feeds, and shorter length of hospital stay.[73,74]

Nutritive Sucking

NS is a complex sensorimotor process and requires precise coordination of suck-swallow and respiratory pattern generators. In both term and preterm infants, swallowing occurs at the expense of rhythmic breathing, interrupts the respiratory cycle, and need to occur at the postinspiratory/expiratory phase of the respiratory cycle with resumption of breathing during the expiratory phase to avoid pulmonary milk aspiration.[75] Because preterm infants breathe irregularly and at rates of 60 breaths or higher ($\geq$1 breath/s) while needing 350 ms to complete a swallow, there is little time to accomplish swallowing during the postinspiratory or expiratory phase. Hence, in preterm infants, apneic swallows are the prominent feature, which decrease with advancing PMA.[76] Apneic swallows are achieved via arrest of respiratory flow, laryngeal adduction, and attenuated diaphragmatic activity. Evolving and established

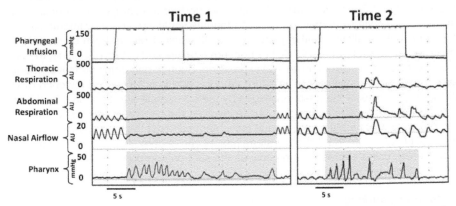

Fig. 4. Maturational changes in respiratory and pharyngeal rhythms.Representative recording demonstrating maturational effect on respiratory and pharyngeal rhythms in an infant at time-1 (younger age) exhibits increased number of pharyngeal peaks, duration, and variability between peaks, with prolonged deglutition apnea in contrast with maturation from the same infant at time-2. From Hasenstab KA, Sitaram S, Lang IM, et al. Maturation modulates pharyngeal-stimulus provoked pharyngeal and respiratory rhythms in human infants. Dysphagia, 33(1), 2018, 63-75.

pulmonary disorders including BPD result in decreased integration of respiratory and feeding rhythms leading to increased apneic swallows and decreased coordination of swallowing-breathing rhythms and hypoxemic episodes.[77]

IMPACT OF PREMATURITY ON AERODIGESTIVE DISORDERS
Pathophysiology of the Coordination of Suck-Swallow-Breathe Sequence

Because both FBM and fetal swallowing are observed ~11 to 14 weeks PMA, it is likely that the overlapping central respiratory and swallowing pattern generators begin interneuronal connectivity (synchronization) during the first half of the second trimester. As detailed earlier, fetal swallowing is initially observed between 10 and 14 weeks PMA and more consistently by 24 weeks PMA, and healthy infants can co-ordinate suck-swallow-breathe sequence at approximately 32 weeks PMA. FBM also get organized in epochs with advancing gestational age and coincide with active (non-rapid eye movement) sleep. Furthermore, bursts and pause pattern of lingual movements represents ontogenic maturation from morphologic and neurologic perspectives. In a preterm piglet model, the animals could coordinate sucking and swallowing but were not able to coordinate swallowing and breathing.[78] Preterm infants, born at 28 to 31 weeks PMA and studied between 32 and 36 weeks, exhibited apneas during (swallows apnea) until 35 weeks PMA and postinspiratory swallows thereafter.[32,76,79] Thus, it is plausible that preterm delivery occurring during the critical window of development disrupts the development and maturation of swallowing skills.[70]

Impact of Pulmonary Insufficiency/Chronic Lung Disease on the Suck-Swallow-Breathe Sequence

Pulmonary insufficiency and chronic lung disease

Because of the immature respiratory system and neural circuitry, preterm infants may need respiratory support. Invasive and prolonged respiratory support with endotra-cheal intubation and assisted mechanical ventilation[80] might lead to lung injury and CLD.[80] Despite recent advances in neonatal-perinatal care, more than 40% of very-low-birth-weight infants develop BPD,[81] which is associated with reduced pulmonary functions, high emergency room visits, increased use of bronchodilators/glucocorti-coids, and neurologic deficits.[82–95] In the absence of an effective therapeutic interven-tion,[85,96–99] noninvasive ventilation (nCPAP and/or heated humidified high-flow nasal cannula [HHFNC]) is the mainstay for attenuating lung injury.[90,100,101]

Suck-swallow-breathe sequence

Oral feeding is a major challenge for preterm infants, which becomes magnified in in-fants with chronic lung disease. Gewolb and Vice demonstrated that although apneic swallows decreased over time in infants with chronic lung disease, at 35 weeks PMA, infants with CLD had significantly higher number of apneic swallows and swallow-breathe phase relationship involving apneas compared with infants without CLD, indi-cating decreased integration of respiratory and swallowing motor activities.[32,76] Miz-uno and colleagues[77] observed that preterm infants with BPD had lower sucking pressure and frequency and decreased feeding efficiency and longer swallow apneas compared with those without CLD (**Fig. 5**).

Implications of delayed initiation of oral feeds

Infants born less than 28 weeks PMA have marked delay in achieving full oral feeds as they receive 4- to 5-fold more respiratory support compared with more mature infants, and there is hesitancy in initiating oral feeds on nCPAP and HHFNC. Jadcherla and colleagues[16,18,29,102,103] compared the timing of initiating and progress of oral feeds to achieving full feeds and observed that the age of infant at first feed correlated with both the age of achieving full gavage and full oral feedings. It is plausible that the shorter gastric emptying time in preterm infants on respiratory support with CPAP compared with preterm infants off CPAP could be one of the factors that positively affects the progress to full gavage feeding, which may result in earlier oral full feeding. In an elegant series of studies, Jadcherla's group demonstrated that early introduction of oral feeding accelerated the transition time from tube to all oral feeding.[16,18,29,102,103] Thus, despite the fact that preterm infants are highly likely to benefit from targeted oromotor feeding therapies,[104] little work has been performed in this important area of infant care.

DILEMMAS OF CURRENT ORAL-FEEDING PRACTICES IN PRETERM INFANTS

Eating is a neurodevelopmental process and achieving full oral feeding competency is a significant challenge to infants who are born prematurely.[115] This challenge is exacerbated for those infants who are less mature at birth and those who have a greater number of medical comorbidities.[18,105,106] Successful eating without cardiorespiratory compromise is an NICU discharge criterion.[107] Historically, NICU health care professionals have prioritized the achievement of full oral feeds as quickly as possible for premature infants in order to accomplish the earliest discharge home. This effort has erroneously been based on expectations of gestational age rather than individualized neurodevelopment and feeding performance.[108,109] An outdated NICU practice of "trial and error" feeding opportunities may contribute to altered development and worse clinical outcomes[110] because the random approach does not support a safe, ordered, and competency-based progression of feeding skills. Evidence suggests that implementation of a standardized feeding protocol for infants weighing less than 1500 g at birth was associated with faster time to reach full feeds, improved growth,[111] and earlier discharge from the hospital.[112]

Another disconcerting consequence of NICU feeding practices is the prevalence of feeding difficulties that develop after NICU discharge,[9] long-term neurodevelopmental outcome, language skill acquisition, resource utilization, and parental distress.

In the NICU, evidence-informed, successful progression to full oral eating is shaped by consistent, infant-focused feeding management practices that include, attention to oral and respiratory control (adequate oral motor control and coordination with suck, swallow, breathe), frequency of opportunity (repetition), and development of predictability (volumes, times, flow). Premature infant swallowing is entrained by the sucking pattern, with coordination of respiration last to be established in the suck-swallow-breathe rhythm.[76] Suck/swallow/breathe coordination is prolonged for those infants born at a younger gestational age.[18,105] Oral feeding milestones are a function of postconceptual age and further delayed for those with medical conditions such as necrotizing enterocolitis, patent ductus arteriosus requiring treatment, or neurologic risk.[106] In addition to the challenges of prematurity, infants with respiratory morbidity such as BPD are further delayed by irregular respiratory pattern, including tachypnea, shorter suck-swallow runs during feeding,[32] and inefficient feeding due to weak sucking pressure[77] (Fig. 5).

Establishing safe feeding for infants with respiratory compromise may be achieved by using vigilant monitoring and attention to cues.[113,114] Ensuring adequate oral motor control and state control during oral feeding with attention to stress signals is key to ensuring a state of oral feeding readiness and essential to ensure quality feeding performance.[108,115] For example, infants who are active and awake at the time of the feed

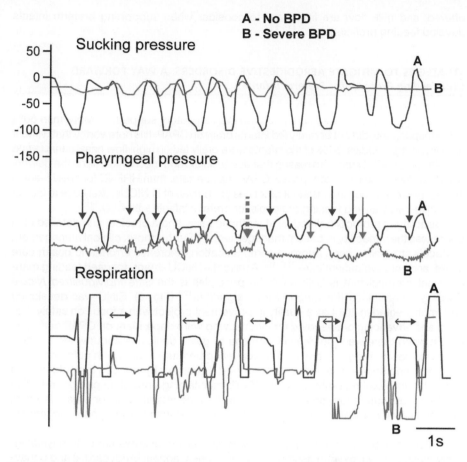

Fig. 5. Impact of pulmonary insufficiency on sucking and pharyngeal pressures. Tracings of sucking pressure (expression: upward), pharyngeal pressure (mmHg), and nasal airflow (inspiration downward and expiration upward) in an infant with (A; *red* waveform) no bronchopulmonary dysplasia (BPD) and with (B; *blue* waveform) with severe BPD. The arrow indicates the onset of swallowing. X-axis, time (seconds); y-axis, pressure (mm Hg). The infant without BPD demonstrates regular sucking pattern, and the infant with severe BPD demonstrated weak negative pressure and low sucking frequency. The dotted (*blue*) arrow indicates swallowing followed by 1.8 seconds of deglutition apnea. (*Adapted from* Mizuno K, Nishida Y, Taki M, et al. Infants with bronchopulmonary dysplasia suckle with weak pressures to maintain breathing during feeding. Pediatrics. ePub 2007 Oct;120(4):e1035-42; with permission.)

consume more feed volume than those who are quietly alert.[108,116] There is well-established evidence that both the quality and quantity of feeding experience may play a role in feeding transition from gavage to nipple feeding. Preterm infants offered earlier and more frequent nipple feeding opportunities may attain independent nipple feeds in a shorter time period.[110,113,117,118] A combination of delayed and oral experience and pulmonary insufficiency is likely the harbinger for oral feeding difficulties and speech problems in infants born prematurely. In addition, predictability regarding such factors as the feeding technique, volume offered, duration of time the meal will be offered, and milk flow are important to consider when supporting preterm infants develop feeding proficiency.[109,115,117]

STRATEGIES TO MITIGATE AERODIGESTIVE DISORDERS: A WAY FORWARD
Oral-Feeding Protocol for Preterm Infants

A recent survey demonstrated that 80% of the NICUs and PICUs did not have a written oral-feeding protocol for infants on noninvasive respiratory support.[119] More than 50% of the respondents did not or rarely fed infants orally on CPAP. It is noteworthy that without any physiologic studies, 54% of the infants were orally fed on high-flow nasal cannula and only 4% on CPAP. It stands to reason that due to fluidic and mechanical flip in the delivery of airflow during the expiratory phase, CPAP may be safer than HHFNC for orally feeding infants. However, such inconsistent practices are prevalent in NICUs, likely due to lack of physiologic studies and feeding protocols for preterm infants with CLD.[119]

Availability of protocol defined as algorithmic rules, and a precise, and detailed plan decreases the variability in patient management.[120] Furthermore, clinical management protocols streamline care, improve communication, decrease errors and health care costs, and improve patient care.[120–122] A validated NICU-infant–focused feeding management protocol that is built on these principles is the *Safe Individualized Nipple Feeding Competence (Feeding in SINC)* algorithm[123] (**Fig. 6**). SINC was developed and implemented in 2014 as a quality improvement project with a focus on safely initiating and advancing oral feeding for infants, who were dependent on CPAP during an epoch when there were no definitive criteria to guide decisions about when to introduce and how to progress oral feeding for very premature infants with pulmonary disease requiring noninvasive respiratory support. It was our hypothesis that infants who were able to breathe comfortably on CPAP, maintaining normal respiratory rate and stable oxygen saturation, could be offered small amounts of bottle or breast feeding, provided cardiorespiratory and state control were maintained throughout the feeding session.

In *Feeding in SINC*, infant signals of homeostasis and distress are both physiologically monitored (eg, oxygen desaturation, tachypnea, apnea, bradycardia) and behaviorally monitored (eg, arching, spitting, choking, weak suck, "shutting down"). Using the SINC algorithm, NICUs have been able to offer oral feeding opportunities to fragile feeders, supported on various modes of noninvasive respiratory support, with an aim to provide feed volumes and feed techniques that are matched to each infant's physiologic stability and feeding skill level. For some infants SINC may be limited to nonnutritive feeding; others achieve full bottle feeding while on continuous positive end expiratory pressure (CPAP) support. Infants following the SINC algorithm are fed by highly skilled nurses and carefully coached parents.[123] The infants may bottle or breast feed depending on parental preference and attendance in the NICU.

At each stage of the *Feeding in SINC* strategy, oral feed volume, maximum feed duration, and feeding technique are specified. Feeding opportunities are offered every time the infant is cueing while monitoring carefully for both engagement and stress cues. At any sign of distress, the feed would be stopped and the infant may return to NNS with a pacifier if still cueing to suck.[123] As the infant progresses through the stages, the infant gains competence by safely eating increased volumes and feeding for increasingly longer time periods.

Initial feeds in stages B and C are offered to a cueing infant at an appropriately pumped breast or by giving a single drop of milk at a time besides a pacifier (see **Fig. 6**). Stage B limits the feed to a maximum of 5% of the feed volume, with the maximum feeding duration of 5 minutes. At all stages, the remainder of the feed

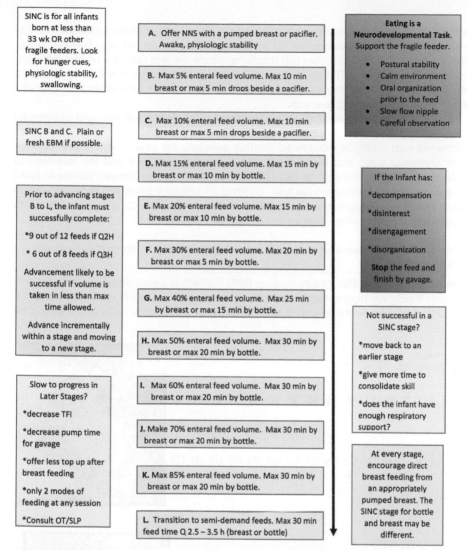

SINC is for all infants born at less than 33 wk OR other fragile feeders. Look for hunger cues, physiologic stability, swallowing.

SINC B and C. Plain or fresh EBM if possible.

Prior to advancing stages B to L, the infant must successfully complete:

*9 out of 12 feeds if Q2H

* 6 out of 8 feeds if Q3H

Advancement likely to be successful if volume is taken in less than max time allowed.

Advance incrementally within a stage and moving to a new stage.

Slow to progress in Later Stages?

*decrease TFI

*decrease pump time for gavage

*offer less top up after breast feeding

*only 2 modes of feeding at any session

*Consult OT/SLP

A. Offer NNS with a pumped breast or pacifier. Awake, physiologic stability

B. Max 5% enteral feed volume. Max 10 min breast or max 5 min drops beside a pacifier.

C. Max 10% enteral feed volume. Max 10 min breast or max 5 min drops beside a pacifier.

D. Max 15% enteral feed volume. Max 15 min by breast or max 10 min by bottle.

E. Max 20% enteral feed volume. Max 15 min by breast or max 10 min by bottle.

F. Max 30% enteral feed volume. Max 20 min by breast or max 5 min by bottle.

G. Max 40% enteral feed volume. Max 25 min by breast or max 15 min by bottle.

H. Max 50% enteral feed volume. Max 30 min by breast or max 20 min by bottle.

I. Max 60% enteral feed volume. Max 30 min by breast or max 20 min by bottle.

J. Make 70% enteral feed volume. Max 30 min by breast or max 20 min by bottle.

K. Max 85% enteral feed volume. Max 30 min by breast or max 20 min by bottle.

L. Transition to semi-demand feeds. Max 30 min feed time Q 2.5 – 3.5 h (breast or bottle)

Eating is a Neurodevelopmental Task. Support the fragile feeder.

- Postural stability
- Calm environment
- Oral organization prior to the feed
- Slow flow nipple
- Careful observation

If the Infant has:

*decompensation

*disinterest

*disengagement

*disorganization

Stop the feed and finish by gavage.

Not successful in a SINC stage?

*move back to an earlier stage

*give more time to consolidate skill

*does the infant have enough respiratory support?

At every stage, encourage direct breast feeding from an appropriately pumped breast. The SINC stage for bottle and breast may be different.

Fig. 6. Safe Individualized Nipple-Feeding Competence (SINC) algorithm. Feeding protocol for preterm infants younger than or equal to 33 weeks PMA. Stages A–L include nonnutritive sucking to semidemand oral breast/bottle feeds. Stacey Dalgleish. (Adapted from Dalgleish SR, Kostecky LL, Blachly N. Eating in "SINC": Safe Individualized Nipple-Feeding Competence, a Quality Improvement Project to Explore Infant-Driven Oral Feeding for Very Premature Infants Requiring Noninvasive Respiratory Support. Neonatal Netw 2016;35(4): 217-227.)

volume is given by gavage. An attempt at breastfeeding with any transfer of milk would be considered an equivalent or successful feeding opportunity at the SINC stage. Stages D through L are offered in a closed bottle with a slow-flow nipple or an appropriately pumped breast. At each stage the volume advances by a specified percentage until the neonate is exclusively breast and/or nipple fed by bottle. At the final stage, L, the infant is eating with a semidemand schedule of 2.5 to 3.5 hours.

To ensure stamina and skill development, advancement in the algorithm requires the infant to successfully take 9/12 feeds in a 2 hourly schedule or 6/8 feeds in a 3 hourly schedule. In that way advancement in feeding is individualized to the infant's ability. For example, the most fragile neonate could spend several weeks in Stage B while convalescing from other comorbidities and practicing nipple-feeding skills in a predictable environment. Occupational Therapy or Speech Language Pathology consultation is sought if an infant is not progressing with nipple feeding as expected or if the infant demonstrates any symptoms of feeding aversion.

As with the *Feeding in SINC* strategy, others have described safe and successful oral feeding sessions for infants on CPAP.[114,124,125] Oral feeding success was achieved with cautious, structured feeding sessions for infants who demonstrated oral readiness cues and physiologic stability during the feed and the intention to stop the feeding at any sign of distress. *Feeding in SINC* has allowed infants to learn to eat as a neurodevelopmental task, building on previous skills and strengths. Each feed and overall progress are monitored closely so that feeds are conducted with safety and stability rather than ending in fatigue or distress.

Rationale and Implementation and Safety of Oral Feeding in Preterm Infants on Respiratory Support

A large number of VLBW infants develop BPD,[81] which is associated with reduced pulmonary functions, high emergency room visits, increased use of bronchodilators/glucocorticoids, and neurologic deficits.[82–95] In the absence of an effective therapeutic

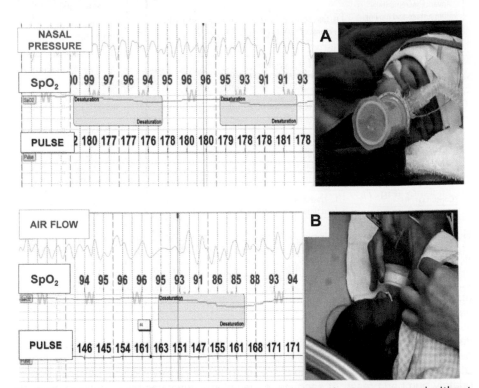

Fig. 7. Respiratory control in an infant on continuous positive airway pressure and without respiratory support. Representative tracings of nasal pressure, pulse oximetry, and pulse (heart rate) in an infant during oral feeding on CPAP (*A*) and without any respiratory support (*B*). Similar oxygen desaturation was observed during feeding in infants on CPAP and room air breathing spontaneously.

intervention,[85,96–99] noninvasive ventilation remains the mainstay for attenuating lung injury.[100,101] Both nCPAP and HHFNC aim to maintain pulmonary functional residual capacity but there are differences how they achieve this goal.[126–128] CPAP (distending pressure 4–$\geq$8 cm H_2O) delivers a positive distending pressure with a fluidic expiratory flip, which decreases the resistance during expiratory phase. HHFNC flushes the airway with high flows (2–8 L per min) with unpredictable pressures and may increase expiratory resistive work of breathing.

Because of the (1) concern of aspiration and consequent cardiorespiratory events,[119] (2) discrepant results, and (3) paucity of well-designed studies, physicians are reluctant to initiate oral-feeding, while the infants are on nCPAP therapy.[114,129,130] Because nCPAP is the most common mode for noninvasive respiratory support, delayed nipple feeding may lead to oral aversion, delayed oromotor skill development,[131] speech impairment, and prolonged hospital stay resulting in parental stress and increased economic costs.[132–135] An infant optimally supported to breathe with noninvasive techniques will be able to suck and swallow more effectively. Despite the likelihood that that preterm infants would benefit from targeted oromotor feeding therapies,[18,104] little work has been performed in this important area of infant care; 80% of the NICUs do not even have a feeding-protocol, whereas infants are supported on noninvasive ventilation.[119]

Animal studies[136] have demonstrated that application of nCPAP in full-term lambs neither had deleterious effect on feeding safety, efficiency, and overall nutritive swallowing-breathing coordination[136–139] nor altered the nutritive esophagodeglutition. Furthermore, nCPAP, and not HHFNC, increased the rate of milk ingestion in both term and preterm lambs.[139,140] Thus, there is robust experimental evidence from animal[136,139,140] and *term* human infant[114] studies that support the authors' proposition that positive effects of nCPAP compared with HHFNC on cardiorespiratory stability result from protective effects on swallowing and laryngeal chemoreflexes, shorter gastric emptying time, and elevation of the gastroesophageal sphincter tone. However, limited data exist on the safety of feeding infants orally while on noninvasive respiratory support. Using the SINC[123] feeding protocol, the authors performed proof of principle studies to investigate the effect of oral feeding on cardiorespiratory variables. The authors' preliminary data (Hasan et al, 2019, unpublished observation) suggest that it is safe to orally feed preterm infants receiving CPAP for pulmonary insufficiency (**Fig. 7**).

Orosensory Stimulation

A recent review by Jadcherla and a large number of studies have suggested that targeted and personalized orosensory stimulation and oral feeding experience improved suck-swallow-breathe coordination leading to transition to full oral feeds.[20,141–144]

In summary, both BPD and aerodigestive disorders are increasing and are associated with prolonged hospital stay, feeding difficulties, and adverse pulmonary and neuro developmental outcomes. A concerted effort to develop and implement evidence-informed and personalized protocols is vital to prevent/treat aerodigestive disorders.

ACKNOWLEDGMENTS

We thank Marie Abrosimova for performing preliminary studies to establish the feasibility and safety of oral feeding on CPAP and Dolma Dejikhangsar for editorial assistance. Financial support by the Canadian Institutes of Health Research (PJT-16880) is gratefully acknowledged.

DISCLOSURE

All authors attest that they have no commercial or financial conflicts of interest or funding resources to disclose.

REFERENCES

1. Greer JJ, Funk GD, Ballanyi K. Preparing for the first breath: prenatal maturation of respiratory neural control. J Physiol 2006;570(Pt 3):437–44.
2. Chou PJ, Ullrich JR, Ackerman BD. Time of onset of effective ventilation at birth. Biol Neonate 1974;24(1):74–81.
3. Hasan SU, Rigaux A. Arterial oxygen tension threshold range for the onset of arousal and breathing in fetal sheep. Pediatr Res 1992;32(3):342–9.
4. Jain L, Dudell GG. Respiratory transition in infants delivered by cesarean section. Semin Perinatol 2006;30(5):296–304.
5. Hillman NH, Kallapur SG, Jobe AH. Physiology of transition from intrauterine to extrauterine life. Clin Perinatol 2012;39(4):769–83.
6. Hooper SB, Te Pas AB, Lang J, et al. Cardiovascular transition at birth: a physiological sequence. Pediatr Res 2015;77(5):608–14.
7. Chan SH, Johnson MJ, Leaf AA, et al. Nutrition and neurodevelopmental outcomes in preterm infants: a systematic review. Acta Paediatr 2016;105(6): 587–99.
8. Kumar RK, Singhal A, Vaidya U, et al. Optimizing nutrition in preterm low birth weight infants-consensus summary. Front Nutr 2017;4:20.
9. Thoyre SM. Feeding outcomes of extremely premature infants after neonatal care. J Obstet Gynecol Neonatal Nurs 2007;36(4):366–75 [quiz: 376].
10. Jensen EA, Schmidt B. Epidemiology of bronchopulmonary dysplasia. Birth Defects Res A Clin Mol Teratol 2014;100(3):145–57.
11. Keszler M, Sant'Anna G. Mechanical ventilation and bronchopulmonary dysplasia. Clin perinatology 2015;42(4):781–96.
12. Shalish W, Anna GM. The use of mechanical ventilation protocols in Canadian neonatal intensive care units. Paediatr Child Health 2015;20(4):e13–9.
13. Vliegenthart RJS, Onland W, van Wassenaer-Leemhuis AG, et al. Restricted ventilation associated with reduced neurodevelopmental impairment in preterm infants. Neonatology 2017;112(2):172–9.
14. Vliegenthart RJS, van Kaam AH, Aarnoudse-Moens CSH, et al. Duration of mechanical ventilation and neurodevelopment in preterm infants. Arch Dis Child FetalNeonatal Ed 2019;104(6):F631–5.
15. Jadcherla S. Dysphagia in the high-risk infant: potential factors and mechanisms. Am J Clin Nutr 2016;103(2):622s–8s.
16. Jadcherla SR. Pathophysiology of aerodigestive pulmonary disorders in the neonate. Clin Perinatol 2012;39(3):639–54.
17. Jadcherla SR. Challenges to eating, swallowing, and aerodigestive functions in infants: a burning platform that needs attention! J Pediatr 2019;211:7–9.
18. Jadcherla SR, Wang M, Vijayapal AS, et al. Impact of prematurity and comorbidities on feeding milestones in neonates: a retrospective study. JPerinatol 2010;30(3):201–8.
19. Lau C. Development of suck and swallow mechanisms in infants. Ann Nutr Metab 2015;66(Suppl 5):7–14.
20. Lau C. Development of infant oral feeding skills: what do we know? Am J Clin Nutr 2016;103(2):616s–21s.

21. Lau C, Sheena HR, Shulman RJ, et al. Oral feeding in low birth weight infants. J Pediatr 1997;130(4):561–9.

22. Barlow SM. Oral and respiratory control for preterm feeding. Curr Opin Otolaryngol Head Neck Surg 2009;17(3):179–86.

23. Dutschmann M, Morschel M, Reuter J, et al. Postnatal emergence of synaptic plasticity associated with dynamic adaptation of the respiratory motor pattern. Respir Physiol Neurobiol 2008;164(1–2):72–9.

24. Bavis RW, MacFarlane PM. Developmental plasticity in the neural control of breathing. Exp Neurol 2017;287(Pt 2):176–91.

25. Fuller DD, Mitchell GS. Respiratory neuroplasticity - overview, significance and future directions. Exp Neurol 2017;287(Pt 2):144–52.

26. Greer JJ, Martin-Caraballo M. Developmental plasticity of phrenic motoneuron and diaphragm properties with the inception of inspiratory drive transmission in utero. Exp Neurol 2017;287(Pt 2):137–43.

27. Gauda EB, McLemore GL. Premature birth, homeostatic plasticity and respiratory consequences of inflammation. Respir Physiol Neurobiol 2020;274:103337.

28. Hocker AD, Stokes JA, Powell FL, et al. The impact of inflammation on respiratory plasticity. Exp Neurol 2017;287(Pt 2):243–53.

29. Jadcherla SR, Khot T, Moore R, et al. Feeding methods at discharge predict long-term feeding and neurodevelopmental outcomes in preterm infants referred for gastrostomy evaluation. J Pediatr 2017;181:125–30.e1.

30. Johnson S, Matthews R, Draper ES, et al. Eating difficulties in children born late and moderately preterm at 2 y of age: a prospective population-based cohort study. Am J Clin Nutr 2016;103(2):406–14.

31. Simpson C, Schanler RJ, Lau C. Early introduction of oral feeding in preterm infants. Pediatrics 2002;110(3):517–22.

32. Gewolb IH, Vice FL. Abnormalities in the coordination of respiration and swallow in preterm infants with bronchopulmonary dysplasia. Dev Med Child Neurol 2006;48(7):595–9.

33. Fucile S, McFarland DH, Gisel EG, et al. Oral and nonoral sensorimotor interventions facilitate suck-swallow-respiration functions and their coordination in preterm infants. Early Hum Dev 2012;88(6):345–50.

34. Fucile S, Gisel EG. Sensorimotor interventions improve growth and motor function in preterm infants. Neonatal Network 2010;29(6):359–66.

35. Fucile S, Gisel EG, Lau C. Effect of an oral stimulation program on sucking skill maturation of preterm infants. Dev Med Child Neurol 2005;47(3):158–62.

36. Fucile S, Gisel E, Lau C. Oral stimulation accelerates the transition from tube to oral feeding in preterm infants. J Pediatr 2002;141(2):230–6.

37. Jadcherla SR, Dail J, Malkar MB, et al. Impact of process optimization and quality improvement measures on neonatal feeding outcomes at an all-referral neonatal intensive care unit. JPEN J Parenter Enteral Nutr 2016;40(5):646–55.

38. Miller AJ. The neurobiology of swallowing and dysphagia. DevDisabil Res Rev 2008;14(2):77–86.

39. Smith JC, Butera RJ, Koshiya N, et al. Respiratory rhythm generation in neonatal and adult mammals: the hybrid pacemaker-network model. Respir Physiol 2000; 122(2–3):131–47.

40. Samson N, Praud JP, Quenet B, et al. New insights into sucking, swallowing and breathing central generators: a complexity analysis of rhythmic motor behaviors. Neurosci Lett 2017;638:90–5.

41. Bautista TG, Sun QJ, Pilowsky PM. The generation of pharyngeal phase of swallow and its coordination with breathing: interaction between the swallow and respiratory central pattern generators. Prog Brain Res 2014;212:253–75.
42. Jean A. Brain stem control of swallowing: neuronal network and cellular mechanisms. Physiol Rev 2001;81(2):929–69.
43. Prabhakar V, Hasenstab KA, Osborn E, et al. Pharyngeal contractile and regulatory characteristics are distinct during nutritive oral stimulus in preterm-born infants: implications for clinical and research applications. Neurogastroenterol Motil 2019;31(8):e13650.
44. Fitting JW. From breathing to respiration. Respiration 2015;89(1):82–7.
45. BuSha BF, Banis G. A stochastic and integrative model of breathing. Respir Physiol Neurobiol 2017;237:51–6.
46. Miller AJ. The search for the central swallowing pathway: the quest for clarity. Dysphagia 1993;8(3):185–94.
47. Smith JC, Ellenberger HH, Ballanyi K, et al. Pre-Botzinger complex: a brainstem region that may generate respiratory rhythm in mammals. Science 1991; 254(5032):726–9.
48. Kam K, Worrell JW, Janczewski WA, et al. Distinct inspiratory rhythm and pattern generating mechanisms in the preBotzinger complex. J Neurosci 2013;33(22): 9235–45.
49. Anderson TM, Ramirez JM. Respiratory rhythm generation: triple oscillator hypothesis. F1000Res 2017;6:139.
50. Patrick J, Fetherston W, Vick H, et al. Human fetal breathing movements and gross fetal body movements at weeks 34 to 35 of gestation. Am J Obstet Gynecol 1978;130(6):693–9.
51. Patrick J, Challis J. Measurement of human fetal breathing movements in healthy pregnancies using a real-time scanner. Semin Perinatol 1980;4(4): 275–86.
52. Patrick J. Fetal breathing movements. Clin Obstet Gynecol 1982;25(4):787–807.
53. Dawes GS. The central control of fetal breathing and skeletal muscle movements. J Physiol 1984;346:1–18.
54. Fox HE, Moessinger AC. Fetal breathing movements and lung hypoplasia: preliminary human observations. Am J Obstet Gynecol 1985;151(4):531–3.
55. Han RN, Mawdsley C, Souza P, et al. Platelet-derived growth factors and growth-related genes in rat lung. III. Immunolocalization during fetal development. Pediatr Res 1992;31(4 Pt 1):323–9.
56. Souza P, Tanswell AK, Post M. Different roles for PDGF-alpha and -beta receptors in embryonic lung development. Am J Respir Cell Mol Biol 1996;15(4): 551–62.
57. Liu J, Tseu I, Wang J, et al. Transforming growth factor beta2, but not beta1 and beta3, is critical for early rat lung branching. Dev Dyn 2000;217(4):343–60.
58. Liu M, Tanswell AK, Post M. Mechanical force-induced signal transduction in lung cells. Am J Physiol 1999;277(4):L667–83.
59. Hasan SU, Bamford OS, Hawkins RL, et al. The effects of brain-stem section on the breathing and behavioural response to morphine in the fetal sheep. J Dev Physiol 1990;13(3):147–55.
60. Wong KA, Bano A, Rigaux A, et al. Pulmonary vagal innervation is required to establish adequate alveolar ventilation in the newborn lamb. J Appl Physiol (1985) 1998;85(3):849–59.

61. Lalani S, Remmers JE, Green FH, et al. Effects of vagal denervation on cardio-respiratory and behavioral responses in the newborn lamb. J Appl Physiol (1985) 2001;91(5):2301–13.

62. Lalani S, Remmers JE, Hasan SU. Breathing patterns, pulmonary mechanics and gas exchange: role of vagal innervation in neonatal lamb. Exp Physiol 2001;86(6):803–10.

63. Lumb KJ, Schneider JM, Ibrahim T, et al. Afferent neural feedback overrides the modulating effects of arousal, hypercapnia and hypoxaemia on neonatal cardio-respiratory control. J Physiol 2018;596(23):6009–19.

64. Hasan SU, Bharadwaj B, Remmers JE, et al. Pulmonary feedback and gesta-tional age-dependent regulation of fetal breathing movements. Canadian journal of physiology and pharmacology 2008;86:691–9.

65. Bolser DC, Gestreau C, Morris KF, et al. Central neural circuits for coordination of swallowing, breathing, and coughing: predictions from computational modeling and simulation. Otolaryngol Clin North Am 2013;46(6):957–64.

66. Feroah TR, Forster HV, Fuentes CG, et al. Contributions from rostral medullary nuclei to coordination of swallowing and breathing in awake goats. J Appl Phys-iol (1985) 2002;93(2):581–91.

67. Zemlan FP, Behbehani MM, Beckstead RM. Ascending and descending projec-tions from nucleus reticularis magnocellularis and nucleus reticularis gigantocel-lularis: an autoradiographic and horseradish peroxidase study in the rat. Brain Res 1984;292(2):207–20.

68. Arvedson JC, Lefton-Greif MA. Anatomy, physiology, and development of feeding. Semin Speech Lang 1996;17(4):261–8.

69. Weckmueller J, Easterling C, Arvedson J. Preliminary temporal measurement analysis of normal oropharyngeal swallowing in infants and young children. Dysphagia 2011;26(2):135–43.

70. Delaney AL, Arvedson JC. Development of swallowing and feeding: prenatal through first year of life. DevDisabil Res Rev 2008;14(2):105–17.

71. Reynolds EW, Grider D, Caldwell R, et al. Swallow-breath interaction and phase of respiration with swallow during nonnutritive suck among low-risk preterm in-fants. Am J Perinatol 2010;27(10):831–40.

72. Bingham PM, Ashikaga T, Abbasi S. Prospective study of non-nutritive sucking and feeding skills in premature infants. Arch Dis Child FetalNeonatal Ed 2010; 95(3):F194–200.

73. Barlow SM, Lee J, Wang J, et al. Frequency-modulated orocutaneous stimula-tion promotes non-nutritive suck development in preterm infants with respiratory distress syndrome or chronic lung disease. J Perinatol 2014;34(2):136–42.

74. Foster JP, Psaila K, Patterson T. Non-nutritive sucking for increasing physiologic stability and nutrition in preterm infants. Cochrane Database Syst Rev 2016;(10):CD001071.

75. Barlow SM. Central pattern generation involved in oral and respiratory control for feeding in the term infant. Curr Opin Otolaryngol Head Neck Surg 2009;17(3): 187–93.

76. Gewolb IH, Vice FL. Maturational changes in the rhythms, patterning, and coor-dination of respiration and swallow during feeding in preterm and term infants. Dev Med Child Neurol 2006;48(7):589–94.

77. Mizuno K, Nishida Y, Taki M, et al. Infants with bronchopulmonary dysplasia suckle with weak pressures to maintain breathing during feeding. Pediatrics 2007;120(4):e1035–42.

78. Mayerl CJ, Gould FDH, Bond LE, et al. Preterm birth disrupts the development of feeding and breathing coordination. J Appl Physiol (1985) 2019;126(6):1681–6.

79. Mizuno K, Ueda A. The maturation and coordination of sucking, swallowing, and respiration in preterm infants. J Pediatr 2003;142(1):36–40.

80. Rutkowska M, Hozejowski R, Helwich E, et al. Severe bronchopulmonary dysplasia - incidence and predictive factors in a prospective, multicenter study in very preterm infants with respiratory distress syndrome. J Matern Fetal Neonatal Med 2019;32(12):1958–64.

81. Stoll BJ, Hansen NI, Bell EF, et al. Trends in care practices, morbidity, and mortality of extremely preterm neonates, 1993-2012. JAMA 2015;314(10):1039–51.

82. Asztalos EV, Church PT, Riley P, et al. Neonatal factors associated with a good neurodevelopmental outcome in very preterm infants. Am J Perinatol 2017;34(4):388–96.

83. Cazzato S, Ridolfi L, Bernardi F, et al. Lung function outcome at school age in very low birth weight children. Pediatr Pulmonol 2013;48(8):830–7.

84. Davidson LM, Berkelhamer SK. Bronchopulmonary dysplasia: chronic lung disease of infancy and long-term pulmonary outcomes. J Clin Med 2017;6(1) [pii:E4].

85. Hasan SU, Potenziano J, Konduri GG, et al. Effect of inhaled nitric oxide on survival without bronchopulmonary dysplasia in preterm infants: a randomized clinical trial. JAMA Pediatr 2017;171(11):1081–9.

86. Isayama T, Lee SK, Yang J, et al. Revisiting the definition of bronchopulmonary dysplasia: effect of changing panoply of respiratory support for preterm neonates. JAMA Pediatr 2017;171(3):271–9.

87. Jobe AH, Bancalari EH. Controversies about the definition of bronchopulmonary dysplasia at 50 years. Acta Paediatr 2017;106(5):692–3.

88. Jobe AH, Steinhorn R. Can we define bronchopulmonary dysplasia? J Pediatr 2017;188:19–23.

89. Keller RL, Feng R, DeMauro SB, et al. Bronchopulmonary dysplasia and perinatal characteristics predict 1-year respiratory outcomes in newborns born at extremely low gestational age: a prospective cohort study. J Pediatr 2017;187:89–97.e3.

90. Kennedy KA, Cotten CM, Watterberg KL, et al. Prevention and management of bronchopulmonary dysplasia: lessons learned from the neonatal research network. Semin Perinatol 2016;40(6):348–55.

91. Kinsella JP, Greenough A, Abman SH. Bronchopulmonary dysplasia. Lancet 2006;367(9520):1421–31.

92. Korhonen P, Laitinen J, Hyodynmaa E, et al. Respiratory outcome in school-aged, very-low-birth-weight children in the surfactant era. Acta Paediatr 2004;93(3):316–21.

93. Lodha A, Seshia M, McMillan DD, et al. Association of early caffeine administration and neonatal outcomes in very preterm neonates. JAMA Pediatr 2015;169(1):33–8.

94. Twilhaar ES, Wade RM, de Kieviet JF, et al. Cognitive outcomes of children born extremely or very preterm since the 1990s and associated risk factors: a meta-analysis and meta-regression. JAMA Pediatr 2018;172(4):361–7.

95. Shennan AT, Dunn MS, Ohlsson A, et al. Abnormal pulmonary outcomes in premature infants: prediction from oxygen requirement in the neonatal period. Pediatrics 1988;82(4):527–32.

96. Mobius MA, Thebaud B. Bronchopulmonary dysplasia: where have all the stem cells gone?:Origin and (potential) function of resident lung stem cells. Chest 2017;152(5):1043–52.

97. O'Reilly M, Thebaud B. Stem cells for the prevention of neonatal lung disease. Neonatology 2015;107(4):360–4.

98. Bhandari A, Carroll C, Bhandari V. BPD following preterm birth: a model for chronic lung disease and a substrate for ARDS in childhood. Front Pediatr 2016;4:60.

99. Nelin LD, Bhandari V. How to decrease bronchopulmonary dysplasia in your neonatal intensive care unit today and "tomorrow. F1000Res 2017;6:539.

100. Schmolzer GM, Kumar M, Pichler G, et al. Non-invasive versus invasive respiratory support in preterm infants at birth: systematic review and meta-analysis. BMJ 2013;347:f5980.

101. Shah V, Hodgson K, Seshia M, et al. Golden hour management practices for infants <32 weeks gestational age in Canada. PaediatrChild Health 2018;23(4): e70–6.

102. Jadcherla SR, Hasenstab KA, Sitaram S, et al. Effect of nasal noninvasive respiratory support methods on pharyngeal provocation-induced aerodigestive reflexes in infants. Am J Physiol Gastrointest Liver Physiol 2016;310(11): G1006–14.

103. Jadcherla SR, Peng J, Moore R, et al. Impact of personalized feeding program in 100 NICU infants: pathophysiology-based approach for better outcomes. J Pediatr Gastroenterol Nutr 2012;54(1):62–70.

104. Shetty S, Hunt K, Douthwaite A, et al. High-flow nasal cannula oxygen and nasal continuous positive airway pressure and full oral feeding in infants with bronchopulmonary dysplasia. Arch Dis Child FetalNeonatal Ed 2016;101(5):F408–11.

105. Dodrill P, Donovan T, Cleghorn G, et al. Attainment of early feeding milestones in preterm neonates. J Perinatol 2008;28(8):549–55.

106. Park J, Knafl G, Thoyre S, et al. Factors associated with feeding progression in extremely preterm infants. Nurs Res 2015;64(3):159–67.

107. Jefferies AL. Going home: facilitating discharge of the preterm infant. Paediatr Child Health 2014;19(1):31–42.

108. Pickler RH, Best AM, Reyna BA, et al. Prediction of feeding performance in preterm infants. Newborn Infant Nurs Rev 2005;5(3):116–23.

109. Howe TH. Should extremely low birthweight premature infants be breastfed exclusively? MCN Am J Matern Child Nurs 2007;32(1):9.

110. Pickler RH, Best A, Crosson D. The effect of feeding experience on clinical outcomes in preterm infants. J Perinatol 2009;29(2):124–9.

111. Thoene MK, Lyden E, Anderson-Berry A. Improving nutrition outcomes for infants < 1500 grams with a progressive, evidenced-based enteral feeding protocol. Nutr Clin Pract 2018;33(5):647–55.

112. McCallie KR, Lee HC, Mayer O, et al. Improved outcomes with a standardized feeding protocol for very low birth weight infants. J Perinatol 2011;31(Suppl 1): S61–7.

113. McCain GC, Del Moral T, Duncan RC, et al. Transition from gavage to nipple feeding for preterm infants with bronchopulmonary dysplasia. Nurs Res 2012; 61(6):380–7.

114. Hanin M, Nuthakki S, Malkar MB, et al. Safety and efficacy of oral feeding in infants with BPD on nasal CPAP. Dysphagia 2015;30(2):121–7.

115. Browne JV, Ross ES. Eating as a neurodevelopmental process for high-risk newborns. Clin Perinatol 2011;38(4):731–43.

116. Pickler RH, McGrath JM, Reyna BA, et al. Effects of the neonatal intensive care unit environment on preterm infant oral feeding. Res Rep Neonatal 2013; 2013(3):15–20.

117. Howe TH, Sheu CF, Holzman IR. Bottle-feeding behaviors in preterm infants with and without bronchopulmonary dysplasia. Am J Occup Ther 2007;61(4): 378–83.

118. Pickler RH. Understanding, promoting, and measuring the effects of mother-infant attachment during infant feeding. J ObstetGynecolNeonatal Nurs 2009; 38(4):468–9.

119. Canning A, Fairhurst R, Chauhan M, et al. Oral feeding for infants and children receiving nasal continuous positive airway pressure and high-flow nasal cannula respiratory supports: a survey of practice. Dysphagia 2019. [Epub ahead of print].

120. Chang SY, Sevransky J, Martin GS. Protocols in the management of critical illness. Crit Care 2012;16(2):306.

121. Fessler HE, Brower RG. Protocols for lung protective ventilation. Crit Care Med 2005;33(3 Suppl):S223–7.

122. Morris AH. Treatment algorithms and protocolized care. Curr Opin Crit Care 2003;9(3):236–40.

123. Dalgleish SR, Kostecky LL, Blachly N. Eating in "SINC": safe individualized nipple-feeding competence, a quality improvement project to explore infant-driven oral feeding for very premature infants requiring noninvasive respiratory support. Neonatal Network 2016;35(4):217–27.

124. Davidson E, Hinton D, Ryan-Wenger N, et al. Quality improvement study of effectiveness of cue-based feeding in infants with bronchopulmonary dysplasia in the neonatal intensive care unit. J Obstet Gynecol Neonatal Nurs 2013;42(6): 629–40.

125. Jadcherla SR, Bhandari V. "Pressure" to feed the preterm newborn: associated with "positive" outcomes? Pediatr Res 2017;82(6):899–900.

126. Manley BJ, Owen LS. High-flow nasal cannula: mechanisms, evidence and recommendations. Semin Fetal Neonatal Med 2016;21(3):139–45.

127. Manley BJ, Roberts CT, Froisland DH, et al. Refining the use of nasal high-flow therapy as primary respiratory support for preterm infants. J Pediatr 2018;196: 65–70.e1.

128. Wilkinson D, Andersen C, O'Donnell CP, et al. High flow nasal cannula for respiratory support in preterm infants. Cochrane Database Syst Rev 2016;(2):CD006405.

129. Ferrara L, Bidiwala A, Sher I, et al. Effect of nasal continuous positive airway pressure on the pharyngeal swallow in neonates. J Perinatol 2017;37(4): 398–403.

130. Slain KN, Martinez-Schlurmann N, Shein SL, et al. Nutrition and high-flow nasal cannula respiratory support in children with bronchiolitis. Hosp Pediatr 2017; 7(5):256–62.

131. Zhang X, Zhou M, Yin H, et al. The predictive value of early oral motor assessments for neurodevelopmental outcomes of moderately and late preterm infants. Medicine 2017;96(50):e9207.

132. Cuevas KD, Silver DR, Brooten D, et al. The cost of prematurity: hospital charges at birth and frequency of rehospitalizations and acute care visits over the first year of life: a comparison by gestational age and birth weight. Am J Nurs 2005;105(7):56–64 [quiz: 65].

133. McCormick MC, Litt JS, Smith VC, et al. Prematurity: an overview and public health implications. Annu Rev Public Health 2011;32:367–79.
134. Ramachandrappa A, Jain L. Health issues of the late preterm infant. Pediatr Clin North Am 2009;56(3):565–77. Table of Contents.
135. Lim G, Tracey J, Boom N, et al. CIHI survey: hospital costs for preterm and small-for-gestational age babies in Canada. Healthc Q 2009;12(4):20–4.
136. Bernier A, Catelin C, Ahmed MA, et al. Effects of nasal continuous positive-airway pressure on nutritive swallowing in lambs. J Appl Physiol (1985) 2012; 112(12):1984–91.
137. Djeddi D, Cantin D, Samson N, et al. Nasal continuous positive airway pressure inhibits gastroesophageal reflux in newborn lambs. PLoS One 2014;9(9): e107736.
138. Djeddi D, Cantin D, Samson N, et al. Absence of effect of nasal continuous positive airway pressure on the esophageal phase of nutritive swallowing in newborn lambs. J Pediatr Gastroenterol Nutr 2013;57(2):188–91.
139. Samson N, Michaud A, Othman R, et al. Nasal continuous positive airway pressure influences bottle-feeding in preterm lambs. Pediatr Res 2017;82(6):926–33.
140. Samson N, Nadeau C, Vincent L, et al. Effects of nasal continuous positive airway pressure and high-flow nasal cannula on sucking, swallowing, and breathing during bottle-feeding in lambs. Front Pediatr 2017;5:296.
141. Rustam LB, Masri S, Atallah N, et al. Sensorimotor therapy and time to full oral feeding in <33weeks infants. Early Hum Dev 2016;99:1–5.
142. Lessen BS. Effect of the premature infant oral motor intervention on feeding progression and length of stay in preterm infants. Adv Neonatal Care 2011;11(2): 129–39.
143. Jadcherla SR. Advances with neonatal aerodigestive science in the pursuit of safe swallowing in infants: invited review. Dysphagia 2017;32(1):15–26.
144. Barlow SM, Burch M, Venkatesan L, et al. Frequency modulation and spatiotemporal stability of the sCPG in preterm infants with RDS. Int J Pediatr 2012;2012: 581538.

Congenital Diarrheal Diseases

Mira Younis, MD[a,b], Radhika Rastogi, MD, MPH[b], Ankur Chugh, MD[c],
Shantanu Rastogi, MD, MMM[d,1], Hany Aly, MD, MSHS[a,b,*,1]

KEYWORDS

- Congenital • Diarrhea • Enzyme deficiency • Parenteral nutrition
- Intestinal transplant • Stem cell transplant

KEY POINTS

- Congenital diarrheal diseases are rare; therefore, caregivers should first rule out the more common acquired causes for diarrhea.
- Indicators in history, examination, and simple stool tests may suggest the presence of congenital diarrheal diseases.
- A final diagnosis of congenital diarrheal diseases is made by intestinal biopsy and molecular genetic studies to detect specific mutations.
- Management of congenital diarrheal diseases could be as simple as avoidance of certain nutrients or as complex as life-long parenteral nutrition.
- Newer research conducted on organoids could be promising for better diagnosis of congenital diarrheal diseases. New treatments may include intestinal, liver, and stem cell transplantation.

INTRODUCTION

Diarrhea, especially in neonates, is a major cause for neonatal mortality worldwide. Each year, almost one-half of a million deaths are attributed to diarrhea. The case fatality rate of neonatal diarrhea may reach 100% in certain areas of the world.[1,2] This high mortality is related to immaturity of the immune system and inability to finely regulate body electrolytes.[3] Early diagnosis is critical to prevent progression of the disease that would otherwise lead to poor outcomes. Therefore, there is a need to better understand neonatal diarrhea. Indeed, the knowledge of diarrhea is mostly gained from

[a] Department of Neonatology, Cleveland Clinic Children's, 9500 Euclid Avenue, M31-37, Cleveland, OH 44195, USA; [b] Cleveland Clinic Lerner's College of Medicine, EC-10 Cleveland Clinic, 9501 Euclid Ave, Cleveland, OH 44195, USA; [c] Pediatric Gastroenterology, Medical College of Wisconsin, 9000 W. Wisconsin Av, 6th Floor Clinics, Suite 610, Milwaukee, WI 53226, USA; [d] Newborn Services, George Washington University Hospital, Children's National Medical Center, 900 23rd Street, NW G2092, Washington, DC 20037, USA
[1] Both authors are senior authors.
* Corresponding author. 9500 Euclid Avenue, M31-37, Cleveland, OH 44195.
E-mail address: alyh@ccf.org

Clin Perinatol 47 (2020) 301–321
https://doi.org/10.1016/j.clp.2020.02.007
0095-5108/20/© 2020 Elsevier Inc. All rights reserved.
perinatology.theclinics.com

the lower income countries and may not be applicable to the disease observed in the high-income countries.[1]

Multiple case reports described prolonged and retracted diarrhea in high-income countries; however, regional and national reports are lacking. A countrywide study from Italy reported the incidence of diarrhea in the newborn to be around 6.72 in 1000 hospitalized infants.[4] The study could not provide accurate estimates for the incidence of diarrhea in neonatal intensive care units as less than 50% of neonatal intensive care units participated in the data collection. However, the study was helpful in providing significant insights into the nature of diarrhea among neonatal intensive care unit population in a high-income country. Of the neonates presenting with diarrhea, only 75% had defined etiologies with more than 50% requiring parenteral rehydration; the mortality rate was 8%. There was a wide variety of etiologies; allergy and infections were responsible for about 40% of the cases.

DEFINITIONS

Diarrhea is defined by the World Health Organization as 3 or more loose or liquid stools per day or an increase in frequency. It does not include the passage of loose, pasty stools by breastfed babies.[2] However, the lack of details or variability in clinical information can result in variable definitions; thus, a recent definition has classified diarrhea in neonates as stool volume of more than 20 mL/kg/d.[5] Any deviation from the routine stool pattern, increased stool volume, and associated clinical evidence of dehydration and electrolyte abnormalities remain clinically useful in making the diagnosis of diarrhea.

Chronic Diarrhea

Chronic diarrhea is defined as presence of diarrhea for more than 14 days. Persistent diarrhea is also defined as diarrhea for 14 days, but usually results from enteric dysfunction related to infection.[2,6] The World Health Organization defines diarrhea that continues for more than 14 days as persistent, the majority of which across the world is caused by viral and bacterial infections. Previously, the terms intractable or protracted diarrhea were used for prolonged diarrheal duration, but they are not used as definitions any longer, because their use was highly variable.[7,8]

Osmotic Diarrhea

Osmotic diarrhea is used to describe unabsorbed or partially absorbed nutrients exerting osmotic pressure, increasing the intraluminal solute load and causing diarrhea. More recently, osmotic diarrhea caused by a particular nutrient intake is referred to as diet-induced diarrhea.[5] The characteristics of this type of diarrhea is an elevated osmotic gap of more than 100 mOsm. It is calculated as $290 - 2 \times$ (stool Na^+ + stool K^+). It is reflective of the role of nutrients in providing the osmolality as diarrhea usually has the same osmolality of the serum. The malabsorption of carbohydrate and fat are common causes of osmotic diarrhea and can be tested as follows.

1. Carbohydrate malabsorption is a typical finding in osmotic diarrhea. When reducing substances in the stool is greater than 0.5%, it usually indicates malabsorption of monosaccharides that get fermented in the large intestine and form short chain fatty acids, which decrease the pH of the stool to less than 5.3.
2. Fat malabsorption occurs when fat loss in stool exceeds 15% to 20%, which is the usual percentage of the fat lost in the stool among normal neonates. A spot test for fecal fat provides the clue for further workup, such as quantitative fecal fat estimation and typing of the fat. If neutral fats are increased, pancreatic insufficiency is

more likely, whereas if split fats are increased, intestinal fat malabsorption is more likely.

Secretory Diarrhea

Secretory diarrhea is used to describe diarrhea that is caused by active ion secretion into the intestinal lumen of the intestine. It does not differentiate between the diarrheas associated with high salt wasting and does not encompass all low osmotic diarrheas of less than 50 mOsm. Hence, some authors have referred to it as electrolyte transport-related diarrhea.[5] The characteristics of this type of diarrhea are low osmotic load of less than 50 mOsm, or high α-1 antitrypsin concentrations in the stool. This protein is resistant to proteases and hence when increased, it reflects the condition of increased secretion such as protein losing enteropathy. Low elastase concentrations in the stool is another possible characteristic of this type of diarrhea. Dietary elastase is not usually digested and becomes diluted in increased secretory states.

Diarrhea in newborns can be stratified into 2 major categories: acquired diarrhea and congenital diarrhea.

ACQUIRED DIARRHEA

Most of the causes of diarrhea during the neonatal period belong to this category. Allergies and infections cause the majority of diarrheal diseases in which the etiology was identified.[4] The timing of diarrhea gives a clue to the cause: those occurring soon after birth, or within a few weeks of birth, could be related to congenital anomalies, necrotizing enterocolitis (especially in preterm neonates), or congenital diarrheal diseases (CDDs). However, those occurring later during infancy, which are usually milder in presentations, are related to infections and allergies both to cow's milk protein or other food proteins. These diseases are described in detail elsewhere.[9–12]

The focus of this review is on CDD, which are also known as congenital diarrhea and enteropathies.

CONGENITAL DIARRHEAL DISEASE
Introduction and Nature of Problem

This group of diseases is also known as congenital diarrhea and enteropathies. This group of diseases until recently were described anecdotally in isolated case reports with confusions in their classification. It was not clear whether CDD referred to multiple disease processes that led to a common clinical presentation or to a single disease that might have varied presentations. More recently, with the rapid advancement in genetic diagnostics, there is a better understanding of these diseases with respect to their presentations and pathophysiology. The majority of CDD present with a single gene involvement, consequently they are reported as "monogenic diarrhea." In some CDD, epithelial cells of the intestine are affected and in others the immune system is affected, making the neonate susceptible to infections.

The clinical presentation of CDD may vary. It can present antenatally with dilated intestinal loops in ultrasound studies and with polyhydroamnios.[13] An important differentiation for acquired diarrhea is the onset of the disease very soon after birth. Because many cases of CDD are related to a single gene defect, its incidence is particularly increased in societies wherein consanguineous marriages are common and in some specific geographic areas related to the founder effect of the gene. The founder effect is exemplified in congenital chloride diarrhea that is mainly diagnosed in Finland, Saudi Arabia, Kuwait, and Poland, whereas it is very sporadic elsewhere.[14] Other examples are the diagnosis of lactase deficiency in Finland,[13] maltase-isomaltase deficiency in Greenland and Canada,[15] and lysinuric protein intolerance in Finland and Japan.[16]

Normal Intestinal Epithelial Function

Because the classification of CDD is based on alterations of certain functions, it is important to review the normal function of the intestinal lining and the epithelial cells.[17] Healthy enterocytes line the mucosa and originate from stem cells in the crypts of Lieberkühn. It takes 3 to 4 days for these cells to migrate from the crypts to the tip of the villus. They are arranged as a polarized monolayer and have a basal side facing the basement membrane and the tissues. Enterocytes are supported by an actin filament meshwork that protrudes to form the brush border. This brush border or microvillus increases the absorptive surface area and increase the epithelial and microbial interactions. The plasma membrane of the brush border has enzymes and transporter proteins that are involved with the metabolism, absorption, and secretion of nutrients, metabolites, and electrolytes to and from the gut lumen, cell interior, and body tissue. The polarization of these enzymes and proteins is important because it facilitates intracellular sorting and trafficking via the Golgi apparatus and endosomes.[18] Tight junctions between the apical domain of the lateral surfaces of the enterocytes provide tight intracellular adhesion, which limits protein diffusion and controls electrolyte transport. Junctions in the lateral domain mediate cell to cell adhesion strength.[19] The presence of both the intercellular adhesions and the polarity of the proteins on cell surface and interior of the enterocyte form a selectively permeable barrier (**Fig. 1**).

Depending on which area of epithelial cell function is affected, Canani and Terrin[20] proposed a classification that has been used with slight modification by others[5]; both have described the groups in detail. There are 4 major groups of disorders: (1) defects in digestion, absorption, and transport of nutrients and electrolytes; (2) disorders of enterocyte differentiation and polarization; (3) defects of enteroendocrine cell differentiation; and (4) dysregulation of the intestinal immune response. Most recently a new group has been added: (5) dysfunction of the immune system, which results in a wide spectrum of both intestinal and extraintestinal manifestations.

A. Defects of digestion, absorption, and transport of nutrients and electrolytes
   Alterations of the epithelial transport proteins represent some of the better known CDD or congenital diarrhea and enteropathies (see **Fig. 1**; **Table 1**).
   1. *Disorders of brush border membranes* usually present as osmotic diarrhea with low pH.
      a. Congenital lactase deficiency: an autosomal recessive (AR) disease with a high incidence in Finland. The lactase (*LCT*) gene is affected, leading to decreased mucosal *lactase-phlorizin hydrolase* enzyme.[21] Neonates develop severe, watery, and osmotic diarrhea soon after starting breast milk or formula feeds, resulting in dehydration. Some may have associated hypercalcinosis and nephrolithiasis. Stringent lactose-free diet rapidly improves the symptoms. Diagnosis is made by duodenal biopsy and measuring lactase enzyme activity or mutation analysis of the *LCT* gene.
      b. Congenital sucrose-isomaltase deficiency is an AR disease with 1:5000 incidence in the European population. *Sucrase-isomaltase* (*SI*) gene loss lead to absence of SI enzyme and inability to digest sucrose and other carbohydrates leading to osmotic diarrhea.[22] Congenital sucrose-isomaltase deficiency presents when sucrose and starch are started during weaning in infants and, in many infants, it remains a mild disease. Strict fructose-reduced diet cures the disease and the use of oral replacement therapy

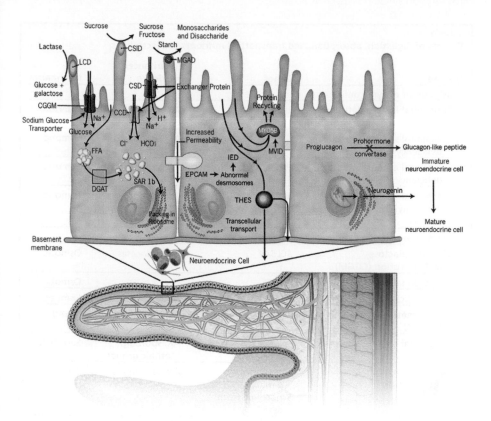

Fig. 1. Normal enterocyte function. (1) Defects in digestion, absorption, and transport of nutrients and electrolytes. CCD, congenital chloride diarrhea; CGGM, congenital glucose -galactose malabsorption; CSD, congenital sodium diarrhea; CSID, congenital sucrose isomaltase deficiency; DGAT, diacyl glycerol transferase; FFA, free fatty acid; LCT, lactase deficiency; MGAD, congenital maltase-glucoamylase deficiency; *SAR1B, SAR1* gene homolog B protein deficiency. (2) Disorders of enterocyte differentiation and polarization. EPCAM, epithelial cell adhesion molecule abnormality; IED, intestinal epithelial dysplasia or tufting enteropathy; MVID, microvillus inclusion disease; MYO5B, myosin type B motor protein B deficiency; THES, trichohepatoenteric syndrome. (3) Defects of enteroendocrine cell differentiation. *NEUROG3*, neurogenin 3 gene mutation; X, prohormone convertase 1/3 deficiency; Y, inflammatory cell/autoimmune cell-related enteropathies.

by yeast-derived sucrose enzyme can be helpful. Diagnosis is confirmed by biopsy demonstrating reduced enzyme activity for sucrase, maltase, and isomaltase, with normal lactase activity. The use of H_2 during sucrose breath test and SI gene mutation detection also helps in the diagnosis.[22]

c. Congenital maltase-glucoamylase deficiency: Causal mutations in the *MGAD* gene have not been described.[23] This enzyme is helpful for final digestion of starch. Maltase-glucoamylase deficiency is treated by elimination diet. Diagnosis is suggested by the presence of glucose in the stool, insufficient increase of glucose after starch diet, and C^{13} starch and starch oligomer breath test.[24]

Table 1
Defects of digestion, absorption, and transport of nutrients or electrolytes

Disease	Genes	Inheritance/ Incidence	Mechanism
Brush border enzyme deficiencies			
Congenital lactase deficiency (CLD)	*LCT*	AR, 1:60.000 in Finland	Osmotic
Congenital sucrase-isomaltase-deficiency (SID)	*SI*	AR, Greenland, Alaska, Canada	Osmotic
Congenital enteropeptidase deficiency (CEP)	*Proenteropeptidase*	AR, very rare	Osmotic
Congenital maltase-glucoamylase-deficiency (CMGD)	*MGAM*	very rare	Osmotic
Defects of membrane carriers			
Glucose-galactose-malabsorption (CGGM)	*SCL5A1*	AR, few cases	Osmotic
Fructose-malabsorption (FM)	*GLUT5*		Osmotic
Fanconi Bickel syndrome (FBS)	*GLUT2*	AR	Osmotic
Acrodermatitis enteropathica (AE)	*SLC39A4*	AR, 1:500.000	Mixed
Congenital chloride diarrhea (CCD, DIAR1)	*SLC26A3*	AR, sporadic/ ethnic groups	Secretory
Congenital sodium diarrhea (CSD, DIAR3)	Classic forms: GUCY2C, SLC9A3 Syndromic form: SPINT2	AR, very rare	Secretory
Lysinuric protein intolerance (LPI)	*SLC7A7*	AR, 1:60.000 in Finland, few worldwide	Osmotic
Primary biliary malabsorption (PBAM)	*SLC10A2*	AR	Secretory
Cystic fibrosis (CF)	*CFTR*	AR, 1:2500	Osmotic
Pancreatic enzyme deficiencies			
Hereditary pancreatitis (HP)	*PRSS1, SPINK1 CFTR, PRSS1,* PRSS2	AD	Osmotic
Congenital pancreas lipase deficiency (PNLIP)	*PNLIP*		Osmotic
Defects in lipid/lipoprotein metabolism			
Chylomicron retention disease (CRD)	*SAR1B*	AR, very rare	Osmotic
Hypobetalipoproteinemia (HLP)	*APOB*	autosomal co-dominant	Osmotic
Abetalipoproteinemia (ALP)	*MTP*	AR, 100 cases, frequent in Ashkenazi	Osmotic
Defective ribosomal proteins			
Shwachman Diamond syndrome (SDS)	*SBDS*	AR, 1:10.000–200.000	Osmotic

(continued on next page)

Table 1 (continued)			
Disease	Genes	Inheritance/ Incidence	Mechanism
Mitochondrial DNA deficiencies			
Pearson syndrome	Mitochondrial DNA deletions		Osmotic

Abbreviation: AD, autosomal dominant.

Adapted from Posovszky C. Congenital intestinal diarrheal diseases: A diagnostic and therapeutic challenge. *Best Pract Res Clin Gastroenterol*. 2016;30(2):187-211. https://doi.org/10.1016/j.bpg.2016.03.004

    d. Congenital enterokinase/enteropeptidase deficiency is caused by a mutation of the *proenteropeptidase* gene. It leads to decreased conversion of trypsinogen to active trypsin, which in turn results in the decreased activation of pancreatic enzymes.[25] This lack leads to protein-losing osmotic diarrhea associated with anemia, hypoproteinemia, and failure to thrive.

2. *Disorders of membrane carriers* usually present as osmotic diarrhea

    a. Congenital glucose-galactose malabsorption is an AR disease with a few hundred cases described. It presents with life-threatening diarrhea and severe dehydration. Mutation of *SLC5A1* gene leads to an alteration of the sodium glucose cotransporter abnormality and insufficient absorption of glucose and galactose.[26] It responds to a glucose- and galactose-free diet. Because fructose is independently absorbed by a GLUT5 transporter, it can be added to a carbohydrate-free formula. The diagnosis is confirmed by glucose in the stool, glucose H_2 breath test, and genetic mutation in the *SLC5A1* gene.

    b. Acrodermatitis enteropathica is caused by a mutation in the *SLC39A4* gene, which encodes a zinc-specific transporter protein expressed in the duodenum and jejunum. Acrodermatitis enteropathica presents with diarrhea, alopecia, perioral and acral dermatitis, and failure to thrive. It is treated by zinc supplementation of 1 to 3 mg/kg/d that typically causes dramatic improvement in a few days.[27]

    c. Congenital chloride diarrhea is an AR disease related to mutations in *SLC26A3* (solute carrier family 26 member 3) leading to abnormal HCO^-_3 and Cl^- exchange especially in the duodenum, ileum, and colon.[14] It has an incidence of 1:3200 in the Middle East and 1:35,000 in Finland.[28] It clinically presents as intrauterine growth restriction and polyhydramnios associated with an distended abdomen. Neonates with this disease typically present with a large volume of watery diarrhea that has high a chloride content (>90 mmol/L) and associated hyponatremia, hypokalemia, hypochloremia, and metabolic alkalosis. Although there is no therapy for this disease, supplementation of chloride, sodium, and potassium prevents dehydration and electrolyte abnormalities; it also prevents the associated renal and developmental complications. In certain subtypes, butyrate decreases fecal ion and stool losses. Although chloride in the stool is diagnostic, the collection of an accurate sample is difficult. Genetic testing for *SLC26A3* mutation provides a definitive diagnosis.

    d. Congenital sodium diarrhea is a rare inherited disorder with abnormalities of *SLC9A3* and *GUCY2C*.[28] Congenital sodium diarrhea presents with large amount of watery diarrhea with associated metabolic acidosis, and hyponatremia with associated large amount of sodium loss (>90 mmol/L). Pregnancy is usually complicated with polyhydramnios and newborns may have large dilated loops of bowel that are filled with fluid and may require enterostomy.[29] Biopsy may show duodenal villous atrophy. Patients present with other anomalies, including bilateral choanal atresia and corneal erosions. Treatment consists of enteral and parenteral nutrition for correction of water and electrolyte imbalance and metabolic acidosis.

e. Lysinuric protein intolerance is an AR aminoaciduria associated with mutation of solute carrier family 7A member 7 (SCLCA7). It has an incidence of 1:60,000 in Finland.[16] It is due to a defect in the transport of lysine, arginine, and ornithine from the basolateral membrane of epithelial cells; therefore, it causes impairment of the urea cycle. Patients develop periodic vomiting and diarrhea, hepatomegaly, mild leukopenia, failure to thrive, and postprandial increase of ammonium after consuming protein-rich food. An increase in ammonia concentrations after ingestion of a protein-rich food impacts neurologic function and development.[16] The disease varies with the protein intake and lysinuric protein intolerance can be treated with low protein intake, preventing and treating hyperammonemia and substitution of citrulline, lysine, and carnitine. If this disease remains unrecognized or inadequately treated, it may be associated with alveolar proteinosis and renal diseases.

f. Primary bile acid malabsorption is an AR disease with mutation of the SCL10A2 gene.[30] Primary biliary malabsorption presents as chronic watery secretory diarrhea with steatorrhea soon after birth requiring parenteral nutrition. It is diagnosed by 24-hour stool bile salt quantification. Primary biliary malabsorption is treated by oral cholestyramine, which binds bile salts.[31]

3. Pancreatic enzyme deficiency

a. Hereditary pancreatitis an autosomal dominant disease related to mutations in cationic trypsinogen (PRSS1), which leads to activation of trypsinogen to trypsin, causing intrapancreatic proteolytic activity and chronic pancreatitis. It can also be related to a mutation in protease inhibitor gene (SPINK1), which decreases activity of SPINK1, which prevents intrapancreatic trypsinogen activation.[32,33] It is a very rare disease with an incidence of 3 per million. Hereditary pancreatitis usually presents in childhood as an acute pancreatitis-like picture followed by steatorrhea and osmotic diarrhea. The disease should be suspected based on family history and confirmed by gene analysis. It is treated by pancreatic enzyme replacement, nutritional support, pain management, and the treatment of complications like pancreatic pseudocysts and bile duct obstruction.[34]

b. Selective exocrine pancreatic failure

i. Congenital pancreatic lipase (PL) deficiency: Only a few cases of PL have been reported. PL activity is regulated by cofactor protein colipase, which helps the attachment of PL to lipid surface. This deficiency of any of these functions leads to fatty stools and osmotic diarrhea. Owing to alternative digestion pathways, failure to thrive is rarely observed. Treatment consists of enzyme replacement.

ii. Defects in lipid and lipoprotein transport and metabolism: Familial hypercholesteremia is a rare AR disease that presents as deficiency of fat-soluble vitamins, failure to thrive, and abnormal serum lipid profile.

4. Defects in lipid and lipoprotein deficiency
   a. Chylomicron retention disease: It is an AR disease related to intracellular trafficking of chylomicron owing to *SAR1B* mutation.[17] Patients present with severe lipid malabsorption, failure to thrive, and diarrhea. Infants with this disease have normal triglyceride levels but low cholesterol, low-density lipoprotein cholesterol, high-density lipoprotein cholesterol, and apolipoproteins along with fat-soluble vitamin deficiency (especially vitamin E) and fatty liver disease.[35] Infants improve with a diet low in long chain fatty acids that is enriched in essential fatty acids and medium chain triglycerides with vitamin E supplementation to prevent neurologic and ophthalmic complications related to its deficiency.
5. Defects in ribosomal proteins
   a. Schwachman-Diamond syndrome is an AR disease with an incidence of about 1:75,000. The mutations alter ribosomal proteins and is associated with bone marrow failure, skeletal abnormalities, and pancreatic exocrine dysfunction. Patients present with variable osmotic diarrhea and fatty stools leading to fat-soluble vitamin deficiency. It can be diagnosed by fecal fat analysis and treated with pancreatic enzyme replacement and fat-soluble vitamin replacement.[36]
6. Defects of mitochondrial DNA
   a. Pearson's syndrome is caused by deletions of mitochondrial DNA and therefore, affects all systems.[37] Specifically, patients have affected bone marrow and exocrine pancreas, presenting as steatorrhea and sideroblastic anemia. Affected respiratory chain complexes cause metabolic and lactic acidosis. Diagnosis is confirmed by molecular analysis and the disease is often fatal in infancy.

B. Defects of enterocyte differentiation or polarization
   These defects manifest early after birth and long-term parenteral nutrition and eventual bowel transplant may be required. They could be isolated or within a group of syndromes such as hemophagocytic lymphohistiocytosis and trihepaticenteric syndrome (see **Fig. 1**; **Table 2**).
   1. Microvillous atrophy or microvillous inclusion disease is an AR disease owing to defective polarization of enterocytes, resulting in abnormal intracellular protein transport. Different mutations have been described, but *MYO5B* is the most common.[17] It is a rare disease with inherited life-threatening diarrheal disease, usually early after birth, occasionally presenting in a few weeks in the late-onset variety. Biopsy shows periodic acid-Schiff–positive granules with atrophic bands of the apical pole. Electron microscopy of epithelial cells, including those from rectal biopsies, show atrophy of microvilli along with accumulation of granules containing typical inclusion bodies.[38] It is associated with poor long-term outcome. Complications associated with prolonged parenteral nutrition and central line access are high. Early intestinal transplant provides a chance for long-term survival.
   2. Intestinal epithelial dysplasia or tufting enteropathy is caused by an *EPCAM* mutation and associated loss of membrane glycoprotein *EPCAM*.[39] This process results in desmosome alteration associated with increased expression of protein desmoglein. The incidence is about 1:50,000 to 1:100,000 in Western Europe, with a higher incidence in the Middle East. Biopsy shows partial villous atrophy with crypt hyperplasia along with disorganized enterocyte that crowd at the villous tips resembling tufts. Patients usually present with severe life-threatening diarrhea nonresponsive to alteration of enteral feeds and

Table 2
Defects of enterocyte differentiation or polarization

Disease	Genes	Inheritance and Incidence	Mechanism
Microvillous atrophy (MVID, DIAR2)	MYO5B	AR, very rare, frequent in Navajo	Mixed
	STX3	AR, very rare	
Variant MVID			
Intestinal epithelial dysplasia (IED, DIAR5)/Tufting enteropathy	EPCAM, SPINK2	AR, frequent in Arabia	Secretory
Trichohepatoenteric syndrome (THES)		AR, 1:400.000	Secretory
THES-1	TTC37		
THES-2	SKIV2L		
Defect of cellular polarization			
Familiar hemophagocytic lymphohistiocytosis type 5 (FHL 5)	STXBP2 (Munc18–2)	AR, very rare	Osmotic

Adapted from Posovszky C. Congenital intestinal diarrheal diseases: A diagnostic and therapeutic challenge. *Best Pract Res Clin Gastroenterol.* 2016;30(2):187-211. https://doi.org/10.1016/j.bpg.2016.03.004

parenteral nutrition. Some patients may present with milder disease where long-term parenteral nutrition and intestinal transplant are required.
3. Trichohepatoenteric syndrome is an AR disease associated with mutation in the *THES37* gene. Loss of this gene leads to defective trafficking and decreased expression of the apical transport protein.[40] Incidence is about 1:500,000. Neonates usually show intrauterine growth restriction with abnormal facial features, including a prominent forehead, flat nasal bridge, and wooly fragile hair. Many patients present with secretory diarrhea a few weeks after birth and failure to thrive. One-half of the patients have chronic liver disease, hypogammaglobinemia, and a poor response to the vaccines. There are no specific histologic findings and the diagnosis is made with mutation in *THES37* gene. Treatment consists of life-long parenteral nutrition and immunoglobin supplementation. Combined intestinal and liver transplant may be considered if parenteral nutrition is complicated by liver failure.[40]

C. Defects of neuroendocrine cells

The gut is one of the largest hormone-producing organs in the body and produces hormones that regulate food intake, glucose homeostasis, and efficient nutrient digestion and absorption. The absence of neuroendocrine cells are associated with this subtype of congenital diarrhea (see **Fig. 1; Table 3**).

1. Congenital malabsorption diarrhea or enteric anendocrinosis is a very rare AR disorder owing to defective enteroendocrine cell differentiation. Mutation of the *neurogenin 3* gene leads to the arrest of maturation of neuroendocrine cells.[41] Biopsy shows normal anatomy with an absence of neuroendocrine cells. Patients present with severe malabsorption diarrhea without dehydration because water absorption is preserved and presents as neonatal diabetes. It is treated with long-term enteral nutrition with partial enteral feeding.
2. Proprotein convertase 1/3 deficiency is a very rare AR disease where there is a defect in the L cells of the enteroendocrine system. L cells produce

Table 3
Defects of enteroendocrine cells

Disease	Genes	Inheritance/Incidence	Mechanism
Congenital malabsorptive diarrhea, anendocrinosis (CMD, DIAR4)	NEUROG3	AR, very rare	Osmotic
Protein-convertase 1/3 deficiency	PCSK1	AR	Osmotic

Adapted from Posovszky C. Congenital intestinal diarrheal diseases: A diagnostic and therapeutic challenge. *Best Pract Res Clin Gastroenterol.* 2016;30(2):187-211. https://doi.org/10.1016/j.bpg.2016.03.004

proprotein convertase 1/3, which converts proglucagon to glucagon-like peptides 1 and 2. Proprotein convertase 1/3 is found in the hypothalamus and pancreas, and its deficiency leads to the patient presenting with obesity, diabetes associated with severe malabsorption, and osmotic diarrhea with dehydration and metabolic acidosis. There is a general malabsorption of most elemental nutrients, such as amino acids and monosaccharides. Despite initial poor growth there is a significant increase in weight and patients become obese. Intestinal biopsy demonstrates morphologic changes with focally increased intraepithelial lymphocytes, shortened villi, edema, irregularity, and vacuolization of the mucosal intestinal epithelium.[42] Generalized malabsorption increases the risk of mortality within the first 2 years of life, similar to congenital malabsorptive diarrhea, and requires parenteral nutrition.

D. Defects of immune system affecting the intestine

Many immunodeficiency disorders present with chronic diarrhea, malabsorption, and inflammatory bowel disease; the gut is the largest lymphoid organ. Primary immunodeficiency affects the gut by autoimmune, infectious, and inflammatory reactions.[43] Physicians should have a high index of suspicion for an immune system disorder based on history of serious and atypical infections; the diagnosis can be confirmed by immunologic and genetic investigations. Treatment is difficult because the diseases are systemic; however, immunoglobulin replacement, antibiotics, immunomodulation, and stem cell transplantation are used to improve the patient's condition or for complete cure for certain diseases. There are myriad groups of immunologic disorder and they are summarized in **Table 4**.

The approach to diagnose a case with neonatal diarrhea is illustrated in **Fig. 2** that includes 4 algorithms.[5,17,20,44] The first algorithm presents the key points to identify whether the diarrhea is congenital or acquired and whether it is osmotic or secretory diarrhea (see **Fig. 2**A). The second algorithm (see **Fig. 2**B) elaborates on the differential diagnosis of secretory diarrhea, and **Fig. 2**C provides the diagnostics of isolated osmotic diarrhea and osmotic diarrhea with other organ systems involved.

CHALLENGES AND FUTURE IMPLICATIONS

The challenges related to better understanding, diagnosis, and management of CDD hinge on expeditious suspicion of CDD. The development of newer models can help to better understand disease mechanism and interventions. The improvement of management options is contingent on knowledge of pathophysiology, as many are monogenic diseases and cannot be addressed by modification of enteral intake or nutrient supplementation.

Table 4
Defects of the immune system affecting the intestine

Disease	Genes	Inheritance/Incidence	Mechanism
Defects of tolerance induction/regulatory T cells			
Autoimmune candidiasis polyendocrinopathy ectodermal dystrophy (APECED)/APS1	AIRE	AR (AD in 1 family), frequent in Finland	Osmotic
Immunodysfunction, polyendocrinopathy, enteropathy, X-linked (IPEX)	FOXP3	X-linked (autosomal)	Mixed, inflammatory
		Very rare	
IPEX-like syndrome		Very rare	Secretory, autoimmune, infectious
CD25 deficiency	CD25	AR	
STAT5b deficiency	STAT5b	AR	
STAT1 gain of function	STAT1	AD	
ITCH deficiency	ITCH	AR	
Immune regulation defects			
Early-onset IBD (IBD28)	IL10RA	AR, very rare	Secretory, inflammatory
IL10R1 deficiency			
Early-onset IBD (IBD25)	IL10RB	AR, very rare	Secretory, inflammatory
IL10R2 deficiency			
IL10 deficiency	IL10	AR, very rare	Inflammatory
Defect in epithelial barrier and response			
X-linked hypohidrotic ectodermal dysplasia with immunodeficiency	IKBKG(NEMO)	X-linked recessive, very rare	Secretory, inflammatory
TTC7A deficiency	TTC7A,	AR, very rare	Mixed
ADAM17 deficiency	ADAM17	AR, very rare	Osmotic
Kindler syndrome	KIND1	AR	Inflammatory

Dysfunction of neutrophil granulocytes, phagocytes and neutropenia

Chronic granulomatous disease (CGD)			1:250,000, rare	Secretory
X-linked, p91phox	CYBB	AR		Inflammatory CD-like
AR cytochrome b negative	CYBA	AR		
AR cytochrome b positive type I	NCF1	AR		
AR cytochrome b positive type II	NCF2	AR		
AR cytochrome b positive type III	NCF4	AR		
Leukocyte adhesion deficiency (LAD1)	ITGB2	AR		
Glycogen storage disease I b (GSD1b)	SLC37A4	AR		Inflammatory
Severe congenital neutropenia	G6PC3	AR		Inflammatory
Combined T-cell, B-cell, and antibody defects				
SCID	RAG1/2, JAK3, PTPRC, CD3D/E/Z chain, ZAP79, CORO IA, DCLREI C, LIG 4, NHEJI, IL-2RG, IL-7RA, ADA, PNP, AK2		1:100.000	
Wiskott-Aldrich syndrome (WAS)	WASP	X-linked recessive		Mixed
B-cell and antibody defects				
Selective IgA deficiency (IGAD)				Secretory, inflammatory
IGAD 1	Chr.6p21	AR, IC, AD		
IGAD 2	TNFRSF13 B			
Agammaglobulinemia				Secretory, inflammatory IBD-like
X-linked (XLA)	BTK, XLR			
AR (AGM1-6)	M Heavy chain, I5, IgA, IgB, BLNK			
Hyper-IgM syndrome				Secretory, inflammatory IBD-like
HIGM1	CD40 L	XLR		
HIGM2	AICDA	AR		

(continued on next page)

Table 4
(continued)

Disease	Genes	Inheritance/Incidence	Mechanism
HIGM3	*CD40*	AR	
HIGM5	*UNG*	AR1:25.000–50.000	Secretory, inflammatory, IBD/celiac-like
CVID			
CVID type 1	*ICOS*	AR	
CVID type 2	*TNFRSF13 B*	AR, AD	
CVID type 3	*CD19*	AR	
CVID type 4	*BAFFR*	AR	
CVID type 5	*CD20*	AR	
CVID type 6	*CD81*	AR	
CVID type 7	*CD21*	AR	
CVID type 8	*LRBA*	AR	
Hyper- and auto-inflammatory defects			
Mevalonate kinase deficiency (MKD)	*MVK*	AR	
Hyper-IgD syndrome (HIGD)			
Mevalonate aciduria (MEVA)			
Familial Mediterranean fever (FMF)	*MEFV*	AR	Inflammatory
X-linked lymphoproliferative syndrome type 2 (XLP-2)	*XIAP*	X-linked	Inflammatory
Hermanskye Pudlak syndrome (HPS)			
HPS-1	*HPS-1*	AR	
HPS-2	*HPS-2*	AR	
HPS-6	*HPS-6*		

Abbreviations: AD, autosomal dominant; AR, autosomal recessive; IBD, inflammatory bowel disease; IC, isolated cases.
Adapted from Posovszky C. Congenital intestinal diarrhoeal diseases: A diagnostic and therapeutic challenge. Best Pract Res Clin Gastroenterol. 2016;30(2):187-211. https://doi.org/10.1016/j.bpg.2016.03.004

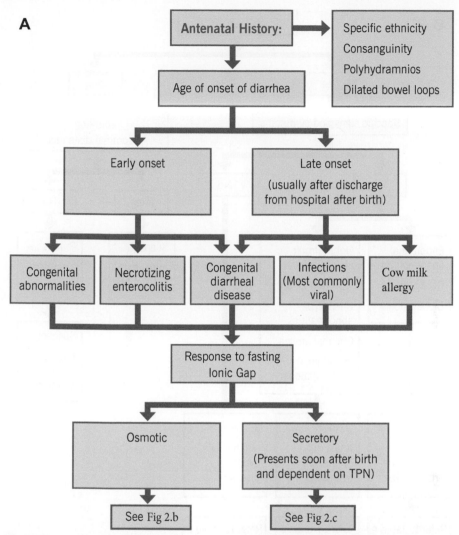

Fig. 2. Diagnostic approach to infants with diarrhea. (*A*) Key points to identify whether the diarrhea is congenital or acquired and whether it is osmotic or secretory diarrhea. (*B*) The differential diagnosis of secretory diarrhea. (*C*) Diagnostics of osmotic diarrhea. IPEX, immunodysfunction, polyendocrinopathy, enteropathy, X-linked; TPN, total parenteral nutrition.

A high index of suspicion based on a high-risk history and simple stool tests should guide the clinician toward these possible diagnoses, which can be confirmed based on intestinal epithelial biopsy and molecular genetic diagnostic testing.

Many models, including single cell culture, have been developed to further understand disease mechanisms and methods to change the effects of abnormal protein function. Creation of patient-specific disease models can be achieved using the organoid technique from the intestinal stem cells, which produces 3-dimensional cultures from stem cells derived from intestinal cells resembling intestinal tissue close to an in vivo model. Although some of these models recapitulate the phenotype well, the

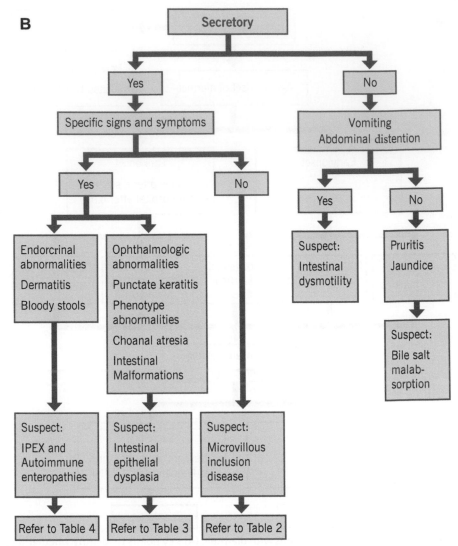

Fig. 2. (*continued*).

confounding effects of environment, diet, and treatment are challenging to replicate. Organoids provide the opportunity to use gene editing tools such as CRISPR to study genotype–phenotype correlations.[17]

Early and consistent removal of specific nutrients in patients whose disease responds to such management can result in treatment of the disease, resulting in improved outcomes and a potentially normal life. For those CDD that are associated with dependence on parenteral nutrition, patients need to be monitored for deterioration of liver function and repeated central line infections, both of which are associated with high morbidity and decreased life expectancy. Such cases are also amenable to management by intestinal and liver transplant.[45] The results of these transplants are variable, although they do increase survival of the recipients. Lifelong immunosuppression secondary to transplantation is associated with a higher risk for acute and chronic

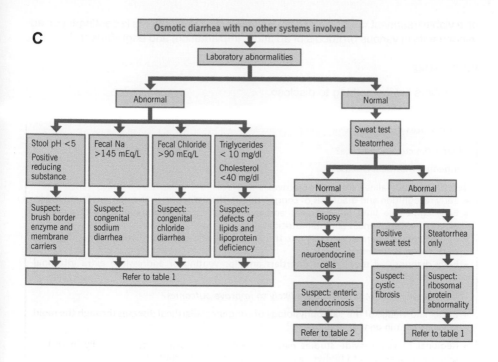

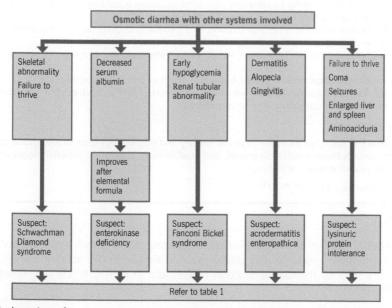

Fig. 2. (*continued*).

opportunistic infections, graft rejection and loss, and the development of secondary malignancy. Stem cell transplantation using CRISPR/Cas-9–corrected intestinal stem cells and autologous epithelial cell transplantation is being increasingly recognized as a viable treatment method for CDD. However, its use in patients is contingent on advancements in various protocols of ablation, implantation, and engraftment.[46]

DISCLOSURE

The authors having nothing to disclose.

Best Practices Box

What is the current practice?

Congenital Diarrheal Diseases

Best practice/guideline/care path objectives
- Early recognition and diagnosis of congenital diarrheal diseases in the neonatal population
- Early aggressive fluid management and nutritional support to prevent life threatening electrolyte disturbances and malnutrition
- Classification of diarrhea according to the underlying etiology and treating different groups of disorders accordingly
- Early diagnosis of multisystem disorders and (preventing or addressing) extra intestinal complications

What changes in current practice are likely to improve outcomes?

- Better knowledge of the pathophysiology of congenital diarrheal diseases through the rapid advancement in genetic diagnostics

- Regional or countrywide studies may delineate the epidemiology, especially in certain geographical areas with higher incidence of congenital diarrheal diseases.

Major Recommendations
- Classify diarrhea according to secretory and osmotic causes according to antenatal history, specific signs and symptoms, blood test and stool tests
- Perform further lab tests, intestinal biopsies and genetic testing to confirm the underlying etiology according to the clinical approach described above
- Early implementation of elimination diet to ensure improved outcomes and potentially a normal life
- Early supplementation with deficient nutrients, enzymes and immunoglobulins.
- Monitor for complications associated with parenteral nutrition and central line access. Intestinal and liver transplant may be considered

Summary statement

A high index of suspicion based on high risk history and simple stool tests should guide the clinician towards these possible diagnoses, and confirm with intestinal epithelial biopsy and molecular genetic diagnostic testing.

Data from References.[5,14,17,20,21,43–45]

REFERENCES

1. Troeger C, Blacker BF, Khalil IA, et al. Estimates of the global, regional, and national morbidity, mortality, and aetiologies of diarrhoea in 195 countries: a systematic analysis for the Global Burden of Disease Study 2016. Lancet Infect Dis 2018;18(11):1211–28.

2. World Health Organization. Diarrhoeal disease. Available at: https://www.who.int/news-room/fact-sheets/detail/diarrhoeal-disease. Accessed March 30. 2020.

3. Sherman PM, Mitchell DJ, Cutz E. Neonatal enteropathies: defining the causes of protracted diarrhea of infancy. J Pediatr Gastroenterol Nutr 2004;38(1):16–26.

4. Passariello A, Terrin G, Baldassarre ME, et al. Diarrhea in neonatal intensive care unit. World J Gastroenterol 2010;16(21):2664–8.

5. Thiagarajah JR, Kamin DS, Acra S, et al. Advances in evaluation of chronic diarrhea in infants. Gastroenterology 2018;154(8):2045–59.e6.

6. Keusch GT, Denno DM, Black RE, et al. Environmental enteric dysfunction: pathogenesis, diagnosis, and clinical consequences. Clin Infect Dis 2014;59(Suppl 4):207–12.

7. Walker-Smith JA. Intractable diarrhea of infancy. Saudi J Gastroenterol 1995;1(3):152–6.

8. Fagundes-Neto U, Wehba J, Viaro T, et al. Protracted diarrhea in infancy. J Pediatr Gastroenterol Nutr 1985;4(5):714–22.

9. Morris G, Kennedy A Jr, Cochran W. Small bowel congenital anomalies: a review and update. Curr Gastroenterol Rep 2016;18(4):16.

10. Neu J, Modi N, Caplan M. Necrotizing enterocolitis comes in different forms: historical perspectives and defining the disease. Semin Fetal Neonatal Med 2018;23(6):370–3.

11. Vandenplas Y. Prevention and management of cow's milk allergy in non-exclusively breastfed infants. Nutrients 2017;9(7):731.

12. Ochoa TJ, Salazar-Lindo E, Cleary TG. Management of children with infection-associated persistent diarrhea. Semin Pediatr Infect Dis 2004;15(4):229–36.

13. Canani RB, Terrin G, Cardillo G, et al. Congenital diarrheal disorders: improved understanding of gene defects is leading to advances in intestinal physiology and clinical management. J Pediatr Gastroenterol Nutr 2010;50(4):360–6.

14. Wedenoja S, Pekansaari E, Höglund P, et al. Update on SLC26A3 mutations in congenital chloride diarrhea. Hum Mutat 2011;32(7):715–22.

15. Swallow DM, Poulter M, Hollox EJ. Intolerance to lactose and other dietary sugars. Drug Metab Dispos 2001;29:513–6.

16. Sebastio G, Sperandeo MP, Andria G. Lysinuric protein intolerance: reviewing concepts on a multisystem disease. Am J Med Genet C Semin Med Genet 2011;157(1):54–62.

17. Overeem AW, Posovszky C, Rings EH, et al. The role of enterocyte defects in the pathogenesis of congenital diarrheal disorders. Dis Model Mech 2016;9(1):1–12.

18. Weisz OA, Rodriguez-Boulan E. Apical trafficking in epithelial cells: signals, clusters and motors. J Cell Sci 2009;122(23):4253–66.

19. Giepmans BNG, van IJzendoorn SCD. Epithelial cell-cell junctions and plasma membrane domains. Biochim Biophys Acta Biomembr 2009;1788(4):820–31.

20. Canani RB, Terrin G. Recent progress in congenital diarrheal disorders. Curr Gastroenterol Rep 2011;13(3):257–64.

21. Kuokkanen M, Kokkonen J, Enattah NS, et al. Mutations in the translated region of the lactase gene (LCT) underlie congenital lactase deficiency. Am J Hum Genet 2006;78(2):339–44.

22. Lücke T, Keiser M, Illsinger S, et al. Congenital and putatively acquired forms of sucrase-isomaltase deficiency in infancy: effects of sacrosidase therapy. J Pediatr Gastroenterol Nutr 2009;49(4):485–7.

23. Nichols BL, Avery SE, Karnsakul W, et al. Congenital maltase-glucoamylase deficiency associated with lactase and sucrase deficiencies. J Pediatr Gastroenterol Nutr 2002;35(4):573–9.

24. Lebenthal E, Khin-Maung-U, Zheng BY, et al. Small intestinal glucoamylase deficiency and starch malabsorption: a newly recognized alpha-glucosidase deficiency in children. J Pediatr 1994;124(4):541–6.
25. Holzinger A, Maier EM, Bück C, et al. Mutations in the proenteropeptidase gene are the molecular cause of congenital enteropeptidase deficiency. Am J Hum Genet 2002;70(1):20–5.
26. Abad-Sinden A, Borowitz S, Meyers R, et al. Nutrition management of congenital glucose-galactose malabsorption: a case study. J Am Diet Assoc 1997;97(12): 1417–21.
27. Schmitt S, Küry S, Giraud M, et al. An update on mutations of the SLC39A4 gene in acrodermatitis enteropathica. Hum Mutat 2009;30(6):926–33.
28. Lechner S, Ruemmele FM, Zankl A, et al. Significance of molecular testing for congenital chloride diarrhea. J Pediatr Gastroenterol Nutr 2011;53(1): 48–54.
29. Müller T, Rasool I, Heinz-Erian P, et al. Congenital secretory diarrhoea caused by activating germline mutations in GUCY2C. Gut 2016;65(8):1306–13.
30. Oelkers P, Kirby LC, Heubi JE, et al. Primary bile acid malabsorption caused by mutations in the ileal sodium-dependent bile acid transporter gene (SLC10A2). J Clin Invest 1997;99(8):1880–7.
31. Pattni S, Walters JRF. Recent advances in the understanding of bile acid malabsorption. Br Med Bull 2009;92(1):79–93.
32. Rosendahl J, Bödeker H, Mössner J, et al. Hereditary chronic pancreatitis. Orphanet J Rare Dis 2007;2:1.
33. Whitcomb DC, Gorry MC, Preston RA, et al. Hereditary pancreatitis is caused by a mutation in the cationic trypsinogen gene. Nat Genet 1996;14(2):141–5.
34. Witt H, Luck W, Hennies HC, et al. Mutations in the gene encoding the serine protease inhibitor, Kazal type 1 are associated with chronic pancreatitis. Nat Genet 2000;25(2):213–6.
35. Peretti N, Sassolas A, Roy CC, et al. Guidelines for the diagnosis and management of chylomicron retention disease based on a review of the literature and the experience of two centers. Orphanet J Rare Dis 2010;5:24.
36. Dror Y, Donadieu J, Koglmeier J, et al. Draft consensus guidelines for diagnosis and treatment of Shwachman-Diamond syndrome. Ann N Y Acad Sci 2011; 1242(1):40–55.
37. Pearson HA, Lobel JS, Kocoshis SA, et al. A new syndrome of refractory sideroblastic anemia with vacuolization of marrow precursors and exocrine pancreatic dysfunction. J Pediatr 1979;95(6):976–84.
38. Ruemmele FM, Schmitz J, Goulet O. Microvillous inclusion disease (microvillous atrophy). Orphanet J Rare Dis 2006;1:22.
39. Ko JS, Seo JK, Shim JO, et al. Tufting enteropathy with EpCAM mutations in two siblings. Gut Liver 2010;4(3):407–10.
40. Hartley JL, Zachos NC, Dawood B, et al. Mutations in TTC37 cause trichohepatoenteric syndrome (phenotypic diarrhea of infancy). Gastroenterology 2010; 138(7):2388–98.e2.
41. Wang J, Cortina G, Wu SV, et al. Mutant neurogenin-3 in congenital malabsorptive diarrhea. N Engl J Med 2006;355(3):270–80.
42. Farooqi IS, Volders K, Stanhope R, et al. Hyperphagia and early-onset obesity due to a novel homozygous missense mutation in prohormone convertase 1/3. J Clin Endocrinol Metab 2007;92(9):3369–73.

43. Agarwal S, Mayer L. Diagnosis and treatment of gastrointestinal disorders in patients with primary immunodeficiency. Clin Gastroenterol Hepatol 2013;11(9): 1050–63.
44. Posovszky C. Congenital intestinal diarrhoeal diseases: a diagnostic and therapeutic challenge. Best Pract Res Clin Gastroenterol 2016;30(2):187–211.
45. Fishbein TM. Intestinal transplantation. N Engl J Med 2009;361(10):998.
46. Hong SN, Dunn JC, Stelzner M, et al. Concise review: the potential use of intestinal stem cells to treat patients with intestinal failure. Stem Cells Transl Med 2017; 6(2):666–76.

Intestinal Failure
A Description of the Problem and Recent Therapeutic Advances

Ethan A. Mezoff, MD[a],*, Peter C. Minneci, MD[b],
Molly C. Dienhart, MD[a]

KEYWORDS

- Short bowel syndrome • Pediatric intestinal failure • Parenteral nutrition

KEY POINTS

- Intestinal failure occurs when gut function is chronically insufficient to meet the nutrient and hydration needs of the growing neonate.
- Care of the neonate with intestinal failure seeks to achieve enteral autonomy and mitigate associated comorbidity.
- Prognosis is favorable and, in many patients, can be approximated through use of nomograms detailing likelihood of enteral autonomy by bowel length and a sober assessment of comorbid conditions.
- Impactful advancements in care have included coalescence of multidisciplinary intestinal rehabilitation teams, new parenteral lipid formulations and strategies of use, and improved care of the central venous catheter.

INTRODUCTION: NATURE OF THE PROBLEM
Definition and Classification of Pediatric Intestinal Failure

Pediatric intestinal failure (IF) occurs in infants or children whose intestinal digestive and absorptive function is insufficient to meet fluid, electrolyte, and nutrient requirements.[1] Clinically, this is observed when parenteral nutrition (PN) is required for a prolonged period. Definitions of IF vary in the literature.[2–5] The authors identify IF in infants or children who have required 60 consecutive days of PN for a primary bowel disorder or surgical outcome.

[a] Division of Gastroenterology, Hepatology & Nutrition, The Ohio State University College of Medicine, Center for Intestinal Rehabilitation and Nutrition Support, Nationwide Children's Hospital, 700 Children's Drive, Columbus, OH 43205, USA; [b] Department of Surgery, The Ohio State University College of Medicine, Center for Surgical Outcomes Research, Abigail Wexner Research Institute, Nationwide Children's Hospital, 700 Children's Drive, Columbus, OH 43205, USA
* Corresponding author.
E-mail address: Ethan.Mezoff@nationwidechildrens.org

Clin Perinatol 47 (2020) 323–340
https://doi.org/10.1016/j.clp.2020.02.008
0095-5108/20/© 2020 Elsevier Inc. All rights reserved.

The ability to study and classify IF has been limited by its rarity. The incidence and prevalence in North America are not known. The prevalence of chronic PN use among pediatric patients in Italy was recently reported to be 14 cases per million inhabitants, with an overall incidence of 1.41 cases per million inhabitant years.[6]

The causes of IF can be grouped into 3 categories: (1) short bowel syndrome (SBS) caused by bowel resection or loss; (b) dysmotility caused by neuropathic, myopathic, paraneoplastic, autoimmune, or idiopathic processes that result in signs and symptoms of mechanical obstruction in the absence of a specific lesion; and (3) mucosal enteropathies, which are rare, generally monogenic, and present early in life with severe diarrhea.[2,7,8] SBS is the most common cause of IF, with a North American incidence reported to be 24.5 cases per 100,000 live births.[2] Combining many recent studies reporting the frequency of causes, necrotizing enterocolitis accounts for 26% of cases, gastroschisis 19%, intestinal atresia 14%, and volvulus 14% (Table 1). Mucosal enteropathy and primary bowel dysmotility are rare causes of IF.

Adaptation

In patients with SBS, the reduction in absorptive and digestive capacity stimulates the remnant bowel to undergo a process of adaptation, characterized by elongation of villi and crypt deepening.[9] Grossly, the bowel dilates and lengthens. This process begins in the first days after resection and can continue for 5 years or longer.[4,10] As adaptation occurs, children tolerate larger proportions of daily nutrient and fluid needs through the gut, with many reaching enteral autonomy. Mechanisms to augment the process of intestinal adaptation are actively under investigation.

Many clinically relevant mediators of adaptation have been described. Use of enteral nutrition and the nutrient source and its components, such as human milk or long chain fats, are known to stimulate adaptation.[11,12] Pancreaticobiliary secretions are also important to mucosal proliferation in the adaptive process.[13] Additional candidates being studied as potential therapeutic targets include epidermal growth factor, insulinlike growth factor, growth hormone, and glucagonlike peptide 2 (GLP-2).[14-18]

Prognosis

Important outcomes to the families of neonates with IF include the probability of achieving enteral autonomy, the development of comorbid disease, and the associated mortality. Although variability in anatomy and adaptation at the patient level requires individualized management strategies, reports have identified several factors that influence these outcomes.

Remnant bowel anatomy and length are predictive of ability to achieve enteral autonomy, with several published nomograms available to assign probability (Fig. 1).[3,19,20] In addition, presence of the ileocecal valve or colon, which acts to slow transit and facilitate improved fluid, electrolyte, and caloric reclamation, are associated with an improved probability of achieving enteral autonomy.[3,19,21-23] The cause of IF, timing of initiation of enteral feedings, and availability of human milk or an amino acid–based formula are also known to modify outcomes.[3,19,21]

Dramatic improvement in survival of patients with IF has occurred, with survival beyond the first few years of life increasing from 70% during the last 2 decades of the twentieth century to 94% to 97% in recent reports.[24-27] Mortality risk is greatest in the first 2 years following diagnosis and has been associated with development of IF-associated liver disease (IFALD), prematurity, and care at a center without multidisciplinary intestinal rehabilitation.[4,25,28-30]

Table 1
Causes of intestinal failure

Author	Location	Years	Definition	Subjects	Men, n (%)	NEC, n (%)	Gastro-schisis, n (%)	Atresia, n (%)	Volvulus, n (%)	HD, n (%)	Dysmotility, n (%)	Enteropathy, n (%)	Other, n (%)
Quiros-Tejeira et al,[22] 2004	Los Angeles, CA	1975–2000	≥90 d PN and ≤75% predicted small bowel length	78	49 (63)	16 (21)	16 (21)	19 (24)	15 (19)	NR	NR	NR	12 (15)
Demehri et al,[98] 2015[a]	Ann Arbor, MI	1988–2013	≥60 d PN or ≤50% predicted small bowel length	171	103 (60)	82 (44)	42 (23)	40 (21)	34 (18)	NR	NR	NR	26 (14)
Merras-Salmio & Pakarinen,[26] 2015[a]	Helsinki, Finland	1988–2014	≥90 d PN or ≤25% predicted small bowel length	48	28 (58)	22 (46)	7 (15)	11 (23)	11 (23)	NR	20[b]	NR	NR
Nucci et al,[99] 2008	Pittsburgh, PA	1996–2006	Evaluation at international referral center	389	239 (61)	74 (19)	78 (20)	47 (12)	58 (15)	31 (8)	35 (9)	8 (2)	58 (15)
Wales et al,[2] 2004	Toronto, Canada	1997–2001	≥42 d PN or ≤25% predicted small bowel length	40	22 (55)	14 (35)	5 (13)	4 (10)	4 (10)	1 (3)	NR	NR	12 (30)
Abi Nader et al,[27] 2016	Paris, France	2000–2013	≥90 d PN	251	137 (55)	31 (12)	30 (12)	16 (6)	42 (17)	25 (10)	23 (9)	25 (10)	68 (27)

(continued on next page)

Table 1
(continued)

Author	Location	Years	Definition	Subjects	Men, n (%)	NEC, n (%)	Gastro-schisis, n (%)	Atresia, n (%)	Volvulus, n (%)	HD, n (%)	Dysmotility, n (%)	Enteropathy, n (%)	Other, n (%)
Squires et al,[4] 2012	Multisite	2000–2007	60 of 74 d consecutive PN	272	156 (57)	71 (26)	44 (16)	27 (10)	24 (9)	11 (40)	NR	3 (1)	91 (33)
Fullerton et al,[100] 2016	Boston, MA	2002–2014	≥90 d PN	313	175 (56)	95 (30)	72 (23)	52 (17)	33 (11)	NR	39 (12)	8 (3)	14 (4)
Total[c]	—	—		1562	909 (58)	405 (26)	294 (19)	216 (14)	221 (14)	68 (4)	117 (7)	44 (3)	281 (18)

Abbreviations: NR not reported; HD Hirschsprung disease.

[a] Causes not mutually exclusive (patients double counted).

[b] Dysmotility disorders counted separately.

[c] Includes some studies in which patients are double counted because of coexisting causes.

Data from Refs.[2,4,22,26,27,98–100]

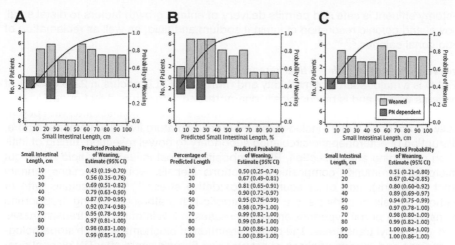

Fig. 1. Nomogram showing predicted probability of weaning from PN based on remnant bowel length. (*A*) Predicted probability based on small intestinal length. (*B*) Predicted probability based on percentage of predicted small intestinal length. (*C*). Predicted probability based on small intestinal length excluding patients who underwent bowel-lengthening procedures. The curved black line indicates predicted probability. Patients who died (n = 8) or underwent transplant (n = 4) were excluded. CI, confidence interval. (*From* Fallon EM, Mitchell PD, Nehra D, et al. Neonates with short bowel syndrome: an optimistic future for parenteral nutrition independence. JAMA Surg. 2014;149(7):663-670; with permission.)

Rehabilitation Strategy

Goals of caring for infants with IF are to achieve enteral autonomy and mitigate associated comorbidity. The cornerstone of this care is nutrition management using available age-specific nutrient dose recommendations.[31] Initially, infants require all or most of their nutrition and fluid parenterally. With increasing enteral nutrition tolerance, and with growth, PN is weaned and eventually discontinued. Sustained growth without PN supplementation indicates achievement of enteral autonomy and readiness for central line removal.

Relevant Morbidities

Many aspects of the cause and care of infants with IF can alter their morbidity, mortality, health-related quality of life, and neurodevelopment. Management strategies should anticipate and mitigate modifiable comorbid conditions and sequelae of care. Maintenance of sufficient growth is critical to avoiding morbidity. Daily calorie provisions should be determined both by estimated needs and the short-term and long-term growth trajectory of the individual patient. The calorie source can be shifted from parenteral to enteral sources as tolerance builds. Growth failure with seemingly sufficient calorie provisions should prompt an evaluation of tolerance/absorption of enteral calories (frequency and consistency of stools, diaper dermatitis). Next, sodium depletion should be evaluated by measuring urine sodium level. A deficiency of whole-body sodium, as indicated by a urine sodium level less than 30 mEq/L, has been associated with growth failure despite sufficient calorie provision.[32] Supplementation with up to 10 mEq/kg of sodium per day may be required.[33] In children with bowel discontinuity in whom a mucus fistula is easily accessible, refeeding of ostomy effluent is safe and permits delivery of enteral growth factors to distal small bowel and colonic resorption of luminal sodium and fluid, as well as reclamation of additional calories.[23,34]

Intestinal failure–associated liver disease

IFALD is a major source of morbidity and mortality. IFALD occurs in 22% to 50% of patients with IF and is biochemically characterized with serum direct or conjugated bilirubin levels greater than 2 mg/dL.[35–37] Pathogenesis is multifactorial, with potentially contributing factors including prematurity, immature liver and immune factors, disruption of enterohepatic circulation secondary to bowel resection, timing of initiation of feeding after resection, PN composition (most influentially, lipid type), gut microbial community composition, infections (sepsis, wound infections, urinary tract infections), and other sources of oxidative stress.[38–42] Cholestasis with or without fibrosis or cirrhosis is a characteristic histopathologic finding. Supporting signs include portal hypertension and increases in levels of hepatic transaminases and γ-glutamyl transferase. The poor correlation of biochemical and histopathologic findings and reports of cases of progressive fibrosis years after PN discontinuation support a strategy of risk-factor modification and frequent monitoring.[43] The choleretic, ursodeoxycholic acid, may improve biochemical indices of IFALD but its effects on histologic changes and changing pathogenesis during growth are unclear.

Complications of central venous access devices

The need for placement and maintenance of a central venous catheter (CVC) for PN place children with IF at risk for insertion site infection, central line–associated blood stream infection (CLABSI), and thrombosis. CLABSI rates in children with IF have recently been reported at between 8.0 and 10.2 infections per 1000 catheter days.[44–46] Notably, probiotic use can lead to contamination of the CVC and should be avoided.[47]

Attempts at CVC salvage are commonly made to avoid CVC loss in patients who may require venous access for life. CVC failure rates increase with replacements, which is associated with venous damage and the development of vascular thrombosis.[48]

Symptoms and medical management

Bowel dysmotility is common and treated symptomatically with prokinetic agents such as erythromycin, amoxicillin–clavulanic acid, and octreotide. Liquid stools related to rapid bowel transit or other causes of malabsorption can lead to substantial fluid and electrolyte losses. Antimotility agents (eg, loperamide, clonidine, and other opioid agonists), antisecretory agents (eg, octreotide, proton pump inhibitors), bile acid binding agents (eg, cholestyramine), and formula additives (eg, soluble fiber) can be used to slow transit and minimize malabsorption. Increased or liquid stool output should prompt assessment for mechanical, ischemic, or infectious problems. In their absence, the medications mentioned earlier can be empirically prescribed with frequent assessment of effectiveness to minimize polypharmacy.

Micronutrient deficiency

Many sources of gut dysfunction associated with IF, including postsurgical anatomy and cholestatic liver disease, may lead to vitamin and mineral malabsorption and, ultimately, insufficiency. Two centers reported a high prevalence of multiple micronutrient insufficiencies, including iron, copper, and fat-soluble vitamins.[49,50]

Insufficiency was observed both during and after transition to enteral autonomy, therefore intestinal rehabilitation programs should practice routine monitoring.

Health-related quality of life and neurodevelopment

Health-related quality of life (HRQOL) and neurodevelopmental outcomes have received heightened attention in the past decade with improved survival.[51] HRQOL may be specifically influenced by the complexity of home PN administration, abdominal pain, loose stools, frequent hospital admissions, and family financial stressors.[52–54] Using the Pediatric Quality of Life Inventory (PedsQL), HRQOL of patients with IF is decreased in physical health, school, and social domains compared with reference data or healthy controls.[55,56] Neurodevelopmental outcomes may be influenced by prematurity at birth, prolonged periods of critical illness, a history of necrotizing enterocolitis or sepsis, multiple sedated procedures, IFALD, micronutrient deficiencies, and lipid restriction.[57–59] Studies specifically evaluating neurodevelopmental outcomes among children with SBS and history of IF used a variety of age-specific assessments and have raised concern for delayed psychomotor and cognitive development.[60–62]

RECENT ADVANCES
Ethanol Locks

Ethanol (ethyl alcohol) has broad-spectrum antiseptic properties and can penetrate and disrupt bacterial biofilm formation.[63,64] Prophylactic use in the form of a lock to minimize blood stream infection (BSI) in pediatric patients generally weighing greater than 5 kg and receiving chronic PN is becoming more common among intestinal rehabilitation centers.[65] A recent meta-analysis showed a reduction in BSI and catheter replacement rates with ethanol use, with a mean decrease in the rate of catheter-related BSI of 6.27 infections per 1000 catheter days (95% confidence interval, 4.89–7.66).[66] When ethanol was implemented as a component of a larger prevention bundle, the BSI rate decreased to less than 1 infection per 1000 catheter days.[67] Potential complications related to ethanol lock therapy include thrombosis/catheter occlusion and breakage.[66]

Lipid Preparations

Currently available intravenous lipid emulsions (IVFEs) used in infants and children in the United States (US Food and Drug Administration [FDA] approved or used off label), include Intralipid, Omegaven, ClinoLipid, and SMOFlipid (**Table 2**). Intralipid is a 20% fat emulsion composed of soybean lipid and for decades was the main lipid emulsion available. With the discovery that phytosterols, a component of this plant-based lipid, contributed to the development of liver disease, alternative strategies were sought to minimize this exposure.[68] Availability of other products led to use of Omegaven, a 10% fish oil emulsion. Proposed benefits include the presence of antiinflammatory fatty acids; α-tocopherol, a known antioxidant; lack of phytosterols; and demonstrable improvement in biochemical markers of cholestasis. Risks with such a product include development of essential fatty acid (EFA) deficiency given lack of omega-6 fatty acids. Composite lipid products also exist; however, none are yet FDA approved for children in the United States. One such product, SMOFlipid (soy, medium-chain triglyceride, olive, and fish oil), has been approved for use in adults in the United States. Potential benefits of this product include a more balanced fat source providing antiinflammatory fatty acid, α-tocopherol, less phytosterol, and presence of EFA. Use of any of the available intravenous lipid emulsions requires monitoring of triglyceride and EFA levels.

Table 2
Composition of available parenteral lipid preparations based on package inserts

Ingredient	Intralipid[a]	Omegaven[a]	SMOFlipid	ClinoLipid
Soybean oil (%)	100	—	30	20
MCT oil (%)	—	—	30	—
Olive oil (%)	—	—	25	80
Fish oil (%)	—	100	15	—
Phytosterols (mg/L)	350–440	3.66	175–200	~275
α-Tocopherol (mg/L)	38	150–300	160–225	32
Linoleic acid (%)	44–62	1.5	14–25	17.9
α-Linolenic acid (%)	4–11	1.1	1.5–3.5	2.35
EPA (%)	0	13–26	1–3.5	0
DHA (%)	0	14–27	1–3.5	0
ARA (%)	0	0.2–2	0	0

Abbreviations: ARA, arachidonic acid; DHA, docosahexaenoic acid; EPA, eicosapentaenoic acid; MCT, medium-chain triglyceride.
[a] FDA approved for pediatric use.

Intestinal Rehabilitation Programs

An important recent advancement is the multidisciplinary intestinal rehabilitation program (IRP) approach. Such a program is composed of, at minimum, a gastroenterologist, surgeon, dietitian, pharmacist, and nurse skilled in the care of a CVC. Collaboration with other specialties, including neonatology and radiology, may be helpful.[69] Care from an IRP has been shown to increase overall survival, reduce septic episodes, improve biochemical indices of IFALD, improve rate of enteral autonomy, and increase rate of removal from bowel transplant listing secondary to clinical improvement.[29,30,70] In addition, rehabilitation programs offer a consolidation of expertise, coordination of management, personalized care, and assistance in transition from pediatric to adult care.[71]

Nontransplant Surgery

Failure to wean from PN should prompt evaluation for surgical therapy. Patients with bowel discontinuity should be considered for early stoma reversal and those that develop dilated bowel and/or bowel dysmotility should be considered for autologous intestinal reconstruction (AIR) surgery, including intestinal tapering or lengthening procedures. The latter include the serial transverse enteroplasty or longitudinal intestinal lengthening procedure and may be performed to address bowel dilatation and dysmotility.[72] Potential complications from AIR include staple-line leak, adhesive or functional bowel obstruction, stricture formation, further dilation, and gastrointestinal bleeding.[72–74]

Intestinal Transplant

Intestinal transplant remains an important treatment modality for irreversible IF. The most common indications for transplant include IFALD, multiple BSIs, and loss of intravenous access.[75] Graft types include small intestine graft, liver–small intestine graft, modified multivisceral graft, and a multivisceral graft, with or without a segment of colon.[76] Among pediatric and adult patients transplanted since 2000, actuarial patient and graft survival at 5 years was 58% and 50%, respectively.[77]

CURRENT CONTROVERSIES
Lipid Management

Over the past 2 decades, the strategy for management of IVFE dosing in IF has changed. Studies from the 1980s showed the contribution of IVFE to the development of cholestasis with improvement in biochemical indices of liver disease with reduction or removal of lipid.[78] In the early 1990s, phytosterols, a major component of soy-based lipids, were implicated in IFALD development, as well as a predominance of proinflammatory fatty acids.[68] These findings favor alternative IVFE preparations. The fish oil–based product, Omegaven, was used as an adjunctive therapy in Europe. Studies showed biochemical improvement in cholestasis, although subsequent studies cautioned that histologic fibrosis may persist in some patients.[79–82]

The observation that withdrawal of lipids resulted in improved biochemical profiles prompted an evaluation of a strategy of lipid dose minimization. Infants receiving 1 g/kg/d of soy emulsion experienced an encouraging improvement, comparable with infants receiving fish oil emulsion, which was confirmed in a randomized controlled trial.[83,84] In addition to supporting a strategy of soy lipid minimization and fish oil use, these observations fueled interest in composite lipid emulsions, which are now available to prescribers in the United States.

At present, the optimal strategy for lipid emulsion dosing is not established and long-term consequences of various strategies on liver health and neurodevelopmental outcome remain unknown. A tailored approach that promotes growth related to the achievement of ideal daily caloric goals using calorie-dense fat and minimizes EFA deficiency with emulsion-specific dosing restrictions, hypertriglyceridemia, and the development of IFALD from excessive use is warranted. Trials are underway to better understand the safety and efficacy of alternative and composite lipid emulsions in the pediatric population.

Feeding Advancement

The optimal approach to neonatal feeding advancement following substantial bowel loss remains under debate. Prompt initiation of enteral feeding following bowel resection has been associated with the achievement enteral autonomy and is advocated when feasible.[3] In the absence of human milk, an amino acid–based formula has been associated with improved tolerance.[19]

A recent survey of 14 US centers reported that many centers prescribe a continuous infusion of human milk or elemental formula in the first 1 to 2 weeks following substantial resection.[85] A European consensus review identifies 3 phases of nutrition management (acute postoperative, early advancement, and late maintenance) but acknowledges that the route of feeding, method or mode of delivery (continuous, bolus, or combination), and overall composition of enteral nutrition remain controversial with regard to relevance, efficiency, and feasibility.[86] Single-center guidelines for feeding advancement of neonates with SBS are available (Fig. 2).[87,88] Such guidelines have been shown to decrease the rate of IFALD and reduce time to enteral autonomy without increasing the incidence of necrotizing enterocolitis.[89]

The authors favor human milk or an amino acid–based formula in the first year of life but consider transition to an intact pediatric formula when tolerance is observed thereafter. We blend continuous feedings overnight and oral or bolus feedings during waking hours to maximize formula contact time with the gut, maintain and develop oromotor skills, and approximate the cyclic physiology of normally fed infants. We also add small-volume oral feedings with fiber-rich infant foods to promote oral skills development and bulk stools.

Feeding Advancement Principles
- Quantify feeding intolerance primarily by stool or ostomy output.
- Assess tolerance no more than twice per 24 h. Advance no more than once per 24-h period.
- Ultimate goals: 150 to 200 mL/kg/d
                            100 to 140 kcal/kg/d
- If ostomy/stool output precludes volume advancement at 20 cal/oz for 7 d, then increasing caloric density of the formula can be performed.
- As feedings are advanced, PN should be reduced such that weight gain velocity is maintained.

Guidelines for feeding advancement

Stool output:
If < 10 mL/kg/d or < 10 stools/d -------------->advance rate by 10 to 20 mL/kg/d
If 10 to 20 mL/kg/d or 10 to 12 stools/d ---> no change
If > 20 mL/kg/d or > 12 stools/d ------------> reduce rate or hold feeds*

Ostomy output:
If < 2 mL/kg/h -------------------->   advance rate by 10 to 20 mL/kg/d
If 2 to 3 mL/kg/h ---------------->   no change
If > 3 mL/kg/h -------------------->   reduce rate or hold feeds*

Stool reducing substances:
If < 1% ------------------------->   advance feeds per stool or ostomy output
If 1% --------------------------->   no change
If > 1% ------------------------->   reduce rate or hold feeds*

Signs of dehydration:
If absent ----------------------->   advance feeds per stool or ostomy output
If present ----------------------->   reduce rate or hold feeds*

Gastric aspirates:
< four times previous h infusion ------> advance feeds
> four times previous h infusion ------> reduce rate or hold feeds*

NB: Oral feeds may be offered as follows:
1. Infant is developmentally able to feed by mouth (PO).
2. One hour's worth of continuous feeds may be offered PO BID-TID after 5 d of continuous feeds. During this time, tube feeds should be held.
3. More than 1 h worth of continuous feeds may be offered PO once the infant has reached full volume of feeds by continuous route and is demonstrating weight gain at least 7 d   have passed on the feeding advancement protocol.

Fig. 2. Example enteral nutrition advancement guidelines for infants with short bowel syndrome. (*From* Gosselin KB, Duggan C. Enteral nutrition in the management of pediatric intestinal failure. J Pediatr. 2014;165(6):1085-1090; with permission.) *Feeds should generally be held for 8 hours, then restarted at 75% of the previous rate.

Challenges and Implications for Practice

The root challenges to progress in intestinal rehabilitation are the rarity and heterogeneity of the disease process. These challenges result in a small number of heterogeneous patients at any single center and have limited available data to mainly single-center studies. Multicenter studies have shed tremendous light but at a high and seemingly unsustainable cost.[4]

FUTURE DIRECTIONS
Multisite Study

Sustained collaborative study of IF will greatly benefit from recent advancements in health information technology and, specifically, the electronic health record. Such advancements make possible the prospect of seamless clinical and research documentation in a single workflow with low funding and little added specialist effort.[90] The path toward this future involves agreement by participating partners on discrete definitions, creation and dissemination of standard data elements forming an IF-specific data dictionary, and the identification of a data coordinating center to receive and analyze information. Subsequently, multisite observational descriptions, collaborative quality improvement, and comparative effectiveness research would be within reach.

Stimulants of Adaptation (Teduglutide)

GLP-2, an amino acid secreted in the distal intestine, enhances nutrient and fluid absorption, increases absorptive surface area, prevents mucosal atrophy, improves barrier function, inhibits gastric emptying, and stimulates intestinal blood flow.[91] Recombinant GLP-2 is approved for use among adult patients with IF (2012) and children 1 year of age or older (2019). Early data have shown a trend toward reductions in PN requirements and advancements in enteral nutrition, with additional studies ongoing (ClinicalTrials.gov, NCT02682381).[92] Limitations include the potential for fluid and electrolyte abnormalities with abrupt cessation of use, the need for daily subcutaneous injections, possible return to PN dependence with drug cessation among those who achieved enteral autonomy, inability to fully wean from PN in many, substantial cost, and the potential for benign or malignant mucosal growth.[91–93] Despite these limitations, GLP-2 holds great promise for a subset of children with IF.

Tissue Engineering

First reported in 1997, tissue engineering small intestine has been an area of ongoing study.[94] Obstacles identified a decade ago, including the expansion of intestinal organoids, the creation of peristalsis, scaling to human dimensions, and regulatory approval, are under scientific scrutiny.[95–97] Nonpharmacologic bowel augmentation through implantation of autologous, engineered tissue promises a novel method of increasing absorptive surface area without exposure to the immune-mediated risks of allogeneic bowel transplant or low donor availability.

SUMMARY

Neonatal IF occurs when long-term gut function is insufficient to meet nutrient and hydration demands. Arising most often following extensive bowel resection, management seeks to avoid comorbid disease, such as IFALD, sepsis, and micronutrient deficiency, while augmenting intestinal adaptation to achieve enteral autonomy in those capable. Important recent developments include the coalescence of dedicated intestinal rehabilitation teams at some centers, nuanced lipid management to avoid hepatotoxicity, attentive CVC management, and pharmacologic augmentation of adaptation. With multidisciplinary care and attention to the individual nuances of each patient with this heterogeneous disorder, the future is bright.

DISCLOSURES

The authors have nothing to disclose.

Best Practices

What is the current practice?

Neonatal IF
  Best practice/guideline/care path objective
  There are recommendations based on expert opinion from individual IRPs, but there are no clear consensus or firm guidelines regarding nutritional practices (both parenteral and enteral), central line management, and surgical approach to care.

What changes in current practice are likely to improve outcomes?

- For infants who have a high likelihood of requiring PN for more than 60 days because of an intestinal disorder, care should be provided in collaboration with an intestinal rehabilitation team.

- The development of electronic health record–based tools to facilitate seamless clinical documentation and data collection, supporting multisite study and the development of evidence-based guidelines.

Major recommendations

- Enteral feedings should be initiated as soon as it is safe to do so with close monitoring of tolerance, which will in turn guide feeding adjustments (grade B).

- Failure to gain weight on presumed adequate calorie support should be promptly investigated to enable appropriate adjustments in care (grade C).

- Careful intravenous fat emulsion management should be initiated at the onset of parenteral support (grade B).

- Lack of progress in enteral feedings should prompt changes in medical approaches and/or consideration of possible surgical interventions (grade C).

- An intestinal rehabilitation team should be involved in the care of infants with IF (grade B).

Summary statement

Care by an intestinal rehabilitation team has been associated with notable improvement in the outcome of infants with IF.

Data from Refs.[1,3,4,19,29,30,69–72,80,83,87,89]

REFERENCES

1. Duggan CP, Jaksic T. Pediatric intestinal failure. N Engl J Med 2017;377(7): 666–75.
2. Wales PW, de Silva N, Kim J, et al. Neonatal short bowel syndrome: population-based estimates of incidence and mortality rates. J Pediatr Surg 2004;39(5): 690–5.
3. Sondheimer JM, Cadnapaphornchai M, Sontag M, et al. Predicting the duration of dependence on parenteral nutrition after neonatal intestinal resection. J Pediatr 1998;132(1):80–4.
4. Squires RH, Duggan C, Teitelbaum DH, et al. Natural history of pediatric intestinal failure: initial report from the Pediatric Intestinal Failure Consortium. J Pediatr 2012;161(4):723–8.e2.
5. Salvia G, Guarino A, Terrin G, et al. Neonatal onset intestinal failure: an Italian Multicenter Study. J Pediatr 2008;153(5):674–6, 676.e1-2.
6. Diamanti A, Capriati T, Gandullia P, et al. Pediatric chronic intestinal failure in Italy: report from the 2016 survey on behalf of Italian Society for Gastroenterology, Hepatology and Nutrition (SIGENP). Nutrients 2017;9(11) [pii:E1217].

7. Canani RB, Castaldo G, Bacchetta R, et al. Congenital diarrhoeal disorders: advances in this evolving web of inherited enteropathies. Nat Rev Gastroenterol Hepatol 2015;12(5):293–302.

8. Passariello A, Terrin G, Baldassarre ME, et al. Diarrhea in neonatal intensive care unit. World J Gastroenterol 2010;16(21):2664–8.

9. Dekaney CM, Fong JJ, Rigby RJ, et al. Expansion of intestinal stem cells associated with long-term adaptation following ileocecal resection in mice. Am J Physiol Gastrointest Liver Physiol 2007;293(5):G1013–22.

10. Helmrath MA, VanderKolk WE, Can G, et al. Intestinal adaptation following massive small bowel resection in the mouse. J Am Coll Surg 1996;183(5):441–9.

11. McManus JP, Isselbacher KJ. Effect of fasting versus feeding on the rat small intestine. Morphological, biochemical, and functional differences. Gastroenterology 1970;59(2):214–21.

12. Feldman EJ, Dowling RH, McNaughton J, et al. Effects of oral versus intravenous nutrition on intestinal adaptation after small bowel resection in the dog. Gastroenterology 1976;70(5 PT.1):712–9.

13. Williamson RC, Bauer FL, Ross JS, et al. Contributions of bile and pancreatic juice to cell proliferation in ileal mucosa. Surgery 1978;83(5):570–6.

14. Chaet MS, Arya G, Ziegler MM, et al. Epidermal growth factor enhances intestinal adaptation after massive small bowel resection. J Pediatr Surg 1994;29(8):1035–8 [discussion: 1038–9].

15. Shin CE, Helmrath MA, Falcone RA Jr, et al. Epidermal growth factor augments adaptation following small bowel resection: optimal dosage, route, and timing of administration. J Surg Res 1998;77(1):11–6.

16. Knott AW, Juno RJ, Jarboe MD, et al. Smooth muscle overexpression of IGF-I induces a novel adaptive response to small bowel resection. Am J Physiol Gastrointest Liver Physiol 2004;287(3):G562–70.

17. Byrne TA, Persinger RL, Young LS, et al. A new treatment for patients with short-bowel syndrome. Growth hormone, glutamine, and a modified diet. Ann Surg 1995;222(3):243–54 [discussion: 254–5].

18. Drucker DJ, Erlich P, Asa SL, et al. Induction of intestinal epithelial proliferation by glucagon-like peptide 2. Proc Natl Acad Sci U S A 1996;93(15):7911–6.

19. Andorsky DJ, Lund DP, Lillehei CW, et al. Nutritional and other postoperative management of neonates with short bowel syndrome correlates with clinical outcomes. J Pediatr 2001;139(1):27–33.

20. Fallon EM, Mitchell PD, Nehra D, et al. Neonates with short bowel syndrome: an optimistic future for parenteral nutrition independence. JAMA Surg 2014;149(7):663–70.

21. Khan FA, Squires RH, Litman HJ, et al. Predictors of enteral autonomy in children with intestinal failure: a multicenter cohort study. J Pediatr 2015;167(1):29–34.e1.

22. Quiros-Tejeira RE, Ament ME, Reyen L, et al. Long-term parenteral nutritional support and intestinal adaptation in children with short bowel syndrome: a 25-year experience. J Pediatr 2004;145(2):157–63.

23. Norsa L, Lambe C, Abi Abboud S, et al. The colon as an energy salvage organ for children with short bowel syndrome. Am J Clin Nutr 2019;109(4):1112–8.

24. Modi BP, Langer M, Ching YA, et al. Improved survival in a multidisciplinary short bowel syndrome program. J Pediatr Surg 2008;43(1):20–4.

25. Hess RA, Welch KB, Brown PI, et al. Survival outcomes of pediatric intestinal failure patients: analysis of factors contributing to improved survival over the past two decades. J Surg Res 2011;170(1):27–31.

26. Merras-Salmio L, Pakarinen MP. Refined multidisciplinary protocol-based approach to short bowel syndrome improves outcomes. J Pediatr Gastroenterol Nutr 2015;61(1):24–9.

27. Abi Nader E, Lambe C, Talbotec C, et al. Outcome of home parenteral nutrition in 251 children over a 14-y period: report of a single center. Am J Clin Nutr 2016; 103(5):1327–36.

28. Squires RH, Balint J, Horslen S, et al. Race affects outcome among infants with intestinal failure. J Pediatr Gastroenterol Nutr 2014;59(4):537–43.

29. Oliveira C, de Silva NT, Stanojevic S, et al. Change of outcomes in pediatric intestinal failure: use of time-series analysis to assess the evolution of an intestinal rehabilitation program. J Am Coll Surg 2016;222(6):1180–8.e3.

30. Stanger JD, Oliveira C, Blackmore C, et al. The impact of multi-disciplinary intestinal rehabilitation programs on the outcome of pediatric patients with intestinal failure: a systematic review and meta-analysis. J Pediatr Surg 2013;48(5): 983–92.

31. A.S.P.E.N. Pediatric assessment and interventions. In: MR Corkins, editor. Pediatric nutrition support handbook. 2nd edition. American Society for Parenteral and Enteral Nutrition; 2015. p. 121–66.

32. Bischoff AR, Tomlinson C, Belik J. Sodium intake requirements for preterm neonates: review and recommendations. J Pediatr Gastroenterol Nutr 2016;63(6): e123–9.

33. Schwarz KB, Ternberg JL, Bell MJ, et al. Sodium needs of infants and children with ileostomy. J Pediatr 1983;102(4):509–13.

34. Elliott T, Walton JM. Safety of mucous fistula refeeding in neonates with functional short bowel syndrome: a retrospective review. J Pediatr Surg 2019; 54(5):989–92.

35. Pichler J, Horn V, Macdonald S, et al. Intestinal failure-associated liver disease in hospitalised children. Arch Dis Child 2012;97(3):211–4.

36. Lauriti G, Zani A, Aufieri R, et al. Incidence, prevention, and treatment of parenteral nutrition-associated cholestasis and intestinal failure-associated liver disease in infants and children: a systematic review. JPEN J Parenter Enteral Nutr 2014;38(1):70–85.

37. Cavicchi M, Beau P, Crenn P, et al. Prevalence of liver disease and contributing factors in patients receiving home parenteral nutrition for permanent intestinal failure. Ann Intern Med 2000;132(7):525–32.

38. Steinbach M, Clark RH, Kelleher AS, et al. Demographic and nutritional factors associated with prolonged cholestatic jaundice in the premature infant. J Perinatol 2008;28(2):129–35.

39. Vileisis RA, Inwood RJ, Hunt CE. Prospective controlled study of parenteral nutrition-associated cholestatic jaundice: effect of protein intake. J Pediatr 1980;96(5):893–7.

40. Tyson JE, Kennedy KA. Trophic feedings for parenterally fed infants. Cochrane Database Syst Rev 2005;(3):CD000504.

41. Lacaille F, Gupte G, Colomb V, et al. Intestinal failure-associated liver disease: a position paper of the ESPGHAN Working Group of Intestinal Failure and Intestinal Transplantation. J Pediatr Gastroenterol Nutr 2015;60(2):272–83.

42. Korpela K, Mutanen A, Salonen A, et al. Intestinal microbiota signatures associated with histological liver steatosis in pediatric-onset intestinal failure. JPEN J Parenter Enteral Nutr 2017;41(2):238–48.

43. Mutanen A, Lohi J, Heikkila P, et al. Persistent abnormal liver fibrosis after weaning off parenteral nutrition in pediatric intestinal failure. Hepatology 2013;58(2): 729–38.

44. Wales PW, Kosar C, Carricato M, et al. Ethanol lock therapy to reduce the incidence of catheter-related bloodstream infections in home parenteral nutrition patients with intestinal failure: preliminary experience. J Pediatr Surg 2011; 46(5):951–6.

45. Jones BA, Hull MA, Richardson DS, et al. Efficacy of ethanol locks in reducing central venous catheter infections in pediatric patients with intestinal failure. J Pediatr Surg 2010;45(6):1287–93.

46. Cober MP, Kovacevich DS, Teitelbaum DH. Ethanol-lock therapy for the prevention of central venous access device infections in pediatric patients with intestinal failure. JPEN J Parenter Enteral Nutr 2011;35(1):67–73.

47. Skljarevski S, Barner A, Bruno-Murtha LA. Preventing avoidable central line-associated bloodstream infections: implications for probiotic administration and surveillance. Am J Infect Control 2016;44(11):1427–8.

48. Barnacle A, Arthurs OJ, Roebuck D, et al. Malfunctioning central venous catheters in children: a diagnostic approach. Pediatr Radiol 2008;38(4):363–78 [quiz: 486–7].

49. Ubesie AC, Kocoshis SA, Mezoff AG, et al. Multiple micronutrient deficiencies among patients with intestinal failure during and after transition to enteral nutrition. J Pediatr 2013;163(6):1692–6.

50. Yang CF, Duro D, Zurakowski D, et al. High prevalence of multiple micronutrient deficiencies in children with intestinal failure: a longitudinal study. J Pediatr 2011;159(1):39–44.e1.

51. Hukkinen M, Merras-Salmio L, Pakarinen MP. Health-related quality of life and neurodevelopmental outcomes among children with intestinal failure. Semin Pediatr Surg 2018;27(4):273–9.

52. Kelly DG, Tappenden KA, Winkler MF. Short bowel syndrome: highlights of patient management, quality of life, and survival. JPEN J Parenter Enteral Nutr 2014;38(4):427–37.

53. Jeppesen PB, Langholz E, Mortensen PB. Quality of life in patients receiving home parenteral nutrition. Gut 1999;44(6):844–52.

54. Winkler MF, Smith CE. Clinical, social, and economic impacts of home parenteral nutrition dependence in short bowel syndrome. JPEN J Parenter Enteral Nutr 2014;38(1 Suppl):32S–7S.

55. Pederiva F, Khalil B, Morabito A, et al. Impact of short bowel syndrome on quality of life and family: the patient's perspective. Eur J Pediatr Surg 2019;29(2): 196–202.

56. Sanchez SE, McAteer JP, Goldin AB, et al. Health-related quality of life in children with intestinal failure. J Pediatr Gastroenterol Nutr 2013;57(3):330–4.

57. Wang X, Xu Z, Miao CH. Current clinical evidence on the effect of general anesthesia on neurodevelopment in children: an updated systematic review with meta-regression. PLoS One 2014;9(1):e85760.

58. Shah DK, Doyle LW, Anderson PJ, et al. Adverse neurodevelopment in preterm infants with postnatal sepsis or necrotizing enterocolitis is mediated by white matter abnormalities on magnetic resonance imaging at term. J Pediatr 2008; 153(2):170–5, 175.e1.

59. Belkind-Gerson J, Carreon-Rodriguez A, Contreras-Ochoa CO, et al. Fatty acids and neurodevelopment. J Pediatr Gastroenterol Nutr 2008;47(Suppl 1):S7–9.

60. Chesley PM, Sanchez SE, Melzer L, et al. Neurodevelopmental and cognitive outcomes in children with intestinal failure. J Pediatr Gastroenterol Nutr 2016; 63(1):41–5.
61. So S, Patterson C, Gold A, et al. Early neurodevelopmental outcomes of infants with intestinal failure. Early Hum Dev 2016;101:11–6.
62. Beers SR, Yaworski JA, Stilley C, et al. Cognitive deficits in school-age children with severe short bowel syndrome. J Pediatr Surg 2000;35(6):860–5.
63. Donlan RM. Biofilm elimination on intravascular catheters: important considerations for the infectious disease practitioner. Clin Infect Dis 2011;52(8):1038–45.
64. McDonnell G, Russell AD. Antiseptics and disinfectants: activity, action, and resistance. Clin Microbiol Rev 1999;12(1):147–79.
65. Opilla MT, Kirby DF, Edmond MB. Use of ethanol lock therapy to reduce the incidence of catheter-related bloodstream infections in home parenteral nutrition patients. JPEN J Parenter Enteral Nutr 2007;31(4):302–5.
66. Rahhal R, Abu-El-Haija MA, Fei L, et al. Systematic review and meta-analysis of the utilization of ethanol locks in pediatric patients with intestinal failure. JPEN J Parenter Enteral Nutr 2018;42(4):690–701.
67. Ardura MI, Lewis J, Tansmore JL, et al. Central catheter-associated bloodstream infection reduction with ethanol lock prophylaxis in pediatric intestinal failure: broadening quality improvement initiatives from hospital to home. JAMA Pediatr 2015;169(4):324–31.
68. Clayton PT, Bowron A, Mills KA, et al. Phytosterolemia in children with parenteral nutrition-associated cholestatic liver disease. Gastroenterology 1993;105(6): 1806–13.
69. Merritt RJ, Cohran V, Raphael BP, et al. Intestinal rehabilitation programs in the management of pediatric intestinal failure and short bowel syndrome. J Pediatr Gastroenterol Nutr 2017;65(5):588–96.
70. Avitzur Y, Wang JY, de Silva NT, et al. Impact of intestinal rehabilitation program and its innovative therapies on the outcome of intestinal transplant candidates. J Pediatr Gastroenterol Nutr 2015;61(1):18–23.
71. Belza C, Wales PW. Impact of multidisciplinary teams for management of intestinal failure in children. Curr Opin Pediatr 2017;29(3):334–9.
72. King B, Carlson G, Khalil BA, et al. Intestinal bowel lengthening in children with short bowel syndrome: systematic review of the Bianchi and STEP procedures. World J Surg 2013;37(3):694–704.
73. Modi BP, Javid PJ, Jaksic T, et al. First report of the international serial transverse enteroplasty data registry: indications, efficacy, and complications. J Am Coll Surg 2007;204(3):365–71.
74. Fisher JG, Stamm DA, Modi BP, et al. Gastrointestinal bleeding as a complication of serial transverse enteroplasty. J Pediatr Surg 2014;49(5):745–9.
75. Kaufman SS, Atkinson JB, Bianchi A, et al. Indications for pediatric intestinal transplantation: a position paper of the American Society of Transplantation. Pediatr Transplant 2001;5(2):80–7.
76. Celik N, Mazariegos GV, Soltys K, et al. Pediatric intestinal transplantation. Gastroenterol Clin North Am 2018;47(2):355–68.
77. Grant D, Abu-Elmagd K, Mazariegos G, et al. Intestinal transplant registry report: global activity and trends. Am J Transplant 2015;15(1):210–9.
78. Allardyce DB. Cholestasis caused by lipid emulsions. Surg Gynecol Obstet 1982;154(5):641–7.

79. Gura KM, Lee S, Valim C, et al. Safety and efficacy of a fish-oil-based fat emulsion in the treatment of parenteral nutrition-associated liver disease. Pediatrics 2008;121(3):e678–86.

80. Puder M, Valim C, Meisel JA, et al. Parenteral fish oil improves outcomes in patients with parenteral nutrition-associated liver injury. Ann Surg 2009;250(3): 395–402.

81. Mercer DF, Hobson BD, Fischer RT, et al. Hepatic fibrosis persists and progresses despite biochemical improvement in children treated with intravenous fish oil emulsion. J Pediatr Gastroenterol Nutr 2013;56(4):364–9.

82. Belza C, Thompson R, Somers GR, et al. Persistence of hepatic fibrosis in pediatric intestinal failure patients treated with intravenous fish oil lipid emulsion. J Pediatr Surg 2017;52(5):795–801.

83. Cober MP, Killu G, Brattain A, et al. Intravenous fat emulsions reduction for patients with parenteral nutrition-associated liver disease. J Pediatr 2012;160(3): 421–7.

84. Nehra D, Fallon EM, Potemkin AK, et al. A comparison of 2 intravenous lipid emulsions: interim analysis of a randomized controlled trial. JPEN J Parenter Enteral Nutr 2014;38(6):693–701.

85. Nucci AM, Ellsworth K, Michalski A, et al. Survey of nutrition management practices in centers for pediatric intestinal rehabilitation. Nutr Clin Pract 2018;33(4): 528–38.

86. Goulet O, Olieman J, Ksiazyk J, et al. Neonatal short bowel syndrome as a model of intestinal failure: physiological background for enteral feeding. Clin Nutr 2013;32(2):162–71.

87. Gosselin KB, Duggan C. Enteral nutrition in the management of pediatric intestinal failure. J Pediatr 2014;165(6):1085–90.

88. Shores DR, Bullard JE, Aucott SW, et al. Implementation of feeding guidelines in infants at risk of intestinal failure. J Perinatol 2015;35(11):941–8.

89. Shores DR, Alaish SM, Aucott SW, et al. Postoperative enteral nutrition guidelines reduce the risk of intestinal failure-associated liver disease in surgical infants. J Pediatr 2018;195:140–7.e1.

90. Mezoff EA, Minneci PC, Hoyt RR, et al. Toward an electronic health record leveraged to learn from every complex patient encounter: health informatics considerations with pediatric intestinal rehabilitation as a model. J Pediatr 2019;215: 257–63.

91. Naberhuis JK, Tappenden KA. Teduglutide for safe reduction of parenteral nutrient and/or fluid requirements in adults: a systematic review. JPEN J Parenter Enteral Nutr 2016;40(8):1096–105.

92. Carter BA, Cohran VC, Cole CR, et al. Outcomes from a 12-week, open-label, multicenter clinical trial of teduglutide in pediatric short bowel syndrome. J Pediatr 2017;181:102–11.e5.

93. Orhan A, Gogenur I, Kissow H. The intestinotrophic effects of glucagon-like peptide-2 in relation to intestinal neoplasia. J Clin Endocrinol Metab 2018; 103(8):2827–37.

94. Choi RS, Vacanti JP. Preliminary studies of tissue-engineered intestine using isolated epithelial organoid units on tubular synthetic biodegradable scaffolds. Transplant Proc 1997;29(1–2):848–51.

95. Dunn JC. Is the tissue-engineered intestine clinically viable? Nat Clin Pract Gastroenterol Hepatol 2008;5(7):366–7.

96. Workman MJ, Mahe MM, Trisno S, et al. Engineered human pluripotent-stem-cell-derived intestinal tissues with a functional enteric nervous system. Nat Med 2017;23(1):49–59.
97. Fuller MK, Faulk DM, Sundaram N, et al. Intestinal crypts reproducibly expand in culture. J Surg Res 2012;178(1):48–54.
98. Demehri FR, Stephens L, Herrman E, et al. Enteral autonomy in pediatric short bowel syndrome: predictive factors one year after diagnosis. J Pediatr Surg 2015;50(1):131–5.
99. Nucci A, Burns RC, Armah T, et al. Interdisciplinary management of pediatric intestinal failure: a 10-year review of rehabilitation and transplantation. J Gastrointest Surg 2008;12(3):429–35 [discussion: 435–6].
100. Fullerton BS, Sparks EA, Hall AM, et al. Enteral autonomy, cirrhosis, and long term transplant-free survival in pediatric intestinal failure patients. J Pediatr Surg 2016;51(1):96–100.

Cholestasis in the Premature Infant

Carol Jean Potter, MD

KEYWORDS

- Cholestasis • Liver dysfunction • Bile acid transport • Premature • Neonatal

KEY POINTS

- The premature liver reacts differently than that of the term infant.
- Comorbidities strongly influence liver function in the preterm infant.
- Imaging is very important in evaluation of the preterm infant.

INTRODUCTION: NATURE OF THE PROBLEM

As advances in medical care have allowed survival of more fragile babies, those cared for in the neonatal intensive care unit (NICU) are smaller in size, more complicated, and more immature. Prematurity not only impairs liver function, but also impairs its ability to respond to the many insults suffered by infants who require care in the NICU. It is often difficult to determine what is primary liver disease and what is a consequence of secondary insults such as sepsis, hypoxia, ischemia, medications, or just the milieu of the premature infant. Diagnostic tools are also limited by blood volume and the baby's ability to tolerate the testing. This article discusses how prematurity affects the liver, how it responds to secondary insults, and sets out approaches to evaluation.

RECENT ADVANCES

Recent advances in hepatology have more clearly defined the process of bile synthesis and flow, including the complex regulation of this process.[1–3] Mechanisms for downregulation by cofactors such as sepsis have been identified.[4,5] At the same time, diagnostic panels with rapid turnaround have been developed that allow testing for genetic variants in liver metabolism and other genetic liver diseases in a time frame that is clinically relevant. This advance has expanded our understanding of the phenotype for variations and their impact on cholestasis in the neonate.[3,6–14] The population being evaluated for liver disease in the NICU has changed dramatically. Babies who are smaller in size, lower in gestational age, and with more complex medical and

Nationwide Children's Hospital, The Ohio State University, 700 Childrens Drive, Columbus, OH 43205, USA
E-mail address: Carol.potter@nationwidechildrens.org

Clin Perinatol 47 (2020) 341–354
https://doi.org/10.1016/j.clp.2020.02.009
perinatology.theclinics.com

Abbreviations	
BSEP	Bile salt export pump
CMV	Cytomegalovirus
GGT	Gamma glutamyl transpeptidase
GLAD	Gestational alloimmune liver disease
NICU	Neonatal intensive care unit
PN	Parenteral nutrition
T4/TSH	Thyroxine/thyroid-stimulating hormone
UTI	Urinary tract infection

surgical problems are surviving. Although we know that not all the bile ducts are formed until after term and that there is developmental regulation of many of the synthesis and transport enzymes of the liver, our understanding is crude.[15–17] At the same time, advances in the management of parenteral nutrition (PN) have allowed us to recognize liver disease previously thought to be from PN or obscured by the changes in the liver of those on PN. All these factors work together to form the clinical picture we see in the premature infant with liver dysfunction.

Prematurity has a profound impact on the liver's ability to synthesize and regulate bile acids.[15] Bile acids are synthesized from cholesterol in the liver in a multistep process. Owing to the immaturity of some steps, the preterm infant makes a smaller quantity of bile acids and the fetus produces some bile acids that are inherently cholestatic and found in much smaller quantities later in life.[17] This factor may add to the cholestasis seen in premature infants. Bile acid synthesis greatly increases in the neonatal period.[18–21] Once made, bile acids are transported out of the liver and into the duct. They are modified by a series of enzymes. Most of these processes are now well-characterized, with identification of mutations that cause disease. These mutations are tested for in genetic cholestasis panels.[6,8–14]

In a separate pathway, bilirubin is transported into the duct and carried to the gut by the bile. The rate-limiting step is the transport of conjugated bilirubin from the hepatocyte into the duct. Neonates have a large heme load to process. If the enzyme is overwhelmed, conjugated bilirubin will back diffuse into the plasma.[4,16]

Fig. 1 demonstrates bile acid synthesis in the liver under the control of FXR. Bile acids are transported into the duct by the bile salt export pump (BSEP), with regulatory help from FIC1 and MDR3. The bile acids are recycled from the circulation to start the

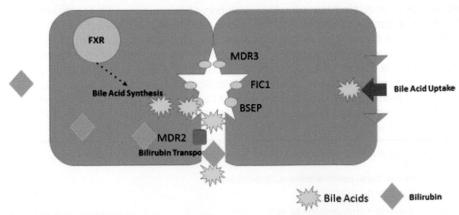

Fig. 1. Demonstrating bile acid synthesis in the liver under the control of FXR.

process again. In a separate pathway, heme is broken down into bilirubin, taken up by the hepatocyte, and transported into the bile by MDR2.

Testing for genetic mutations is now done with large panels rather than testing for a single disease. This strategy decreases cost, improves testing time, and limits the amount of blood needed for testing. As more babies are tested, we are finding expanded phenotypes of mutations. Sequencing in a large cohort of patients with mutations in bile acid transporters including FIC1, BSEP, and MDR3 showed a large number of patients who had previously unrecognized novel mutations as well as mutations that had been previously thought to be normal variants, which can cause disease.[11,12] A diagnosis of a genetic cause of cholestasis is more likely in infants presenting with either low gamma glutamyl transpeptidase (GGT) (suggesting bile acid transport or synthesis problems) or high GGT (suggesting poor bile flow with elevated bile acids in the duct). In studies of post-term infants, there is a greater than 50% chance of finding a genetic diagnosis with this phenotype. In babies without such a phenotype (neonatal cholestasis, prematurity, and PN-associated cholestasis), there remains a 15% chance of diagnosis with genetic panels. Researchers also postulate that other genes modify the effects of these major disease-causing mutations and may add to pathogenesis.[11] There is a growing literature about cholestatic babies with single mutations in more than 1 gene and the possible significance thereof. Multiple mutations in genes that contribute to cholestasis are more common in cholestatic babies than in control babies.[11,13,22] This finding may be particularly true in the premature infant with lower baseline levels of bile acid transporters. We are slowly developing an understanding of the interactions of genes, but presently can only infer the results of interaction by knowing the mechanism of each gene.

Additionally, we know that the clinical situation greatly influences cholestasis. For example, women with cholestasis of pregnancy or contraceptive-induced cholestasis recover once the hormonal downregulation of their transporters is removed.[23] As noted elsewhere in this article, premature infants have very low level of transporters because of immaturity. We currently cannot predict what genetic changes will predispose to cholestasis during this period of developmental downregulation of transporters.

CURRENT CONTROVERSIES

One of the most difficult questions for the hepatologist in the NICU is what constitutes an appropriate evaluation. None of the pathways for the evaluation of neonatal cholestasis that exist in the literature were developed for the preterm infant.[24,25] As noted, most of the enzymes involved in bile synthesis and transport have a developmental ontogeny and are present in low levels in the preterm infant. The understanding of this ontogeny and its clinical implications are somewhat crude. This factor makes it more difficult to discriminate primary liver disease from the interaction of prematurity with secondary insults. Unlike a term 2-month-old infant presenting with cholestasis as an outpatient, these premature babies frequently have comorbidities that influence cholestasis. In addition to these considerations, the evaluation must also take into account the limited blood volume of these babies and the difficulty and stress involved in obtaining specimens.

The first step is a detailed history. Pertinent historical data includes

- Mother's prior pregnancies and outcomes
  - Gestational alloimmune liver disease (GALD) usually does not occur in the first pregnancy and becomes more severe with each subsequent pregnancy.
  - Prenatal deaths may be associated with genetic causes.

- Family history
  - Prolonged neonatal cholestasis in a parent signals genetic disease such as alpha-1 antitrypsin deficiency or a bile acid transport defect.
  - Prenatal or early neonatal deaths may be associated with genetic disease.
  - A genetic diagnosis may have not been suspected in the baby. For instance, the diagnosis of Alagille syndrome is more likely when a prior baby died of pulmonary atresia. Similarly a diagnosis of a bile acid synthesis defect would explain a sibling death from intracranial bleeding.
- Prenatal history
  - Intrauterine growth retardations can cause a paucity of bile ducts.
  - Prenatal growth can signal genetic problems.
  - Cholestasis of pregnancy is associated with bile acid transport defects.[23,26]
  - HELLP syndrome is associated with fatty oxidation defects.
  - A detailed prenatal history is usually available.
- Gestational age at delivery
  - The lower the gestational age, the fewer bile ducts, fewer transport enzymes, a smaller bile acid pool and more cholestatic bile acids there are.[15,17]
- Newborn screen
  - Understand what your state screens for. These results may be able to be expedited.
- Fructose and galactose exposure
  - Galactose should not be given to a baby with liver disease until the newborn screen results are known. Fructose is in most oral medications and the sugar pacifiers are dipped in the help soothe the infant. It is also added to many formulas. Fructose may need to be withdrawn if its introduction preceded the liver dysfunction.
- Thyroxine/thyroid-stimulating hormone (T4/TSH)
  - The newborn screen may be TSH based and miss central hypothyroidism. Premature infants are at higher risk for thyroid dysfunction.
  - Thyroid Dysfunction
    - Congenital hypothyroidism and congenital hypopituitarism are both causes of neonatal cholestasis. The mechanisms are not clear. In a series of patients who had a liver biopsy for cholestasis before the diagnosis of hypopituitarism was made there was decreased staining for the transporter BSEP and the ectoenzyme, GGT, suggesting abnormal membrane fluidity as the issue rather than a problem with 1 bile acid transporter. These baby's liver disease improves with hormone supplementation.[27] Thyroid abnormalities and adrenal insufficiency are common in sick premature infants. Very low birth weight neonates have a steady decrease in T4 levels for the first 2 weeks after birth because of lower levels of TSH. Fetal production of T4 is very low at 20 weeks gestation and then gradually increases. Premature infants also have an immature thyroid–pituitary hormone axis and may have low levels of thyroid hormones and TSH during their NICU stay. There are several other mechanisms for congenital hypothyroidism. Screening should include both a TSH and T4.[28] Small for gestational age may be an additional risk factor for the development of a delayed increase in TSH.[29] It is unclear how much of a role this factor is playing in cholestasis. It is also not clear what the therapy should be. There is some evidence that supplementation of thyroid hormone in some gestational age ranges is associated with worse a developmental outcome. It is not known if this is causative or just an association.

- Size for gestational age
  - Intrauterine growth retardation is associated with paucity of bile ducts at birth.
- Apgar score
  - Low Apgar scores are associated with liver ischemia.
- Cytomegalovirus (CMV)
  - CMV can be acquired through frozen breast milk and cause hepatitis.[30]
- Necrotizing enterocolitis can
  - Cause translocation of bacteria into the portal blood.
  - Interrupt enteral feeds, which is important to normal liver function.
  - Cause ischemia to the liver or thrombosis of portal blood supply.
- Hypoxic–ischemic encephalopathy/shock
  - Liver ischemia results in high transaminases and bilirubin, which gradually decrease, unless there is irreversible liver injury.
  - Infants with an ischemic event in utero close to the time of delivery or at the time of delivery usually present with multiorgan failure, high transaminases that gradually improve, an elevated direct bilirubin, and prolonged coagulation studies that improve over the course of several days with supportive care. In contrast, babies with primary severe liver disease may present with no preceding event, have lower transaminases, and not respond to supportive care. In these babies, coagulation studies can be very helpful in determining how aggressive an evaluation should be.
- Heme load
  - A careful history should be obtained, looking for possible source of a large heme load to process. The rate-limiting step in the excretion of conjugated bilirubin is MDR2, the transport of conjugated bilirubin from the hepatocyte into the bile duct. This enzyme has a limited capacity in the preterm infant. Hemolysis or hemorrhage into the abdomen or head may overwhelm the system, leading to back diffusion of conjugated bilirubin from the hepatocyte into the plasma because of the inability to transport it into the duct. This process is completely separate from bile acid transport, except that it is the bile that carries the bilirubin down the duct and out of the liver. It is important to remember that bilirubin is only a surrogate marker and may be misleading, particularly in the preterm infant. Elevated direct bilirubin may occur without cholestasis or liver injury.
- PN
  - A companion article describes the effects of PN related liver and intestinal failure (see Mezoff and colleagues, Intestinal Failure: A Description of the Problem and Recent Therapeutic Advances, in this issue).
- Growth
  - Poor weight gain with cholestasis owing to fat malabsorption.
  - Some genetic causes are associated with poor growth.
- Cardiac, function and structure
  - Congenital heart disease may be associated with Alagille syndrome and biliary atresia.
  - Right-sided heart failure decreases outflow from the liver.
  - Portosystemic shunts are more common with congenital heart disease.[31–33]
  - A large patent ductus arteriosus may impede liver outflow.
  - Cardiomyopathy occurs with mitochondrial disease, which can also affect the liver.
- Congenital malformations
  - Consider whether there are malformations that are associated with liver disease or may predispose to secondary liver disease. Urogenital malformations predispose to infections that downregulate bilirubin and bile acid excretion.

- Genetics
  - Syndromes, such as trisomy 21, may be associated with cholestasis. Ductal plate malformations may result in renal and liver disease.
- Urinary tract infection (UTI)
  - A UTI can downregulate the transport of bilirubin, causing elevated direct bilirubin without liver dysfunction. Also, a UTI may cause downregulation of bile acid uptake by the hepatocyte, downregulation of transport out of the hepatocyte, and thus retention of bile acids in the hepatocyte leading to liver toxicity.[4,26,34]
- Sepsis
  - Similar mechanisms to UTI but more severe.
  - Infections impact the liver of preterm infants. Endotoxin suppresses MDR2, the transporter of conjugated bilirubin from the hepatocyte to the bile duct. Urinary infections are not uncommon in the NICU and may be asymptomatic and not associated with renal malformations. An *Escherichia coli* UTI may present with elevated direct bilirubin without other signs of liver dysfunction. Sepsis or translocation of bacteria from the gut to the liver though the portal vein during necrotizing enterocolitis may suppress not only MDR2, but also the suppress the uptake of bile acids from the serum into the liver and suppress the transport of bile acids out of the liver via BSEP suppression, leading to bile acid toxicity in the hepatocyte.[4,5] Viral infections such as CMV, enterovirus, and adenovirus may cause significant viral hepatitis and liver dysfunction.
- Timing of liver dysfunction
  - Liver disease immediately after birth is more likely to be primary and genetic.
  - Liver dysfunction occurring latter should be evaluated for secondary causes in addition to primary liver disease.
  - The timing of presentation is often hard to determine, because liver evaluation is often not done.

Most cholestasis in the NICU eventually resolves with variable amount of sequela. It can be difficult to distinguish who will do well at the time of presentation. Genetics probably plays a role in this. Genetic studies enable us to make a diagnosis when the phenotype is not fully developed, is unusual, or complicated by other comorbidities. The role of heterozygote mutations, gene modifiers, the interplay between mutations in multiple genes, and minor mutations at a time of stress and low levels of enzymes, is just beginning to be understood.

CLINICAL RELEVANCE

Once a detailed history and physical examination are completed, recommendations for evaluation should be formulated. Considerations should include the following.

1. How critical is the liver dysfunction? Does the evaluation need to be done rapidly or can it be done in a stepwise fashion?
2. Is there a treatable etiology that would improve the outcome? What is the impact of a delayed diagnosis?
3. Is there a diagnosis that, if made, would stop further invasive testing?
4. What is the blood volume required for testing? Could the information be obtained another way such as genetic panels, urine studies, testing parents, or imaging?
5. How is gestational age influencing the presentation or results?
6. Are there nutritional implications of the cholestasis that need to be addressed?

Before deciding on an evaluation to determine etiology it is important to have a complete set of liver laboratory tests including aspartate aminotransferase, alanine aminotransferase, alkaline phosphatase, GGT, fractionated bilirubin, and coagulation studies. Each have their caveats in this setting, but together can help to form a picture. Hepatocellular evaluation is similar to that of older children. Transaminases signal liver inflammation, necrosis, or hemolysis. Low levels may mean low hepatic mass, such as in GALD. Biliary evaluation in the premature infant is more difficult and requires a detailed understanding of the measurements. Alkaline phosphatase is affected by bone disease and calcium, phosphorous, and vitamin D in the premature infant. GGT is equally problematic. GGT is reported to be high in preterm infants, although we do not know the ontogeny of those findings.[35,36] Processes that affect premature livers often lead to lower than expected GGT. An elevated GGT requires normal membrane fluidity and less GGT is synthesized in premature infants. It also requires bile acids in the duct for the detergent effect to elute the GGT into the serum.[27] Premature infants have a very low bile acid pool and they also have fewer transporters to transport those bile acids into the duct. Infection may also inhibit transport of bile acids, so a low GGT may not have the same implications as it does in the cholestatic term infant who is several weeks old. Bilirubin is complicated by large heme load, as discussed elsewhere in this article. Coagulation studies are difficult to obtain in premature babies because of the volume required in 1 free flowing draw. However, they are very helpful in determining the synthetic function of the liver and the severity of disease.

1. How critical is the liver dysfunction? Does the evaluation need to be done rapidly or can it be done in a stepwise fashion?
   a. A well and stable premature infant who develops elevated direct bilirubin with normal transaminases may only need a urine culture, thyroid studies, an ultrasound examination with doppler to look for duct and blood flow abnormalities, and a urine CMV with repeat liver tests in a week. Obtaining urine bile acids in the initial evaluation may be useful because they are easy to obtain and are not helpful after ursodeoxycholic acid is started.
   b. A sick neonate with multiorgan failure needs a more aggressive and rapid evaluation. Concerning presentations are stated in **Table 1**, and the potential actions that can tackle the aberrant mechanisms of biliary transport are described in **Table 2**.
2. Is there a treatable etiology that would improve the outcome?
   Diagnostic testing is limited by the blood volume that can be safely drawn each day. Some testing, such as hematologic and genetic studies, must be done before transfusion. Priority should be given treatable diagnoses, etiologies that would change clinical care, and monitoring for complications that require intervention. Coagulation studies are difficult to obtain in the premature infant and often require arterial puncture. However, they are one of the few ways to measure the function of the liver and thus important to obtain. It is often not practical to evaluate for every etiology on the differential diagnosis. Infections, thyroid disease, and conditions such as GALD may take priority over genetic conditions that have no therapy. Investigations that use imaging may be better tolerated than drawing large volumes of blood (**Table 3**).
3. Is there a diagnosis that would stop further invasive testing?
   Infants who present with cholestasis at birth are more likely to have genetic liver disease. They are often too small for liver biopsy. Sending genetic panels early in the course of evaluation may be useful because, by the time they are back, the course of the liver disease will be more clear. It is always important to look for infections such as UTI and CMV from breast milk because these infections are both common in the NICU. A cholangiogram via the gallbladder can define

Table 1
Table of critical presentations and associated pathophysiologic relevance

Multiorgan failure	GALD, mitochondrial, amino acids, organic acids, fatty acid oxidation defects, infection
Prolonged coagulation studies that do not correct with vitamin K	Poor synthetic function of liver
Hepatosplenomegaly at birth	Viral, storage, hemophagocytic lymphohistiocytosis, metabolic, heme disease
Elevated direct bilirubin at birth	Intrauterine process
High transaminases	Shock, ischemia, clot in liver inflow or outflow, hemolysis, muscle disease, mitochondrial
Coagulopathy with direct bilirubin and low transaminases	GALD, low liver mass
Acidosis	Metabolic disease, poor perfusion
Altered alertness	Encephalopathy, shunt
Refractory hypoglycemia	Poor liver reserve, GALD, mitochondrial disease, shunt
Prior neonatal death	Genetic disease or GALD
Elevated lactate or NH_3	Metabolic disease
Abnormal ultrasound	Vascular malformations, duct malformations, masses, umbilical venous catheter malposition
High lactate	Mitochondrial, poor liver clearance, ischemia

Table 2
Table of actions to consider for appropriate therapies to normalize liver functions

Normalization of glucose	IV drip to avoid intermittent hypoglycemia
Removal of galactose and fructose	Fructose is in most oral drugs and the sugar used for soothing, Galactose (breast milk) held until galactosemia testing done
Administration of Vitamin K	IV daily
Clotting studies	Correct if bleeding
lactate	Mitochondrial disease or poor liver clearance, supportive care
NH_3	Urea cycle or liver failure
Ferritin	GALD although not specific for this
Amino acids	Metabolic therapy as indicated
Organic acids	Metabolic therapy as indicated
Genetic panel	Multiple diseases with one sample
Microarray	Screen for genetic disease
Cultures	Bacterial and viral sepsis
Viral PCR	Rapid turn around
Acyclovir	HSV is the most common cause of liver failure in the neonate
Ultrasound examination with doppler	Flow to liver, clots or shunts that bypass the liver

Abbreviations: IV, intravenous; PCR, polymerase chain reaction.

Table 3
Causes of liver dysfunction and potential therapies

Cause	Therapy
GALD	Exchange transfusion and IgG infusion, transplantation
Viral (especially herpes)	Antivirals
Hypoxic–ischemic encephalopathy/shock	Supportive care
Tyrosinemia	2-nitro-4-trifluoromethylbenzoyl-1,3-cyclohexanedione
Biliary atresia	Surgical
Bile acid synthesis defects	Cholic acid
Amino acids, organic acids, urea cycle	Metabolic therapy, dialysis
Mitochondrial	supportive
Shunt	supportive

duct patency and structural abnormalities. Scintigraphy is often not helpful in this age group.

4. What is the blood volume required for testing? Could the information be obtained in another way, such as genetic panels, urine studies, testing parents, or imaging?

Alpha-1 antitrypsin deficiency is a part of the first tier evaluation of older term babies. There is, however, no therapy. If genetic causes of cholestasis are a concern, a genetic panel that has a somewhat longer turnaround time, but provides more information for the same amount of blood may be a better choice. Imaging is a valuable part of hepatic evaluation in the NICU. Ultrasound examination can delineate anatomy of the biliary tree even in very tiny infants. Malformation of the ducts can be seen. Doppler evaluation can define blood flow, direction of flow, and clots, as well as detecting congenital shunts. Abnormalities of flow owing to heart disease can be seen and followed. Ultrasound examination can be done at the bedside, while in an isolette, and is tolerated by even the very fragile babies. Limited magnetic resonance can be done without sedation to evaluate iron deposition for the diagnosis of GALD. Computed tomography angiograms are useful for evaluating shunts not clearly delineated by ultrasound examination. Bile duct patency is always a concern in babies with elevated direct bilirubin because of the fear of missing biliary atresia. In the last 4 years at our institution, 20 cholangiograms under ultrasound guidance through the gallbladder to define duct patency or malformations in the NICU. They are not only diagnostic, but also can be therapeutic by clearing sludge. Scintigraphy is usually not helpful in this population. It relies on the transport of the isotope by MDR2, the bilirubin transporter. This transporter is present at low levels in the preterm baby and is already occupied by bilirubin. The study also relies on bile flow to carry to isotope to the gut, once excreted. Bile flow is minimal and slow at this age, so enough isotope may not reach to gut to be detected.[37]

5. How does gestational age influence results?

The liver does not have all its bile ducts until just after term. The ducts start centrally and grow to the periphery. Many enzymes for synthesis and transport are at low levels and gradually increase toward term and in infancy.[15,17] Our understanding of this ontogeny is crude and is extrapolated from animal models. These developmental changes lead to very slow bile flow, which in turns makes secondary insults such as infection more impactful on the liver than they would be in an older child. Minor mutations in the transport of bile acids may become symptomatic because of developmental decrease at baseline. Bilirubin metabolism is also immature at a time when the baby has a very large heme load to process. The rate-limiting step is MDR2 transport of conjugated bilirubin out of the hepatocyte and into the duct. Because the preterm infant has low levels of MDR2 some of the conjugated bilirubin will back diffuse from the hepatocyte and into the plasma, as discussed elsewhere in this article. Once the bilirubin is in the duct, it is carried to the gut by bile, which has a low flow rate compared with older infants.[17] The more premature the baby is, the more pronounced these issues are.

6. Are there nutritional implications of the cholestasis the need to be addressed?

Babies with cholestasis have low luminal bile acids leading to difficulty with fat absorption. They may need supplementation of medium chain triglycerides (MCT), which can be absorbed without bile. This supplement can be added to breast milk or breast milk can be concentrated with a high MCT formula. If breast milk is not being, used a high MCT formula can be chosen. Even with high MCT, these babies may require more calories per kilogram than expected to grow appropriately. They may also require fat-soluble vitamin supplementation. It is important to remember that they may remain cholestatic and require these interventions even after the bilirubin returns to normal.

CHALLENGES AND IMPLICATIONS FOR PRACTICE

Imaging is critical to the hepatic evaluation of premature infants. Skilled technologists and pediatric radiologists are often able to define duct abnormalities and abnormal vasculature that would be otherwise missed. Subtle changes in flow and cardiac function can the impact the liver. Collaboration between the neonatologist, cardiologist and hepatologist is essential to determine optimal timing of interventions. Skilled interventional radiologists can safely do percutaneous cholangiograms through the gall bladder. Although less frequently used, magnetic resonance and computed tomography with 3-dimensional reconstruction may provide valuable information. Integrating these specialists and modalities into a team enhances care.

The understanding of genetic testing in liver disease is progressing rapidly, but is currently one of the biggest challenges in the evaluation of cholestasis in the NICU. We need better tools to evaluate which mutations are important. There is no central database collecting clinical information to correlate with test results with clinical information. We are barely beginning to look at minor mutations and the implications of gene modifiers and gene interactions in older children. We are not studying the course of premature infants with genetic mutations in liver regulation.

FUTURE DIRECTIONS

A better understanding of the ontogeny of liver maturation in the premature infant is needed along with a better understanding of secondary insults on the premature liver. Understanding the role of genetic variants in liver regulation will improve the clinicians' ability to refine testing to include these developmental and genetic considerations. The goal would be to better predict who has secondary disease that may resolve with time, who has primary or secondary liver disease that needs intervention, and to evaluate in a way better tolerated by these fragile infants.

Box 1
Considerations more common in premature than the term infant

- Prenatal insults
  - Viral
  - Genetic
  - Placental
  - Maternal disease
- Delivery complications
- Large heme loads
- Nonhepatic infections
- Vascular malformations
- Comorbidities

SUMMARY

Current pathways for the evaluation of the cholestatic infant are for the term infant who is past the perinatal period. Although all the diseases considered can and do occur in premature infants, other considerations must be included. This article can be used as a guide to the evaluation but unless an answer is readily evident, early involvement of an experienced hepatologist is warranted (**Box 1**).

Although each baby is unique, **Box 2** provides a good starting evaluation for the well-appearing premature infant with liver dysfunction.

It is often difficult to tell if the sick premature infant with liver dysfunction has primary liver disease or systemic disease that is effecting the liver. Thus, evaluation must look for both. **Box 3** provides useful studies, which should be tailored to the situation.

The evaluation of the premature infant with liver disease is very complex and has many components. Each infant is different. A systematic approach should include a careful history; evaluation of comorbidities; consideration of gestationally appropriate liver pathophysiology; consideration of genetic etiologies; an understanding of liver dysfunction; collaboration with neonatologists, radiologists, surgeons, hepatologists, pathologists, and other subspecialists; and prioritization of studies based on medical urgency.

Box 2
Well-appearing premature infant

- Check Newborn Screen
- Urine culture
- T4, TSH
- Coagulation studies
- Ultrasound examination with Doppler
- Consider genetic studies
- Consider urine bile acids
- Consider serum bile acids

> **Box 3**
> **Sick premature evaluation**
>
> Liver evaluation
>   Coagulation studies
>   Aspartate aminotransferase, alanine
>   aminotransferase, GGT, alkaline phosphatase,
>   fractionated bilirubin
>   Genetic studies
>   Lactate, glucose
>   Amino acids, organic acids
>   Newborn Screen
>   Acyl carnitine profile
>   Galactose/fructose history
>   Viral and bacterial studies
>   Ultrasound examination with Doppler
>   Ferritin
>
> Systemic evaluation
>   Head ultrasound examination
>   Heart echocardiography
>   Necrotizing enterocolitis evaluation
>   Hypoxia/shock
>   Urine and blood cultures,
>   cerebrospinal fluid indicated
>   Complete blood count
>   Acid–base studies
>   Pituitary evaluation

DISCLOSURE

The author has nothing to disclose.

REFERENCES

1. Sticova E, Jirsa M, Pawlowska J. New insights in genetic cholestasis: from molecular mechanisms to clinical implications. Can J Gastroenterol Hepatol 2018;2018: 2313675.
2. Heubi JE, Setchell KD, Bove KE. Inborn errors of bile acid metabolism. Semin Liver Dis 2007;27(3):282–94.
3. Knisely AS, Gissen P. Trafficking and transporter disorders in pediatric cholestasis. Clin Liver Dis 2010;14(4):619–33.
4. Chand N, Sanyal AJ. Sepsis-induced cholestasis. Hepatology 2007;45(1): 230–41.
5. Whiting JF, Green RM, Rosenbluth AB, et al. Tumor necrosis factor-alpha decreases hepatocyte bile salt uptake and mediates endotoxin-induced cholestasis. Hepatology 1995;22(4 Pt 1):1273–8.
6. Sambrotta M, Strautnieks S, Papouli E, et al. Mutations in TJP2 cause progressive cholestatic liver disease. Nat Genet 2014;46(4):326–8.
7. Davit-Spraul A, Gonzales E, Jacquemin E. NR1H4 analysis in patients with progressive familial intrahepatic cholestasis, drug-induced cholestasis or intrahepatic cholestasis of pregnancy unrelated to ATP8B1, ABCB11 and ABCB4 mutations. Clin Res Hepatol Gastroenterol 2012;36(6):569–73.
8. Gomez-Ospina N, Potter CJ, Xiao R, et al. Mutations in the nuclear bile acid receptor FXR cause progressive familial intrahepatic cholestasis. Nat Commun 2016;7:10713.
9. Maddirevula S, Alhebbi H, Alqahtani A, et al. Identification of novel loci for pediatric cholestatic liver disease defined by KIF12, PPM1F, USP53, LSR, and WDR83OS pathogenic variants. Genet Med 2019;21(5):1164–72.
10. van Ooteghem NA, Klomp LW, van Berge-Henegouwen GP, et al. Benign recurrent intrahepatic cholestasis progressing to progressive familial intrahepatic cholestasis: low GGT cholestasis is a clinical continuum. J Hepatol 2002;36(3): 439–43.

11. Chen HL, Li HY, Wu JF, et al. Panel-based next-generation sequencing for the diagnosis of cholestatic genetic liver diseases: clinical utility and challenges. J Pediatr 2019;205:153–9.e6.

12. Droge C, Bonus M, Baumann U, et al. Sequencing of FIC1, BSEP and MDR3 in a large cohort of patients with cholestasis revealed a high number of different genetic variants. J Hepatol 2017;67(6):1253–64.

13. Henkel SA, Squires JH, Ayers M, et al. Expanding etiology of progressive familial intrahepatic cholestasis. World J Hepatol 2019;11(5):450–63.

14. Khan HH, Mew NA, Kaufman SS, et al. Unusual cystic fibrosis transmembrane conductance regulator mutations and liver disease: a case series and review of the literature. Transplant Proc 2019;51(3):790–3.

15. Chen HL, Chen HL, Liu YJ, et al. Developmental expression of canalicular transporter genes in human liver. J Hepatol 2005;43(3):472–7.

16. Tomer G, Ananthanarayanan M, Weymann A, et al. Differential developmental regulation of rat liver canalicular membrane transporters Bsep and Mrp2. Pediatr Res 2003;53(2):288–94.

17. Heubi JE. Bile acid metabolism. In: Gluckman PD, Heymann MA, editors. Pediatrics and perinatology. 2nd edition. London: Arnold; 1996. p. 663–8.

18. Heubi JE, Balistreri WF, Suchy FJ. Bile salt metabolism in the first year of life. J Lab Clin Med 1982;100(1):127–36.

19. Watkins JB, Szczepanik P, Gould JB, et al. Bile salt metabolism in the human premature infant. Preliminary observations of pool size and synthesis rate following prenatal administration of dexamethasone and phenobarbital. Gastroenterology 1975;69(3):706–13.

20. Watkins JB, Ingall D, Szczepanik P, et al. Bile-salt metabolism in the newborn. Measurement of pool size and synthesis by stable isotope technic. N Engl J Med 1973;288(9):431–4.

21. Gao B, St Pierre MV, Stieger B, et al. Differential expression of bile salt and organic anion transporters in developing rat liver. J Hepatol 2004;41(2):201–8.

22. Goldschmidt ML, Mourya R, Connor J, et al. Increased frequency of double and triple heterozygous gene variants in children with intrahepatic cholestasis. Hepatol Res 2016;46(4):306–11.

23. Yeap SP, Harley H, Thompson R, et al. Biliary transporter gene mutations in severe intrahepatic cholestasis of pregnancy: diagnostic and management implications. J Gastroenterol Hepatol 2019;34(2):425–35.

24. Dani C, Pratesi S, Raimondi F, et al, Task Force for Hyperbilirubinemia of the Italian Society of Neonatology. Italian guidelines for the management and treatment of neonatal cholestasis. Ital J Pediatr 2015;41:69.

25. Fawaz R, Baumann U, Ekong U, et al. Guideline for the evaluation of cholestatic jaundice in infants: joint recommendations of the North American Society for Pediatric Gastroenterology, Hepatology, and Nutrition and the European Society for Pediatric Gastroenterology, Hepatology, and Nutrition. J Pediatr Gastroenterol Nutr 2017;64(1):154–68.

26. Kubitz R, Droge C, Stindt J, et al. The bile salt export pump (BSEP) in health and disease. Clin Res Hepatol Gastroenterol 2012;36(6):536–53.

27. Grammatikopoulos T, Deheragoda M, Strautnieks S, et al. Reduced hepatocellular expression of canalicular transport proteins in infants with neonatal cholestasis and congenital hypopituitarism. J Pediatr 2018;200:181–7.

28. Schmaltz C. Thyroid hormones in the neonate: an overview of physiology and clinical correlation. Adv Neonatal Care 2012;12(4):217–22.

29. Uchiyama A, Watanabe H, Nakanishi H, et al. Small for gestational age is a risk factor for the development of delayed thyrotropin elevation in infants weighing less than 2000 g. Clin Endocrinol (Oxf) 2018;89(4):431–6.
30. Lanzieri TM, Dollard SC, Josephson CD, et al. Breast milk-acquired cytomegalovirus infection and disease in VLBW and premature infants. Pediatrics 2013; 131(6):e1937–45.
31. Blanc T, Guerin F, Franchi-Abella S, et al. Congenital portosystemic shunts in children: a new anatomical classification correlated with surgical strategy. Ann Surg 2014;260(1):188–98.
32. Gupta P, Sinha A, Sodhi KS, et al. Congenital extrahepatic portosystemic shunts: spectrum of findings on ultrasound, computed tomography, and magnetic resonance imaging. Radiol Res Pract 2015;2015:181958.
33. Bernard O, Franchi-Abella S, Branchereau S, et al. Congenital portosystemic shunts in children: recognition, evaluation, and management. Semin Liver Dis 2012;32(4):273–87.
34. Ruangkit C, Satpute A, Vogt BA, et al. Incidence and risk factors of urinary tract infection in very low birth weight infants. J Neonatal Perinatal Med 2016;9(1): 83–90.
35. Kim DB, Lim G, Oh KW. Determination of reference range of gamma glutamyl transferase in the neonatal intensive care unit. J Matern Fetal Neonatal Med 2017;30(6):670–2.
36. Wang JS, Tan N, Dhawan A. Significance of low or normal serum gamma glutamyl transferase level in infants with idiopathic neonatal hepatitis. Eur J Pediatr 2006; 165(11):795–801.
37. Barseghyan K, Ramanathan R, Chavez T, et al. Utility of hepatobiliary scintigraphy in diagnosing or excluding biliary atresia in premature neonates and full-term infants with conjugated hyperbilirubinemia who received parenteral nutrition. J Matern Fetal Neonatal Med 2018;31(24):3249–54.

Human Milk Supplements
Principles, Practices, and Current Controversies

Muralidhar H. Premkumar, MBBS, DCH, DNB, MRCPCH, MS[a],*,
Leonor Adriana Massieu, RD, LD, CNSC[b],
Diane M. Anderson, PhD, RD, LD[a], Ganga Gokulakrishnan, MD, MS[a]

KEYWORDS

- Breast milk • Human milk fortification • Human milk supplement
- Extrauterine growth restriction • Macronutrients • Fortifier
- Human milk–derived fortifier • Preterm

KEY POINTS

- Although human milk is the most optimal source of nutrition, unsupplemented human milk fails to meet the energy and protein needs of the preterm infant.
- Multinutrient fortification is the most common strategy to enhance the nutritional content of human milk.
- Individual fortification is potentially a superior strategy compared with standard fortification; refinement in strategies of individual fortification is needed to improve its efficacy.
- Human milk–derived fortifier is an exciting new invention; its benefits in exclusively human milk–fed preterm infants are unclear.

INTRODUCTION

Preterm infants have an increased energy need because of deficient energy stores and rapid postnatal growth. The inability to provide optimal nutrition in preterm infants leads to extrauterine growth restriction, defined as growth less than the 10th percentile of the expected value.[1–4] The incidence of extrauterine growth restriction varies between 50% and 86%.[2,3] Postnatal nutrition and growth have a significant impact on long-term neurodevelopmental outcomes.[5,6] In a study of 124 infants, the provision of each 1 g/kg/d in protein and 10 kcal/kg/d of energy were associated with a 4.6-point increase in the Mental Development Index.[6]

Although human milk (HM) is the most optimal source of nutrition to a preterm infant, it often fails to meet the nutritional demands of the premature infant. In a study of nearly 800 breast milk samples, 56% of the samples had protein content less than

[a] Division of Neonatology, Department of Pediatrics, Baylor College of Medicine, Texas Children's Hospital, Houston, TX, USA; [b] Department of Clinical Nutrition Services, Texas Children's Hospital, Houston, TX, USA
* Corresponding author. Texas Children's Hospital, 6621 Fannin, Suite 6104, Houston, TX 77030.
E-mail address: premkuma@bcm.edu

Clin Perinatol 47 (2020) 355–368
https://doi.org/10.1016/j.clp.2020.02.001
0095-5108/20/© 2020 Elsevier Inc. All rights reserved.

1.5 g protein/dL, 79% with a fat content less than 4 g/dL, and 67% with an energy level less than 67 kcal energy/dL.[7] The energy and protein content of breast milk also varies with gestational age at birth and the period of lactation. Preterm breast milk contains higher concentrations of protein and energy compared with term breast milk.[8] After the first few weeks, the protein concentrations have been found to decrease and plateau, whereas the content of carbohydrates and fat remains stable after a gradual increase.[9]

The goal of nutritional support in a preterm infant is to achieve a postnatal weight gain that mirrors the intrauterine growth. The accepted parameters include a postnatal weight gain of greater than 15 g/kg/d, gain in the head circumference of greater than 0.9 cm/wk, and an increase in length by 0.9 cm/wk (**Table 1**).[3,5,10,11] The recommended enteral energy and protein intake to support the optimal growth of a preterm infant are 110 to 135 kcal/kg/d and 3.5 to 4.5 g/kg/d, respectively (**Table 2**).[12–14] Because of the variable and often deficient composition of macronutrients in HM, it is often challenging to meet the nutritional requirements of preterm infants. Nutritional goals are achieved by modifying the content of breast milk with the use of supplements and fortifiers. American Academy of Pediatrics (AAP) recommends routine fortification of breast milk as the standard of care in infants with birth weight less than 1500 g.[15]

CLASSIFICATION OF SUPPLEMENTS AND FORTIFIERS

According to the definitions laid down by the Food and Drug Administration, a supplement is defined as a dietary ingredient, such as a vitamin, mineral, herb or other botanic, or amino acid; dietary substance used to supplement the diet by increasing the total dietary intake; or a concentrate, metabolite, constituent, extract, or combination of the preceding substances.[16] In the literature, the terms "fortifiers" and "supplements" are often used interchangeably. Based on the number of nutrients in the composition the supplements/fortifiers are classified as:

Multinutrient fortifiers
- Bovine milk–derived multinutrient fortifiers
- HM-derived multinutrient fortifiers
- Formula products designed for preterm infants
  ○ Preterm formula
  ○ Transitional formula

Single-nutrient supplements
- Glucose polymers
- Fat emulsions and medium-chain triglyceride (MCT) preparations
- Protein fortifiers/protein concentrates
- Vitamins
- Iron

Table 1 Acceptable growth rates in preterm and term infants			
Age	Weight	Length (cm/wk)	Head Circumference (cm/wk)
Newborn infants (premature and term)			
<2 kg	15–20 g/kg/d[10,75]	0.8–1.0[11,76]	0.8–1.0[11,76]
≥2 kg	20–30 g/d[75,77]		

Data from Refs.[10,11,75–77]

Table 2
Recommended enteral intake of energy and protein in preterm and term infants

	Preterm	Term
Energy (kcal/kg/d)	110–135[12–14]	See below[14,78,a]
Protein (g/kg/d)	3.5–4.5[13,14]	1.5 (healthy)[78] 2–3 (illness/surgery)[79]

[a] 0–3 mo: estimated energy requirements (EER) = (89 × wt [kg] − 100) + 175 kcal (EER = kcal/d). *Data from* Refs.[12–14,78,79]

PRACTICES OF SUPPLEMENTATION AND FORTIFICATION
Multinutrient Fortification

Several strategies have been described for the multinutrient fortification of HM for the preterm infant.

Standard fortification
Standard fortification (SF) is the most widely used method of fortification where a fixed amount of multinutrient fortifier is added to HM. This strategy is based on an assumption of 1.5 g/dL of protein in HM.[17] The advantage of SF is its simplicity and absence of the need for complicated nutritional analyses of breast milk. A recent Cochrane meta-analysis (14 studies; n = 1071) compared SF of breast milk with unfortified breast milk in preterm infants and found that SF showed improved in-hospital growth. There was no conclusive evidence to suggest improvement in long-term growth rates or neuro-developmental outcomes.[18] Because the protein content of breast milk in later stages of lactation is frequently less than the assumed value of 1.5 g/dL, SF often fails to meet the growth demands of the preterm infant.[7,9] In a study of 127 very low birth weight (VLBW) infants, despite SF the proportion of infants with growth restriction increased at discharge from the hospital. This was associated with suboptimal delivery of energy and protein to the premature infant.[19]

Individualized fortification
A more individualized approach to fortification is to enhance the intake of a single macronutrient/fortifier based either on the physiologic response of the infant or on the macronutrient content in breast milk. Two forms of individualized fortification that have been described are adjustable fortification (AF) and targeted fortification (TF).[7,20–22]

Adjustable fortification The strategy of AF is based on the premise of a metabolic response to the protein content in the feeds. This strategy assumes a positive correlation of higher protein intake with blood urea nitrogen (BUN) or urinary urea creatinine ratios.[20,23] Arslanoglu and colleagues[20] modified the protein intake with the addition of single-nutrient protein supplements in addition to the SF to maintain BUN in the target range of 9 to 14 mg/dL. In comparison with SF, infants in the adjustable group demonstrated better weight gain and head circumference. However, BUN may not be a reliable indicator of protein intake in preterm infants because of the high rate of catabolism, and immature synthetic or renal excretory capacity.[24]

Targeted fortification In TF HM is analyzed and adjusted for macronutrients. Bulut and colleagues[24] randomized 32 VLBW infants to either AF or TF. The AF group received additional protein if BUN was less than or equal to 5 mg/dL. In the TF group, protein intakes were calculated based on spectroscopic analysis of HM, and protein supplementation was provided when the calculated intakes were less than 4.5 g/kg/d. The TF group received higher protein (4.5 vs 4.01 g/kg/d; $P = .001$), and demonstrated better weight gain and head circumference.[24] In a recent randomized controlled trial (RCT) Kadıoğlu Şimşek and colleagues[25] compared three fortification strategies of SF, AF, and TF. The weight gain in the AF and TF groups was significantly higher compared with the SF group (23.5 g/kg/d, 25.5 g/kg/d vs 12 g/kg/d; $P<.001$). Although TF seems to be an effective strategy, it requires additional equipment and staff to analyze HM, thus making it labor-intensive, and expensive.

Single Nutrient Fortification

Iron
Preterm infants have higher enteral iron requirements because they are at increased risk for iron deficiency secondary to inadequate iron stores, rapid postnatal growth, and frequent blood draws. The enteral iron requirement in preterm infants is determined to be 2 to 4 mg/kg/d.[26,27] AAP recommends supplementing exclusively and partially breastfed preterm infants with 2 mg/kg/d of iron starting at 2 weeks of age, and continued up to 12 months of age.[27] Those fortifiers, which are iron-fortified, may meet the 2 mg/kg/d of iron requirement. Because preterm formula contains more iron compared with term formula (14.6 mg/L vs 12 mg/L), infants fed exclusively with preterm formula do not require additional iron supplements.[14,26,27] Because term infants are thought to have sufficient iron stores until 4 to 6 months of age, exclusively breastfed or partially breastfed term infants should receive iron supplementation at the dose of 1 mg/kg/d starting at 4 months of age and continued until iron-fortified solid foods are introduced.[26,27]

Vitamin D
The 2008 AAP Clinical Report recommends vitamin D supplementation of 400 IU/day for all breastfed term infants starting in the first few days after birth.[28] Because all formulas in the United States contain at least 400 IU/L of vitamin D_3, formula-fed infants do not require routine vitamin D supplementation. However, infants who receive a mixture of breastfeeds and formula should still receive the full supplementation of vitamin D of 400 IU/day. In VLBW infants, vitamin D intake of 200 to 400 IU/day is recommended. In preterm infants with birth weight greater than 1500 g, the dose of vitamin D is 400 IU/day.[29] Because individual HM fortifiers (HMFs) may vary with their vitamin D content they should be evaluated for the need of additional supplementation.

Carbohydrate
These supplements are usually made of glucose polymers. Glucose polymers increase caloric density without significantly increasing osmolality and do not require lactase for digestion, which is favorable for preterm infants because they are deficient in lactase. These high-energy, low-electrolyte preparations contain maltodextrin, a glucose polymer, as the source of unflavored carbohydrate (1 g = 0.95 g of maltodextrin; 3.84 kcal/g). When this glucose polymer along with MCT oil is added to account for 10% or 20% of total caloric intake, it has been shown to only marginally increase osmolality by 3% (325 mOsm/kg) and 7% (336 mOsm/kg), respectively.[30] In the systematic review by Amissah and colleagues[31] only one very-low-quality study was included, which did not have enough evidence to support the short-term or long-term effects of such supplementation.

Protein
Protein concentrates are usually bovine in origin and contain either intact or hydrolyzed protein. These supplements are often administered in a varied dose along

with another multinutrient fortifier as part of AF or TF strategies as described previously.[20,24] In a Cochrane meta-analysis (6 studies; n = 204; very-low-quality evidence) Amissah and colleagues[32] compared the effectiveness and safety of breast milk supplemented with protein to unsupplemented breast milk in preterm infants. Preterm infants fed with protein-supplemented breast milk showed better in-hospital growth rates. No data were available about long-term neurodevelopmental outcomes. The disadvantages of using protein supplements are the volume displacement of the breast milk and high osmolality. The addition of a single-protein supplement to a multinutrient fortifier has been shown to increase the osmolality as high as 484 mOsm/kg.[33] This strategy of a single protein supplementation is scarcely practiced in isolation but rather prescribed in combination with multinutrient fortifiers.[20,34,35]

Fat

Fat supplements are available as microlipids or MCT oils.[36] Fat supplements serve as a calorie-dense source, without increasing the osmolality of feeds. Combinations of microlipid and fish oil have also been used in the rehabilitation of infants with intestinal failure.[37] Amissah and colleagues[38] performed a systematic review comparing breast milk supplemented with fat to unsupplemented breast milk in preterm infants. Only one small study of very low quality was included where the intervention group received 1 g of HM fat/100 mL. No difference was noted for in-hospital growth rates or feed intolerance. In a study by Hair and colleagues,[39] HM-derived cream supplementation was provided to preterm infants on an exclusive HM-derived diet. The addition of HM-derived cream supplementation resulted in better weight (14.0 ± 2.5 vs 12.4 ± 3.0 g/kg/d; P = .03) and length (1.03 ± 0.33 vs 0.83 ± 0.41 cm/wk; P = .02). Based on currently available evidence, the utility of fat supplement is restricted to the following: as a sole fat supplement in children with intestinal failure and in combination with multinutrient fortification to further increase energy content.

CONTROVERSIES
Use of Hydrolyzed Protein Formula and Fortifiers in Preterm Infants

Hydrolyzed protein formulas were initially developed to treat infants found to have cow's milk protein allergy. These formulas contain protein digested either chemically or enzymatically into oligopeptides.[40] Hydrolyzed protein formulas are generally classified as

1. Partially hydrolyzed formulas: peptides with molecular weights of 3 to 10 kDa
2. Extensively hydrolyzed formulas: peptides with molecular weights of less than 3 kDa
3. Elemental formulas: amino acid–based.

Of note, only extensively hydrolyzed and elemental formulas are considered to be hypoallergenic.[40,41] Such formulas have also been used in the preterm population because it is often perceived to improve feeding tolerance, and as a feeding strategy following necrotizing enterocolitis (NEC) and gastrointestinal surgeries.[42,43] Although its property as a hypoallergenic formula in term infants is well described, the reported usefulness in preterm infants is unclear. A recent Cochrane systematic review by Ng and colleagues[44] reviewed a total of 11 trials comparing preterm infants less than 34 weeks gestational age fed protein hydrolysate feeds with those fed with the standard formula. This review failed to show any difference in either the feeding intolerance or the risk of NEC with the use of hydrolysate feeds in preterm infants. Additionally, the most recent AAP Clinical report has stated that there is a paucity of evidence to support the use of hydrolyzed formulas as a prevention strategy against atopy or cow's milk protein allergy.[45]

There are several commercially available bovine multinutrient milk fortifiers composed of either intact or hydrolyzed protein. When hydrolyzed, the extent of protein digestion varies from partially to extensively hydrolyzed. In the United States, all the powdered multinutrient fortifiers contain intact protein, whereas liquid HMFs contain hydrolyzed protein. As mentioned elsewhere in this review, the use of powdered HMF is discouraged because of concerns for *Cronobacter sakazakii* infection. In studies comparing liquid HMFs containing hydrolyzed protein with intact protein, weight gain and the incidence of feed intolerance was similar between groups.[46,47]

Use of Powdered Versus Liquid Fortifiers

Powdered formula and fortifiers are not commercially sterile; hence they carry a risk of bacterial contamination. Several instances of *C sakazakii* infections have been reported in infants following exposure to the artificial formula.[48,49] In a report published in 2012, 99% of the infants with invasive *Cronobacter* were less than 2 month old. Ninety percent of those cases were exposed to powdered infant formula or HMF, whereas only 23% to 26% were exposed to breast milk or ready-to-feed (RTF) formula.[50] These contaminations have been sourced to the powdered product, and the techniques of preparation at the consumer end. Such events have led to widespread changes to reduce the risk of *Cronobacter* infection globally and nationally. These include minimum standards for formula companies and recommendations to decrease the risk for *C Sakazakii* infection. Kim and colleagues[46] compared the liquid HMF (Abbott Nutrition, Columbus, OH) with powdered intact protein HMF (Similac Human Milk Fortifier, Abbott Nutrition) and found that infants in liquid HMF group received significantly higher protein (3.9 g/kg/d vs 3.3 g/kg/d; $P<.0001$). Both fortifiers were well tolerated and both groups demonstrated adequate growth. Similar findings of safety and noninferiority of liquid HMF over powdered HMF has been shown in other studies.[47] In 2002, the US Centers for Disease Control and Prevention and Food and Drug Administration recommended the use of alternatives to powdered formulas in the neonatal intensive care unit, such as breast milk, liquid fortifiers, or RTF formula.[48]

ACIDIFIED LIQUID HUMAN MILK FORTIFIER VERSUS NONACIDIFIED LIQUID HUMAN MILK FORTIFIER

As a result of concerns of contamination with powdered HMF, several liquid fortifiers were introduced to ensure sterility. Broadly there are two types of liquid HMFs based on the method used for sterilization: acidified liquid HMF (AL-HMF) and nonacidified liquid HMF (NAL-HMF). Both these products also contain higher protein thus minimizing the need for further fortification. In two retrospective studies, it has been shown that the use of an AL-HMF fortifier resulted in significant metabolic acidosis, impaired growth, and possibly increased the risk of NEC.[51,52] In one study, 120 infants received one of the three interventions: powdered HMF, AL-HMF, or NAL-HMF. AL-HMF infants received higher calories and proteins, but demonstrated slower growth compared with powdered HMF and NAL-HMF (median 10.59 vs 15.37, 14.03 g/kg/d; $P<.0001$), respectively. Also, AL-HMF infants demonstrated lower serum bicarbonate levels after Day 14 and 30 compared with NAL-HMF.[52] Schanler and colleagues performed an RCT comparing AL-HMF with NAL-HMF in which 164 infants participated. In this trial, although the weight gain in the first 29 days was similar, the AL-HMF group demonstrated more metabolic acidosis (27% vs 5%; $P<.001$) and feed intolerance.[53] However, it was pointed out that in this nonblinded industry-sponsored trial, there were no differences in the main study outcome of growth. It has been questioned whether biochemical acidosis such as these, a regular feature in the first few days of the life of an extremely low birth weight, is clinically relevant.[54] Currently, AL-HMF and NAL-HMF are commercially available and seem to have comparable growth outcomes. Despite unclear benefits over one another, liquid fortifiers, whether acidified or not, should be used when available given the lower risk for contamination and possible infection. One disadvantage of liquid HMF compared with powdered HMF is the excess amount of displacement of human breast milk, thus diminishing the benefits of breast milk.

INSTANCES WHERE THE STANDARD FORTIFICATION PROCESS MAY BE INADEQUATE

Often because of increased energy demands, preterm infants may not achieve optimal growth despite enteral feeding volumes of 160 to 180 mL/kg/d with SF. Clinicians also resort to fluid restriction with feed volumes restricted to 120 to 150 mL/kg/d in such scenarios as chronic lung disease, patent ductus arteriosus, or intolerance to larger feeding volumes. In such situations, infants' growth needs are not met even with SF strategies, placing them at higher risk for poor growth and metabolic bone disease. Fortification of human breast milk using a higher fortifier to HM ratio, or with RTF preterm formula (30 kcal/oz) is often tried to increase the nutritional content. Replacing breast milk with transitional formula or RTF for a few feeds can also increase the nutrition delivery without the hassle of mixing feeds. With the advent of HM-derived fortifiers and cream, it is possible to concentrate to 24, 26, 28, and 30 kcal/oz.[55,56] However, all these alternative approaches are not extensively studied and carry some risks. Fortification of bovine milk–based fortifiers beyond 24 kcal/oz with different HM to fortifier ratio maintains the balance of nutrients but increases osmolality and renal solute load, and should be used with caution.[57] Single-nutrient additives that are in powdered form are associated with the risk of bacterial contamination. The practice of providing extra feeds of enriched preterm formula displaces HM, thus depleting the benefits of breast milk.

EXCLUSIVE HUMAN MILK–BASED DIET VERSUS BOVINE MILK–BASED DIET

Minimizing the risk of NEC is an important factor taken into consideration when devising feeding strategies for preterm infants. With improved ability to sustain increasingly smaller preterm infants, NEC continues to remain a significant challenge.[39,58–62] In numerous studies, HM feeding has been shown to be the most important nutritional intervention that decreases the risk of NEC.[63,64] Sisk and colleagues[64] have demonstrated HM to have a dose-dependent protective effect against NEC. Infants who received HM greater than 50% of their enteral intake had a significantly lower incidence of NEC compared with those infants who received HM less than 50% intake (10.6% vs 3.2%). In the Cochrane meta-analysis comparing donor HM with formula feeding, the use of formula feeding was associated with an increased risk for NEC (relative risk, 1.87; 95% confidence interval, 1.23–2.85).[65]

To study the effects of an exclusive HM diet, Sullivan and colleagues compared bovine milk–derived multinutrient fortifier with a lactoengineered HM-derived multinutrient fortifier.[61] The HM-derived fortifier group received donor milk if mother's own milk was unavailable and fortification was initiated at either 40 mL/kg/d (HM 40) or 100 mL/kg/d (HM 100). In contrast, those infants who received bovine milk–derived HMF were fed with formula when mother's milk was insufficient, and fortification was initiated at 100 mL/kg/d of feeds (bovine). The incidence of NEC in HM 40, HM 100, and bovine groups were 1.7%, 3.2%, and 15.3%, respectively (P<.05). In this study, the infants who received HM-derived HMF demonstrated a 90% reduction in the incidence of surgical NEC. Studies of similar design have shown similar benefits with the use of HM-derived fortifier.[58,66–68] However, the major criticism of this design was the use of formula in the control group instead of donor milk to supplement the mother's own milk. O'Connor and colleagues[69] conducted a study in which the control and the intervention arms received only HM, either as the mother's own milk or donor milk. The control arm received the bovine milk–derived multinutrient fortifier, whereas the intervention group received HM-derived multinutrient fortifier. In this study of 125 infants, there was no difference in the incidence of NEC (4.9% vs 4.7%; $P = .95$) or feeding intolerance. Thus, although it is clear that HM feeding has a dose-dependent protective effect against NEC, whether HM-derived fortifier has an additional protective effect in decreasing the incidence of NEC in exclusively breast milk–fed preterm infants remains uncertain.

FUTURE DIRECTIONS

As medical advances continue to lower the thresholds of prematurity, the clinicians' ability to optimize nutritional strategies in a preterm neonate has become even more challenging. Advances in technology, diagnostics, and bioengineering have resulted in numerous discoveries and inventions that in turn show immense potential to improve short- and long-term outcomes of this vulnerable preterm population. Next we highlight some of the areas that might benefit from further attention and research.

Rigorous Research of Exclusive Human Milk Diets

Although HM has undoubtedly been shown to benefit preterm infants in myriad ways it must be acknowledged that knowledge gaps exist. There is a need to build a robust evidence base for the use of HM-derived fortifier in preterm infants with high or exclusive use of breast milk. However, such research endeavors might be challenging considering the lack of equipoise concerning HM-derived multinutrient fortifier among neonatal providers and families of preterm infants. Although lactoengineering of HM has resulted in HM-derived multinutrient fortifiers and cream supplements as described previously, the next step is to manufacture a cost-effective version of these supplements so that preterm infants in resource-limited settings can also benefit from the advances in lactoengineering.

Alternate Protein Sources

Concerns regarding sensitization to a bovine protein have spurred the research into search for alternative sources for HM supplements. Investigations are underway in Denmark evaluating the safety and efficacy of bovine colostrum–based products. This research was spurred by encouraging animal data from piglet models where bovine colostrum, when compared with formula feeding, was shown to demonstrate better preservation of gut function and enhanced antibacterial defense when used to fortify donor HM[70]. The notion that the protective qualities of colostrum are species-specific has now been questioned. Investigators from Italy have recently published a study protocol for an RCT of a novel fortifier and protein supplement derived from donkey milk.[71] They hypothesize that when compared with bovine milk, donkey milk is biochemically more similar to HM. If donkey milk–derived fortifiers were shown to be beneficial, neonatal nutrition would be entering an exciting new direction, opening further avenues of research.

Neonatal Nutritional Interventions on Sex-Specific Effects and Long-term Programming

There is emerging evidence to suggest that fetuses and neonates experience sex-specific effects with regard to growth, nutrition, and metabolism.[72,73,74] This is further evidenced by data from investigators in New Zealand who demonstrated that preterm lambs receiving nutritional supplementation exhibited sex-specific differences in glucose tolerance as adults, highlighting the likely programming effects that need to be considered when studying fortification practices.[73] These findings in insulin resistance also correlated with the expression of key genes in β-cell development. Discoveries such as these highlight the paucity of knowledge when it comes to the sex-specific effects of neonatal nutrition including fortification on long-term metabolic health.

Translating and Implementing Best Practices in Resource-Limited Settings

Most clinical studies are performed in resource-rich, higher-income countries in Europe and the Americas. There is a dearth of studies performed on populations in resource-poor and low-income settings, making it difficult to translate these findings

---

Best Practices Box

Fortification of Human Milk

Best practice
- In term infants, exclusive breastfeeding is recommended in the first 6 months[15]
- All preterm infants should receive HM[15]
- Provide fortified HM for infants with birth weight less than 1500 g[15]
- Avoid powdered fortifiers and powdered formula as much as possible in infants less than 2 months[50]
- Supplement vitamins and iron to meet needs when appropriate[14,27]

What changes in current practice are likely to improve outcomes?
- Improved rates of breast milk production and its use
- Increased amount of HM fed to preterm infants
- Better fortification strategies of HM feeds in preterm infants

Major Recommendations:
- Provide the mother's milk to premature infants, using donor HM when maternal milk is not available (Moderate quality evidence; Strong recommendation)
- Fortify HM with HMFs in infants <1500 g (Low quality evidence; Strong recommendation)
- Provide 400 units of vitamin D/day to partially and fully breastfed infants (Low quality evidence; Strong recommendation)
- Provide at least 2 mg/kg/d iron to partially and fully breastfed preterm infants until 1 year of age (Low quality evidence; Strong recommendation)
- Use an individualized fortification strategy (Very low quality evidence; Weak recommendation)
- Avoid the use of powdered fortifiers when possible in premature infants (Very low quality evidence; Strong recommendation)
- Use HM-based fortifier in premature infants fed exclusively with HM (Low quality evidence; Weak recommendation)

Summary Statement:

Supplementation of HM feeds with fortifiers where appropriate in term and preterm infants improves their short-term growth. Additional studies are required to show their impact on long-term growth and neurodevelopment.

Data from Refs.[14,15,27,50]

to such settings. Future research needs to address this issue and broaden the scope of such important interventions.

REFERENCES

1. Clark RH, Thomas P, Peabody J. Extrauterine growth restriction remains a serious problem in prematurely born neonates. Pediatrics 2003;111(5 Pt 1):986–90.
2. Dusick AM, Poindexter BB, Ehrenkranz RA, et al. Growth failure in the preterm infant: can we catch up? Semin Perinatol 2003;27(4):302–10.
3. Griffin IJ, Tancredi DJ, Bertino E, et al. Postnatal growth failure in very low birth-weight infants born between 2005 and 2012. Arch Dis Child Fetal Neonatal Ed 2016;101(1):F50–5.
4. Su BH. Optimizing nutrition in preterm infants. Pediatr Neonatol 2014;55(1):5–13.
5. Ehrenkranz RA, Dusick AM, Vohr BR, et al. Growth in the neonatal intensive care unit influences neurodevelopmental and growth outcomes of extremely low birth weight infants. Pediatrics 2006;117(4):1253–61.
6. Stephens BE, Walden RV, Gargus RA, et al. First-week protein and energy intakes are associated with 18-month developmental outcomes in extremely low birth weight infants. Pediatrics 2009;123(5):1337–43.
7. de Halleux V, Rigo J. Variability in human milk composition: benefit of individualized fortification in very-low-birth-weight infants. Am J Clin Nutr 2013;98(2): 529S–35S.
8. Bauer J, Gerss J. Longitudinal analysis of macronutrients and minerals in human milk produced by mothers of preterm infants. Clin Nutr 2011;30(2):215–20.
9. Maly J, Burianova I, Vitkova V, et al. Preterm human milk macronutrient concentration is independent of gestational age at birth. Arch Dis Child Fetal Neonatal Ed 2019;104(1):F50–6.
10. Fenton TR, Anderson D, Groh-Wargo S, et al. An attempt to standardize the calculation of growth velocity of preterm infants-evaluation of practical bedside methods. J Pediatr 2018;196:77–83.
11. Ehrenkranz RA, Younes N, Lemons JA, et al. Longitudinal growth of hospitalized very low birth weight infants. Pediatrics 1999;104(2 Pt 1):280–9.
12. Agostoni C, Buonocore G, Carnielli VP, et al. Enteral nutrient supply for preterm infants: commentary from the European Society of Paediatric Gastroenterology, Hepatology and Nutrition Committee on Nutrition. J Pediatr Gastroenterol Nutr 2010;50(1):85–91.
13. Koletzko B, Poindexter B, Uauy R. Recommended nutrient intake levels for stable, fully enterally fed very low birth weight infants. World Rev Nutr Diet 2014;110: 297–9.
14. American Academy of Pediatrics Committee on Nutrition. Feeding the infant. In: Kleinman RE, Greer FR, editors. Pediatric nutrition. Itasca (IL): American Academy of Pediatrics; 2019. p. 113–62.
15. Johnston M, Landers S, Noble L, Section on Breastfeeding. Breastfeeding and the use of human milk. Pediatrics 2012;129(3):e827–41.
16. Food and Drug Administration, Dietary supplement products & ingredients. Food/Dietary Supplements 2019 06-19-209. Available at: https://www.fda.gov/food/dietary-supplements/dietary-supplement-products-ingredients.   Accessed October 20, 2019.
17. Adamkin DH, Radmacher PG. Fortification of human milk in very low birth weight infants (VLBW <1500 g birth weight). Clin Perinatol 2014;41(2):405–21.

18. Brown JV, Embleton ND, Harding JE, et al. Multi-nutrient fortification of human milk for preterm infants. Cochrane Database Syst Rev 2016;(5):CD000343.

19. Henriksen C, Westerberg AC, Ronnestad A, et al. Growth and nutrient intake among very-low-birth-weight infants fed fortified human milk during hospitalisation. Br J Nutr 2009;102(8):1179–86.

20. Arslanoglu S, Moro GE, Ziegler EE. Adjustable fortification of human milk fed to preterm infants: does it make a difference? J Perinatol 2006;26(10):614–21.

21. Picaud JC, Houeto N, Buffin R, et al. Additional protein fortification is necessary in extremely low-birth-weight infants fed human milk. J Pediatr Gastroenterol Nutr 2016;63(1):103–5.

22. Rochow N, Fusch G, Choi A, et al. Target fortification of breast milk with fat, protein, and carbohydrates for preterm infants. J Pediatr 2013;163(4):1001–7.

23. Mathes M, Maas C, Bleeker C, et al. Effect of increased enteral protein intake on plasma and urinary urea concentrations in preterm infants born at < 32 weeks gestation and < 1500 g birth weight enrolled in a randomized controlled trial: a secondary analysis. BMC Pediatr 2018;18(1):154.

24. Bulut O, Coban A, Uzunhan O, et al. Effects of targeted versus adjustable protein fortification of breast milk on early growth in very low-birth-weight preterm infants: a randomized clinical trial. Nutr Clin Pract 2019. https://doi.org/10.1002/ncp. 10307.

25. Kadıoğlu Şimşek G, Alyamac Dizdar E, Arayici S, et al. Comparison of the effect of three different fortification methods on growth of very low birth weight infants. Breastfeed Med 2019;14(1):63–8.

26. Baker RD, Greer FR, Committee on Nutrition American Academy of Pediatrics. Diagnosis and prevention of iron deficiency and iron-deficiency anemia in infants and young children (0-3 years of age). Pediatrics 2010;126(5):1040–50.

27. American Academy of Pediatrics Committee on Nutrition. Micronutrients and macronutrients. In: Kleinman RE, Greer FR, editors. Pediatric nutrition. Itasca (IL): American Academy of Pediatrics; 2019. p. 561–90.

28. Wagner CL, Greer RF, The Section on Breastfeeding and The Committee on Nutrition American Academy of Pediatrics. Prevention of rickets and vitamin D deficiency in infants, children, and adolescents. Pediatrics 2008;122(5):1142–52.

29. Abrams SA, Committee on Nutrients. Calcium and Vitamin D requirements of enterally fed preterm infants. Pediatrics 2013;131(5):e1676–83.

30. Pereira-da-Silva L, Dias MP, Virella D, et al. Osmolality of preterm formulas supplemented with nonprotein energy supplements. Eur J Clin Nutr 2008;62(2): 274–8.

31. Amissah EA, Brown J, Harding JE. Carbohydrate supplementation of human milk to promote growth in preterm infants. Cochrane Database Syst Rev 2018;(8):CD000280.

32. Amissah EA, Brown J, Harding JE. Protein supplementation of human milk for promoting growth in preterm infants. Cochrane Database Syst Rev 2018;(6):CD000433.

33. Kreins N, Buffin R, Michel-Molnar D, et al. Individualized fortification influences the osmolality of human milk. Front Pediatr 2018;6:322.

34. Puangco MA, Schanler RJ. Clinical experience in enteral nutrition support for premature infants with bronchopulmonary dysplasia. J Perinatol 2000;20(2):87–91.

35. Rigo J, Hascoet JM, Billeaud C, et al. Growth and nutritional biomarkers of preterm infants fed a new powdered human milk fortifier: a randomized trial. J Pediatr Gastroenterol Nutr 2017;65(4):e83–93.

36. Berseth CL, Harris CL, Wampler JL, et al. Liquid human milk fortifier significantly improves docosahexaenoic and arachidonic acid status in preterm infants. Prostaglandins Leukot Essent Fatty Acids 2014;91(3):97–103.

37. Yang Q, Ayers K, Chen Y, et al. Early enteral fat supplement and fish oil increases fat absorption in the premature infant with an enterostomy. J Pediatr 2013;163(2):429–34.

38. Amissah EA, Brown J, Harding JE. Fat supplementation of human milk for promoting growth in preterm infants. Cochrane Database Syst Rev 2018;(6):CD000341.

39. Hair AB, Blanco CL, Moreira AG, et al. Randomized trial of human milk cream as a supplement to standard fortification of an exclusive human milk-based diet in infants 750-1250 g birth weight. J Pediatr 2014;165(5):915–20.

40. Sampson HA, Bernhisel-Broadbent J, Yang E, et al. Safety of casein hydrolysate formula in children with cow milk allergy. J Pediatr 1991;118(4 Pt 1):520–5.

41. Sampson HA, James JM, Bernhisel-Broadbent J. Safety of an amino acid-derived infant formula in children allergic to cow milk. Pediatrics 1992;90(3):463–5.

42. Hays T, Wood RA. A systematic review of the role of hydrolyzed infant formulas in allergy prevention. Arch Pediatr Adolesc Med 2005;159(9):810–6.

43. Miller M, Burjonrappa S. A review of enteral strategies in infant short bowel syndrome: evidence-based or NICU culture? J Pediatr Surg 2013;48(5):1099–112.

44. Ng DHC, Klassen JR, Embleton ND, et al. Protein hydrolysate versus standard formula for preterm infants. Cochrane Database Syst Rev 2019;(7):CD012412.

45. Greer FR, Sicherer SH, Burks AW, et al. The effects of early nutritional interventions on the development of atopic disease in infants and children: the role of maternal dietary restriction, breastfeeding, hydrolyzed formulas, and timing of introduction of allergenic complementary foods. Pediatrics 2019;143(4) [pii: e20190281].

46. Kim JH, Chan G, Schanler R, et al. Growth and tolerance of preterm infants fed a new extensively hydrolyzed liquid human milk fortifier. J Pediatr Gastroenterol Nutr 2015;61(6):665–71.

47. Moya F, Sisk PM, Walsh KR, et al. A new liquid human milk fortifier and linear growth in preterm infants. Pediatrics 2012;130(4):e928–35.

48. Centers for Disease Control and Prevention. Enterobacter sakazakii infections associated with the use of powdered infant formula—Tennessee, 2001. MMWR Morb Mortal Wkly Rep 2002;51(14):297–300.

49. Centers for Disease Control and Prevention. Cronobacter species isolation in two infants—New Mexico, 2008. MMWR Morb Mortal Wkly Rep 2009;58(42):1179–83.

50. Jason J. Prevention of invasive Cronobacter infections in young infants fed powdered infant formulas. Pediatrics 2012;130(5):e1076–84.

51. Cibulskis CC, Armbrecht ES. Association of metabolic acidosis with bovine milk-based human milk fortifiers. J Perinatol 2015;35(2):115–9.

52. Thoene M, Lyden E, Weishaar K, et al. Comparison of a powdered, acidified liquid, and non-acidified liquid human milk fortifier on clinical outcomes in premature infants. Nutrients 2016;8(8) [pii:E451].

53. Schanler RJ, Groh-Wargo SL, Barrett-Reis B, et al. Improved outcomes in preterm infants fed a nonacidified liquid human milk fortifier: a prospective randomized clinical trial. J Pediatr 2018;202:31–7.e2.

54. Ziegler EE. Equivalence of fortifiers. J Pediatr 2019;205:291.

55. Choi A, Fusch G, Rochow N, et al. Target fortification of breast milk: predicting the final osmolality of the feeds. PLoS One 2016;11(2):e0148941.

56. Fomon SJ, Ziegler EE. Renal solute load and potential renal solute load in infancy. J Pediatr 1999;134(1):11–4.

57. Stoll BJ, Hansen NI, Bell EF, et al. Trends in care practices, morbidity, and mortality of extremely preterm neonates, 1993-2012. JAMA 2015;314(10):1039–51.

58. Cristofalo EA, Schanler RJ, Blanco CL, et al. Randomized trial of exclusive human milk versus preterm formula diets in extremely premature infants. J Pediatr 2013; 163(6):1592–5.e1.

59. Lucas A, Gore SM, Cole TJ, et al. Multicentre trial on feeding low birthweight infants: effects of diet on early growth. Arch Dis Child 1984;59(8):722–30.

60. Lucas A, Morley R, Cole TJ. Randomised trial of early diet in preterm babies and later intelligence quotient. BMJ 1998;317(7171):1481–7.

61. Sullivan S, Schanler RJ, Kim JH, et al. An exclusively human milk-based diet is associated with a lower rate of necrotizing enterocolitis than a diet of human milk and bovine milk-based products. J Pediatr 2010;156(4):562–7.e1.

62. Tyson JE, Lasky RE, Mize CE, et al. Growth, metabolic response, and development in very-low-birth-weight infants fed banked human milk or enriched formula. I. Neonatal findings. J Pediatr 1983;103(1):95–104.

63. Sisk PM, Lambeth TM, Rojas MA, et al. Necrotizing enterocolitis and growth in preterm infants fed predominantly maternal milk, pasteurized donor milk, or preterm formula: a retrospective study. Am J Perinatol 2017;34(7):676–83.

64. Sisk PM, Lovelady CA, Dillard RG, et al. Early human milk feeding is associated with a lower risk of necrotizing enterocolitis in very low birth weight infants. J Perinatol 2007;27(7):428–33.

65. Quigley M, Embleton ND, McGuire W. Formula versus donor breast milk for feeding preterm or low birth weight infants. Cochrane Database Syst Rev 2019;(7):CD002971.

66. Ganapathy V, Hay JW, Kim JH. Costs of necrotizing enterocolitis and cost-effectiveness of exclusively human milk-based products in feeding extremely premature infants. Breastfeed Med 2012;7(1):29–37.

67. Ghandehari H, Lee ML, Rechtman DJ, et al. An exclusive human milk-based diet in extremely premature infants reduces the probability of remaining on total parenteral nutrition: a reanalysis of the data. BMC Res Notes 2012;5:188.

68. Hair AB, Hawthorne KM, Chetta KE, et al. Human milk feeding supports adequate growth in infants </= 1250 grams birth weight. BMC Res Notes 2013;6:459.

69. O'Connor DL, Kiss A, Tomlinson C, et al. Nutrient enrichment of human milk with human and bovine milk-based fortifiers for infants born weighing <1250 g: a randomized clinical trial. Am J Clin Nutr 2018;108(1):108–16.

70. Sun J, Li Y, Pan X, et al. Human milk fortification with bovine colostrum is superior to formula-based fortifiers to prevent gut dysfunction, necrotizing enterocolitis, and systemic infection in preterm pigs. JPEN J Parenter Enteral Nutr 2019; 43(2):252–62.

71. Coscia A, Bertino E, Tonetto P, et al. Nutritional adequacy of a novel human milk fortifier from donkey milk in feeding preterm infants: study protocol of a randomized controlled clinical trial. Nutr J 2018;17(1):6.

72. Alur P. Sex differences in nutrition, growth, and metabolism in preterm infants. Front Pediatr 2019;7:22.

73. Jaquiery AL, Park SS, Phua HH, et al. Brief neonatal nutritional supplementation has sex-specific effects on glucose tolerance and insulin regulating genes in juvenile lambs. Pediatr Res 2016;80(6):861–9.

74. Berry MJ, Jaquiery AL, Oliver MH, et al. Neonatal milk supplementation in lambs has persistent effects on growth and metabolic function that differ by sex and gestational age. Br J Nutr 2016;116(11):1912–25.

75. Ziegler EE. Protein requirements of very low birth weight infants. J Pediatr Gastro-enterol Nutr 2007;45(Suppl 3):S170–4.
76. Moyer-Mileur LJ. Anthropometric and laboratory assessment of very low birth weight infants: the most helpful measurements and why. Semin Perinatol 2007; 31(2):96–103.
77. WHO Multicentre Growth Reference Study Group. WHO Child Growth Standards, in length/height-for-age, weight-for-age, weight-for-length, weight-for-height and body mass index-for-age: methods and development. Geneva (Switzerland): World Health Organization; 2006.
78. Institute of Medicine. Dietary reference intakes for energy, carbohydrate, fiber, fat, fatty acids, cholesterol, protein, and amino acids. Washington, DC: The National Academies Press; 2005.
79. Mehta NM, Compher C, A.S.P.E.N. Board of Directors. A.S.P.E.N. clinical guidelines: nutrition support of the critically ill child. JPEN J Parenter Enteral Nutr 2009; 33(3):260–76.

Gut Injury and the Microbiome in Neonates

Mohan Pammi, MD, PhD[a],*, Emily Hollister, PhD[b], Josef Neu, MD[c]

KEYWORDS

- Gut • Injury • Microbiome • Inflammation • Neonate • Metagenomics • Sequencing

KEY POINTS

- There are many predisposing factors that lead to neonatal intestinal injury. These include ischemia, tissue hypoxia, microbial dysbiosis, and food protein allergy.
- Commensal bacteria in the developing gut microbiome are essential for immune tolerance and the relative role of dysbiosis and inflammation that predispose to intestinal injury remains unclear.
- Optimizing the gut microbiome and strategies to decrease intestinal injury are key to improve neonatal outcomes.

OUTLINE

1. Introduction
2. Neonatal gut injury
   a. Modes of neonatal gut injury
      i. Intestinal ischemia and reperfusion injury
      ii. Food protein–induced enterocolitis syndrome
      iii. Spontaneous intestinal perforation
      iv. Transfusion associated gut injury
   b. Potential mechanisms for gut injury
      i. Vascular mediators
      ii. Defective development of the intestinal microvasculature and impaired microcirculation
      iii. Genetic predilection
      iv. Role of growth factors
3. Infant microbiome and gut injury interactions
4. Recent advances

[a] Section of Neonatology, Department of Pediatrics, Baylor College of Medicine and Texas Children's Hospital, 6621, Fannin, WT 6-104, Houston, TX 77030 USA; [b] Diversigen, Inc, Information Technology and Analytics, 2450 Holcombe Boulevard, Suite BCMA, Houston, TX 77021, USA; [c] Section of Neonatology, Department of Pediatrics, University of Florida, 1600 SW Archer Road, Gainesville, FL 32610, USA
* Corresponding author.
E-mail address: mohanv@bcm.edu

Clin Perinatol 47 (2020) 369–382
https://doi.org/10.1016/j.clp.2020.02.010
0095-5108/20/© 2020 Elsevier Inc. All rights reserved.

5. Current controversies
6. Summary

INTRODUCTION

Several forms of neonatal intestinal injury have been clustered under the term "necro-tizing enterocolitis" (NEC). We are beginning to recognize that what is called "NEC" is likely several different disease entities similar to diabetes.[1] Unfortunately, the different categories of intestinal injury that have been called "NEC" still have not been clearly differentiated, and the disease has not clearly been defined, if in fact a discrete disease does exist. Here, the authors take the opportunity to better delineate some of the categories of intestinal injury that have been classified as "NEC" in order to develop clearer targets for development of more sensitive and specific diagnostic bio-markers and in the same manner preventative and therapeutic strategies.

NEONATAL GUT INJURY

The intestinal mucosa and its innate and adaptive immune systems serve as a defense against intestinal injury initiated by both physical and biological agents, including harmful microbes and other sensitizing antigens.[2] The tight junctions of the epithelial cells act as a barrier to bacterial translocation and entry of bacterial antigens. Mucus (mucin) secreted by the goblet cells of the mucosa also acts as a protective barrier and may influence host-microbe interactions.[3] Immunoglobulins, especially immunoglob-ulin A (IgA), various immune cell types, enzymes such as intestinal alkaline phospha-tase, as well as exogenous factors found in milk (especially, when derived from the babies' own mothers) play important protective roles.[4,5] In preterm infants, the under-development of mucosal barriers and associated dysmotility of the gastrointestinal (GI) tract that leads to stasis and prolonged exposure to antigens and other noxious elements may predispose to intestinal injury.

Modes of Neonatal Gut Injury

Intestinal ischemia and reperfusion injury
Congenital heart disease is a risk factor for intestinal injury in term and preterm infants. Univentricular heart disease, such as hypoplastic left heart syndrome, and those with large left-to-right shunts, such as truncus arteriosus or aorto-pulmonary window, are associated with high risk of intestinal injury.[6–8] Hypoperfusion and ischemic states may trigger a strong innate immune response, which may partly explain the develop-ment of intestinal injury in these conditions.[9] The outcomes in ischemic gut injury owing to cardiac disease are less severe than those of traditional NEC in preterm in-fants.[8] Moreover, the risk of gut injury can be decreased by optimizing splanchnic cir-culation, and there is a good reason to call this gut injury "cardiogenic ischemic necrosis of the intestine."[1]

Food protein–induced enterocolitis syndrome
Many cases have been reported in infants whereby abdominal distension, bloody stools, discoloration of the abdomen, and pneumatosis intestinalis were related to cow's milk protein in the feeds, and the clinical condition got better when food protein was eliminated.[10] Food protein–induced enterocolitis syndrome (FPIES) has likely been called "NEC" in a large number of infants and is likely to be a discrete but yet poorly described form of intestinal injury, especially in preterm infants.

FPIES has been described more commonly in older infants. It appears to be a still poorly understood non–Ig E–mediated syndrome resulting in hypersensitivity to food antigens.[10] Patients with FPIES typically present in the first months after birth with vomiting, diarrhea, hematochezia, or lethargy within 1 to 4 weeks after initial exposure to a triggering antigen. Transforming growth factor-β and IgA in breast milk may be protective for infants who are exclusively breast-fed, but nonetheless FPIES may still occur in breast-fed infants.[11,12]

At this juncture, knowledge about how to best diagnose this entity in preterm infants remains poor. From a causal perspective, if in the future, we are able to discern this as a distinct entity with clear biomarkers, we might be able to better diagnose, prevent, and treat this disease. Although mothers' milk is usually thought of as the ideal food for her baby, it is possible that inciting antigens may still be present and may partially depend on the mother's diet. Because mothers' milk may not always be devoid of the sensitizing agent, it is possible to see this in exclusively breast-fed babies, and at a minimum, temporary treatment with extensively hydrolyzed or amino acid formulas, and/or altering the mother's diet may be the best form of treatment and/or prevention in those infants who are disposed to this form of intestinal injury.

Spontaneous intestinal perforation
Spontaneous intestinal perforation (SIP) is seen more commonly in extremely low-birth-weight infants (born at 1000 g or less) and not accompanied by extensive intestinal inflammation or necrosis. The risk of SIP is increased with the concomitant administration of postnatal steroids and prophylactic indomethacin.[13,14] Whether the proximity of timing between maternal administration of steroids and postnatal administration of indomethacin or ibuprofen increases the risk of this form of intestinal injury is unclear and requires close scrutiny. The pathophysiology of SIP is unclear but often associated with focal thinning or absence of intestinal muscularis propria.[15] SIP is often lumped with an "NEC" diagnosis, especially if a peritoneal drain is placed without visualizing the intestines, creating confusion in outcome estimation.

Transfusion-associated gut injury
Several observational studies have demonstrated an association between blood transfusions and intestinal injury that has been termed "NEC" in preterm infants.[16] It is common practice to withhold feeds during packed red cell blood transfusions in neonatal units. A recent study or metaanalysis has concluded that the association of blood transfusions and NEC is based on low or very low certainty of evidence.[17] Patel and colleagues[18] have demonstrated that the severe anemia that prompted the transfusion may be the culprit in causing the gut injury rather than the transfusion itself. Although the existence of transfusion-associated intestinal injury versus anemia-associated intestinal injury is being debated, we are still far from understanding causality of either phenomenon, if it indeed exists.

Potential Mechanisms Causing Gut Injury

Vascular mediators
Vascular mediators, such as nitric oxide (NO), that cause vasodilation, catecholamines and endothelin (ET), that cause vasoconstriction, regulate neonatal intestinal vascular resistance, and may influence the pathophysiology of gut injury (**Fig. 1**).[19] NO is produced from conversion of arginine to citrulline in a reaction catalyzed in the intestine by 2 NO synthases (NOS). NO is produced constitutively by endothelial NOS or eNOS that persists at low levels and inducible NO synthase (iNOS), which is induced and upregulated during inflammation.[20] eNOS is expressed in the intestinal microcapillaries at low levels and regulates vascular tone and mucosal blood flow. NO may protect from oxidative stress by scavenging oxygen radicals and promote leukocyte adhesion to the endothelium, facilitating leukocyte recruitment. iNOS is upregulated during

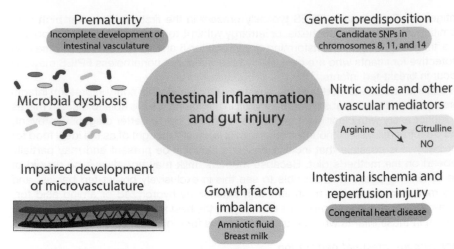

Fig. 1. Potential mechanisms causing gut injury.

inflammation and is responsible for high levels of NO, which dramatically increase blood flow by dilating the capillaries, which may lead to gut barrier failure, increasing translocation and impairing epithelial restitution.[21,22] NO readily reacts with the superoxide ion to form peroxynitrite, a reactive oxygen and nitrogen species that is highly toxic to epithelial cells, which may induce enterocyte apoptosis and inhibit epithelial restitution processes, including enterocyte proliferation and migration.[23] Endothelin-1 is the most important vasoconstrictor of the intestinal microvasculature and acts through its receptors ETR1 and ETR2B.[24,25] ET has been implicated in intestinal ischemia and injury. Catecholamines act through alpha-adrenergic receptors in the mesenteric vessels and cause vasoconstriction.[26] Preterm infants on high doses of epinephrine or norepinephrine are thus at increased risk of intestinal perforation because of intestinal ischemia. Regulation of iNOS expression by bacteria and their pathogen-associated molecular patterns or lipopolysaccharides (LPS) leads to signaling via pattern recognition receptors, and activation of the transcription factors, such as nuclear factor kappa B (NF-κB), which can bind to the iNOS promoter and induce transcription of the iNOS gene.[27,28]

Defective development of the intestinal microvasculature and impaired microcirculation

Defective development of the intestinal microvasculature and impaired microcirculation may lead to intestinal gut injury.[29] Preterm infants are frequently exposed to hypoxic states during or after birth, which causes the vascular endothelial growth factor (VEGF) and the proangiogenic VEGF receptor-2 signaling pathway to be downregulated at a time when the intestinal microvasculature is not completely developed. Postnatal stresses (eg, infection and inflammation) further reduce VEGFR2 signaling and resulting endothelial cell proliferation. Thus, the underdeveloped intestinal microvasculature, while sufficient for a "sterile" fasted intestine, may be inadequate to meet the metabolic demand of postnatal stresses, such as enteral feeding and bacterial colonization, resulting in ischemia and necrosis, thus contributing to neonatal gut injury.

Genetic predilection

Genetic predilection for exaggerated intestinal inflammation and injury that predisposes to gut injury and NEC in some preterm infants has been reported.[30–32] Genetic analysis of a poorly defined disease can be problematic because many forms of gut injury may be grouped under the term NEC. Focused candidate gene approach has identified many single nucleotide polymorphisms (SNPs) in the inflammatory signaling pathways associated with toll-like receptors (TLRs) and nucleotide oligomerization domain (NOD)-like receptors.[30] SNPs in carbamyl phosphate synthetase-1, inter-leukin-12 (IL-12; p40 promoter CTCTAA/GC), VEGF (C-2578A), and NFKB1 have been associated with NEC.[32] Jilling and colleagues[31] performed the first genome-wide association study in NEC in 751 extremely preterm infants (30 with surgical NEC) and identified 35 SNPs significantly associated with NEC. A cluster of SNPs in chromosome 8 (8q23.3) had the strongest association for NEC (odds ratio: 4.72; 95% confidence interval: 2.51–8.88). Other clusters of SNPs identified in chromosomes 14 and 11 also demonstrated significant association. A validation cohort did not have sufficient power to replicate these findings, except for a single SNP found in chromosome 8.

Role of growth factors

The *role of growth factors* in the development of neonatal gut injury has been reviewed.[33,34] Growth factors play an important role in the development, growth, and health of the GI tract by affecting the activities of the intestinal cells, such as pro-liferation, migration, differentiation, and survival. Growth factors present in amniotic fluid and breast milk may help in the prenatal and postnatal development and growth of the intestine, in repair and restitution after intestinal injury. It stands to reason that if growth factors that are normally present at a stage of development are decreased or absent, then those preterm infants may be prone to the development of intestinal injury. Epidermal growth factor and heparin binding epidermal growth factor are the ones that have been most commonly studied.[35,36]

INFANT MICROBIOME AND GUT INJURY INTERACTIONS
The Microbiome in Early Life

The neonatal microbiome undergoes a major transition during the birthing process; in utero the fetal skin is bathed in the amniotic fluid, and after birth, the neonate encoun-ters a gaseous microbe-rich environment. The naïve neonatal microbiome matures and evolves rapidly into an adultlike microbiome during infancy and early child-hood.[37–39] Before birth, the maternal and fetal ecosystems play a role in timing of de-livery. At birth, mode of delivery (vaginal or cesarean) and later feeding, antibiotic exposure, and the environment influence the composition of the developing neonatal microbiome.[40–43] During the neonatal period, microbial dysbiosis has been implicated in neonatal diseases, such as NEC, and dysbiosis in the lung to bronchopulmonary dysplasia.[44,45] The intestinal microbiome (gut)-brain axis has been implicated in neu-rodevelopmental disorders, such as autism.[46,47]

The development of the neonatal microbiome, immunity, and metabolic homeosta-sis may be influenced by *antenatal factors*, which affect the infant (maternal modifiers or maternal determinants).[48,49] Maternal colonization has been shown to affect neonatal microbial colonization and development of neonatal immunity.[50] Animal studies report the effects of maternal microbiota on infants' transcription profiles, including those involved in innate immunity (antibacterial peptides), inflammation, and metabolism of microbial molecules.[50] Maternal IgA in breast milk binds to infant intestinal bacteria (especially Enterobacteriaceae, which are a family of bacteria under the phylum Proteobacteria) and may play a protective role against NEC.[51] Maternal obesity and a high-fat diet during pregnancy may have an effect on the neonate's im-mune system, affect neonatal microbial colonization, and predispose to metabolic disease later in life.[48] The hypothesized mechanisms for this effect may be that the maternal metabolic derangement affects the infant's liver and other end organs by altered metabolite production, altered gut barrier integrity, and hematopoietic immune cells. Maternal programming of the fetal immune system may be affected by maternal antibodies, inflammatory mediators, micronutrients, microbial products, and maternal cells.[49]

The preterm intestinal microbiome is more similar to that of germ-free mice than that of adult mice. Germ-free mice lack the normal immune regulation by commensal bacteria, and accumulation of invariant natural killer T cells (iNKT) in the colon and lung may result in mucosal pathologic condition.[52] An interesting observation is that in *neonatal germ-free mice* (but not adult mice) exposed to conventional microbiota, decreased methylation of the Cxcl16 gene results in decreased expression and decreased accumulation of iNKT. Therefore neonatal exposure to conventional microbiota is critical in immune regulation and may have long-lasting effects.[52] Composition of the gut microbiota in preterm infants shows a predominance of bacteria belonging to the phylum Proteobacteria in contrast to adults and older children whereby members of the Firmicutes predominate.[53,54] La Rosa and colleagues[40] observed an orchestrated patterned progression of gut microbiota toward an abundance of Clostridia with increasing gestational age and predominance of Proteobacteria. Antibiotics, feeding, or mode of delivery caused abrupt shifts in microbiota but did not change this seemingly predestined progression. Intestinal injury classified as NEC using a set of unclear diagnostic criteria is associated with a Proteobacteria bloom[55] and decreased abundances of anaerobic bacterial taxa (especially Negativicutes).[56] Metagenomic evaluation of the intestinal microbiome in intestinal injury has also been shown to be associated with uropathogenic *Escherichia coli* (a member of the class gamma-Proteobacteria and phylum Proteobacteria).[57]

Microbiota and Metabolites Drive Innate Immune Responses and Inflammation

Microbiota on human body surfaces and their metabolites act as environmental triggers that influence mammalian gene expression.[58,59] Recognition of commensal-derived pathogen associated molecular patterns, such as LPS, by the intestinal epithelial cells (IEC) induce secretion of the antimicrobial peptide RegIIIγ, which mediates colonization resistance in the gut.[60] *Microbiota-derived signals*, butyrate, propionate, and acetate (short-chain fatty acids, SCFAs), induce IL-18 production from the IEC through activation of NOD-like family, receptors.[61] Acetate produced by Bifidobacteria promotes epithelial cell barrier function by inducing an antiapoptotic response in the IEC. Thus, microbiota and their metabolites mediate immune response via the IEC and immune cells.[60,62]

Microbiota and Metabolites Influence the Human Epigenome and Expression of Genes Associated with Inflammation

Epigenetics involves the molecular processes that permit changes in gene expression without a change in the genetic code.[63] The most characterized epigenetic mechanisms are DNA methylation and histone modifications, which alter gene transcription in response to environmental triggers. Epigenomic modifications are maintained by the balancing activity of epigenomic modifying enzymes, such as DNA methyltransferases, histone acetyltransferases, and histone methyltransferases.[58,59,63] Animal studies report *repression of proinflammatory genes by microbiota,* and such repression is not seen in germ-free mice. Studies in germ-free mice have shown that DNA methylation of the TLR4 gene in the IECs was lower compared with conventional mice, indicating that TLR4 gene expression is repressed in wild-type mice.[64] Other experiments show that mononuclear phagocytes from conventionally housed mice compared with germ-free mice showed that commensal bacteria increased histone H3 methylation and decreased transcription of inflammatory genes.[65] Increased abundances of Firmicutes and Bacteroidetes are associated with obesity and cardiovascular risk factors possibly because of their effects on glucose absorption, generation of fatty acids, hepatic lipogenesis, and tissue adipocyte deposition.[66,67] Microbial metabolites (ie, metabolites produced by microbiota) may induce changes in the epigenome. It is known that germ-free mice have lower levels of SCFAs compared with conventionally housed animals.[68,69] SCFAs inhibit histone deacetylase activity, which may be a potential target for epigenomic changes.[70,71] SCFAs also have been shown to stimulate histone acetylation of FoxP3 (forehead box P3) locus on naïve CD4$^+$ T cells, increase FoxP3 expression, and promote differentiation of regulatory T cells (anti-inflammatory effects).[61,68,72] Faecalibacterium prausnitzii and Eubacterium rectale/Roseburia species (members of the phylum Firmicutes) are major contributors of butyrate, which regulates gene expression by histone modifications.[73] LPS, an inflammatory marker for cardiovascular disease, may also have a role in epigenetic regulation of intestinal and immune cells.[74]

MECHANISMS OF MICROBIOTA INDUCED NEONATAL GUT INJURY

Normal development of the gut microbiome that is associated with appropriate colonization with commensal bacteria increases immune tolerance and decreases the excessive inflammatory responses.[72,75,76] The absence of disease in animal models of germ-free mice and increased risk after antibiotics that alter microbial community composition point to microbial dysbiosis as a plausible factor in the etiopathogenesis of gut injury.[45,77]

Intestinal inflammation and injury are mediated via immune mechanisms.[3] The interactions of the intestinal epithelium with the developing gut microbiome, including commensal bacteria, may be associated with molecular signaling and involvement of innate and adaptive immune cells. Schirmer and colleagues[78] studied the cytokine expression patterns from intestinal cells in response to different microbiome patterns and their metabolites. Cytokine patterns from the intestinal cells were stimulus specific, and tumor necrosis factor-α (TNF-α) and interferon-γ production are associated with specific microbial metabolic pathways: palmitoleic acid metabolism and tryptophan degradation to tryptophol. Stimulus specific responses may explain why dysbiosis or altered microbiome patterns may lead to different cytokine responses and exaggerated inflammation that may drive the development of NEC.

TLR signaling by bacterial LPS and TLR4 mechanisms that lead to inflammation and neonatal gut injury has been well studied[79] (Fig. 2). Microbes with their microbial-associated molecular patterns and microbial products, such as LPS from gram-negative bacteria and peptidoglycans from gram-positive bacteria, initiate inflammatory signaling pathways, in particular the TLR4 signaling pathway that initiates inflammation and tissue injury. The TLR-4 plays an important role in the phagocytosis and translocation of gram-negative bacteria across the intestinal mucosal barrier, the activation of which leads to activation of NF-κB and caspases. TLR activation leads to a proinflammatory response with secretion of proinflammatory cytokines and IL that leads to intestinal injury. TLR2 is a membrane surface receptor that is activated by bacterial peptidoglycans, which are highly expressed on the outer membranes of gram-positive bacteria and in fungal substances. TLR2 is expressed on microglia and inflammatory cells, such as monocyte/macrophage, dendritic cells, B lymphocytes, and T lymphocytes. In general, the TLR2 signaling pathway leads to production of TNF-α and NF-κB.[80]

The intestinal microbiome and its host recognition elements, such as the TLR, TLR2, TLR4, and their adaptor protein, myeloid differentiation primary-response 88, NO, and

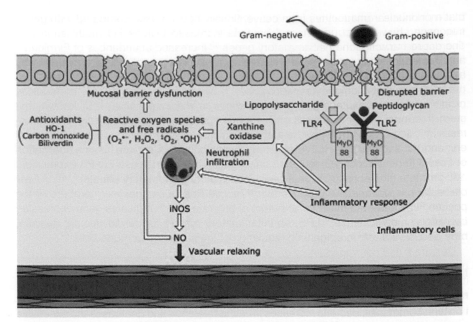

Fig. 2. Mechanisms of microbiome-mediated gut injury. MyD88, myeloid differentiation primary-response 88. (*From* Nadatani Y, Watanabe T, Shimada S, et al. Microbiome and intestinal ischemia/reperfusion injury. J Clin Biochem Nutr. 2018 Jul; 63(1): 26–32; with permission.)

other elements of oxidative stress, may also be involved in *intestinal ischemia reperfusion injury.*[81] Intestinal reperfusion injury is attenuated in germ-free mice and by administration of antibiotics, indicating the importance of the microbiome in the causation of this injury.[82,83]

RECENT ADVANCES

There are likely to be several regulatory, inflammatory, and metabolic pathways involved in the pathogenesis of different forms of intestinal injury. New technologies using multi-omic pathway analyses related to the different categories of intestinal injury will guide us in the future.

Molecular mechanisms from the insults causing injury are being teased out. There has been a growing impetus to redefine NEC, so it is more specific and clinically relevant based on the understanding that gut injury may result from many different insults, all of which lead to the inflammation injury sequence. Redefining NEC is essential to get accurate epidemiologic data that will inform research studies. Growth factor research has increased beyond the most commonly studied epidermal growth factor and heparin-binding epidermal growth factor.[33] Stem cells facilitate repair and restitution and may be important interventions to decrease morbidity and mortality after neonatal gut injury.[84] New anti-inflammatory agents that act on the signaling pathways, for example, TLR4 antagonist C34, are being studied that may ameliorate or prevent intestinal inflammation.[85,86]

CURRENT CONTROVERSIES

In recent years, the perception that the intrauterine environment is sterile has been challenged. Molecular techniques have identified the presence of bacterial DNA in the endometrium of nonpregnant women,[87,88] as well as in the amniotic fluid and placental tissue from healthy pregnancies,[89,90] and the meconium of healthy infants,[89] suggesting that the acquisition of the neonatal microbiome may begin before birth. The degree to which the bacterial signals detected in placental tissues and amniotic fluid represent living bacteria and are capable of seeding the neonatal microbiome acquisition and development is controversial. A large part of this controversy lies in the low (microbial) biomass nature of placental tissue and amniotic fluid and the technical challenges associated with distinguishing true biological signals from noise. Early studies reporting the presence of the placental microbiome have been challenged with respect to their reproducibility, potential for sample contamination during labor, delivery, and the sample collection process, and degree to which thorough extraction and sequencing controls were included as a part of the study design (ie, the reporting the "kit-ome").[91–93] Recently published results refute the widespread presence of a placental microbiome but indicate that *Streptococcus agalactiae* (group B Streptococcus) was detected in ~5% of samples before the onset of labor.[93] Similarly, *Mycoplasma* sp and *Ureaplasma* sp were detected in placental tissue in cases of preterm birth associated with chorioamnionitis.[92]

Despite these controversies, a growing body of evidence suggests that a mother's microbiome has the potential to influence immune development in her offspring,[50] and it is generally agreed that postnatal colonization during and in the days to weeks after birth are likely to have greater influence on microbiome development than potential intrauterine exposure.

SUMMARY

Neonatal gut injury can result from many different insults (ischemia, hypoxia due to anemia, dysbiosis) and the molecular mechanisms of gut injury after these insults are being researched. The developing microbiome is not a bystander but actively participates in the initiation and evolution of the gut injury. Optimizing the microbiome and its downstream effects may help us devise novel therapeutic and preventive strategies against neonatal gut injury, including NEC.

DISCLOSURE

The authors have nothing to disclose.

REFERENCES

1. Neu J, Modi N, Caplan M. Necrotizing enterocolitis comes in different forms: historical perspectives and defining the disease. Semin Fetal Neonatal Med 2018; 23(6):370–3.
2. Lenfestey MW, Neu J. Gastrointestinal development: implications for management of preterm and term infants. Gastroenterol Clin North Am 2018;47(4): 773–91.
3. Mara MA, Good M, Weitkamp JH. Innate and adaptive immunity in necrotizing enterocolitis. Semin Fetal Neonatal Med 2018;23(6):394–9.
4. Zhu J, Dingess KA. The functional power of the human milk proteome. Nutrients 2019;11(8) [pii:E1834].
5. Palmeira P, Carneiro-Sampaio M. Immunology of breast milk. Rev Assoc Med Bras (1992) 2016;62(6):584–93.
6. Pickard SS, Feinstein JA, Popat RA, et al. Short- and long-term outcomes of necrotizing enterocolitis in infants with congenital heart disease. Pediatrics 2009;123(5):e901–6.

7. Carlo WF, Kimball TR, Michelfelder EC, et al. Persistent diastolic flow reversal in abdominal aortic Doppler-flow profiles is associated with an increased risk of necrotizing enterocolitis in term infants with congenital heart disease. Pediatrics 2007;119(2):330–5.

8. McElhinney DB, Hedrick HL, Bush DM, et al. Necrotizing enterocolitis in neonates with congenital heart disease: risk factors and outcomes. Pediatrics 2000;106(5):1080–7.

9. Wu H, Deng YY, Liu L, et al. Intestinal ischemia-reperfusion of macaques triggers a strong innate immune response. World J Gastroenterol 2014;20(41):15327–34.

10. Caubet JC, Cianferoni A, Groetch M, et al. Food protein-induced enterocolitis syndrome. Clin Exp Allergy 2019;49(9):1178–90.

11. Monti G, Castagno E, Liguori SA, et al. Food protein-induced enterocolitis syndrome by cow's milk proteins passed through breast milk. J Allergy Clin Immunol 2011;127(3):679–80.

12. Kaya A, Toyran M, Civelek E, et al. Food protein-induced enterocolitis syndrome in two exclusively breastfed infants. Pediatr Allergy Immunol 2016;27(7):749–50.

13. Paquette L, Friedlich P, Ramanathan R, et al. Concurrent use of indomethacin and dexamethasone increases the risk of spontaneous intestinal perforation in very low birth weight neonates. J Perinatol 2006;26(8):486–92.

14. Stark AR, Carlo WA, Tyson JE, et al. Adverse effects of early dexamethasone treatment in extremely-low-birth-weight infants. National Institute of Child Health and Human Development Neonatal Research Network. N Engl J Med 2001;344(2):95–101.

15. Lai S, Yu W, Wallace L, et al. Intestinal muscularis propria increases in thickness with corrected gestational age and is focally attenuated in patients with isolated intestinal perforations. J Pediatr Surg 2014;49(1):114–9.

16. Kirpalani H, Zupancic JA. Do transfusions cause necrotizing enterocolitis? The complementary role of randomized trials and observational studies. Semin Perinatol 2012;36(4):269–76.

17. Hay S, Zupancic JA, Flannery DD, et al. Should we believe in transfusion-associated enterocolitis? Applying a GRADE to the literature. Semin Perinatol 2017;41(1):80–91.

18. Patel RM, Knezevic A, Shenvi N, et al. Association of red blood cell transfusion, anemia, and necrotizing enterocolitis in very low-birth-weight infants. JAMA 2016;315(9):889–97.

19. Nair J, Lakshminrusimha S. Role of NO and other vascular mediators in the etiopathogenesis of necrotizing enterocolitis. Front Biosci (Schol Ed) 2019;11:9–28.

20. Grishin A, Bowling J, Bell B, et al. Roles of nitric oxide and intestinal microbiota in the pathogenesis of necrotizing enterocolitis. J Pediatr Surg 2016;51(1):13–7.

21. Sorrells DL, Friend C, Koltuksuz U, et al. Inhibition of nitric oxide with aminoguanidine reduces bacterial translocation after endotoxin challenge in vivo. Arch Surg 1996;131(11):1155–63.

22. Kolb E. Current knowledge on the formation of nitric oxide in endothelial cells of blood vessels, in nerve cells and macrophages as well as its significance in vascular dilatation, information transmission and damage of tumor cells. Z Gesamte Inn Med 1991;46(12):431–6 [in German].

23. Ford HR. Mechanism of nitric oxide-mediated intestinal barrier failure: insight into the pathogenesis of necrotizing enterocolitis. J Pediatr Surg 2006;41(2):294–9.

24. Nankervis CA, Schauer GM, Miller CE. Endothelin-mediated vasoconstriction in postischemic newborn intestine. Am J Physiol Gastrointest Liver Physiol 2000;279(4):G683–91.

25. Nankervis CA, Nowicki PT. Role of endothelin-1 in regulation of the postnatal intestinal circulation. Am J Physiol Gastrointest Liver Physiol 2000;278(3):G367–75.
26. Rudner XL, Berkowitz DE, Booth JV, et al. Subtype specific regulation of human vascular alpha(1)-adrenergic receptors by vessel bed and age. Circulation 1999; 100(23):2336–43.
27. Kleinert H, Schwarz PM, Forstermann U. Regulation of the expression of inducible nitric oxide synthase. Biol Chem 2003;384(10–11):1343–64.
28. Farlik M, Reutterer B, Schindler C, et al. Nonconventional initiation complex assembly by STAT and NF-kappaB transcription factors regulates nitric oxide synthase expression. Immunity 2010;33(1):25–34.
29. Bowker RM, Yan X, De Plaen IG. Intestinal microcirculation and necrotizing enterocolitis: the vascular endothelial growth factor system. Semin Fetal Neonatal Med 2018;23(6):411–5.
30. Cuna A, George L, Sampath V. Genetic predisposition to necrotizing enterocolitis in premature infants: current knowledge, challenges, and future directions. Semin Fetal Neonatal Med 2018;23(6):387–93.
31. Jilling T, Ambalavanan N, Cotten CM, et al. Surgical necrotizing enterocolitis in extremely premature neonates is associated with genetic variations in an intergenic region of chromosome 8. Pediatr Res 2018;83(5):943–53.
32. Bhandari V, Bizzarro MJ, Shetty A, et al, Neonatal Genetics Study Group. Familial and genetic susceptibility to major neonatal morbidities in preterm twins. Pediatrics 2006;117(6):1901–6.
33. Shelby RD, Cromeens B, Rager TM, et al. Influence of growth factors on the development of necrotizing enterocolitis. Clin Perinatol 2019;46(1):51–64.
34. Rowland KJ, Choi PM, Warner BW. The role of growth factors in intestinal regeneration and repair in necrotizing enterocolitis. Semin Pediatr Surg 2013;22(2): 101–11.
35. Feng J, El-Assal ON, Besner GE. Heparin-binding epidermal growth factor-like growth factor reduces intestinal apoptosis in neonatal rats with necrotizing enterocolitis. J Pediatr Surg 2006;41(4):742–7 [discussion: 742–7].
36. Feng J, El-Assal ON, Besner GE. Heparin-binding epidermal growth factor-like growth factor decreases the incidence of necrotizing enterocolitis in neonatal rats. J Pediatr Surg 2006;41(1):144–9 [discussion: 144–9].
37. Kim CS, Claud EC. Necrotizing enterocolitis pathophysiology: how microbiome data alter our understanding. Clin Perinatol 2019;46(1):29–38.
38. Baranowski JR, Claud EC. Necrotizing enterocolitis and the preterm infant microbiome. Adv Exp Med Biol 2019;1125:25–36.
39. Underwood MA, Sohn K. The microbiota of the extremely preterm infant. Clin Perinatol 2017;44(2):407–27.
40. La Rosa PS, Warner BB, Zhou Y, et al. Patterned progression of bacterial populations in the premature infant gut. Proc Natl Acad Sci U S A 2014;111(34): 12522–7.
41. Stewart CJ, Embleton ND, Marrs ECL, et al. Longitudinal development of the gut microbiome and metabolome in preterm neonates with late onset sepsis and healthy controls. Microbiome 2017;5(1):75–PMC5508794.
42. Stewart CJ, Embleton ND, Marrs EC, et al. Temporal bacterial and metabolic development of the preterm gut reveals specific signatures in health and disease. Microbiome 2016;4(1):67.
43. Shao Y, Forster SC, Tsaliki E, et al. Stunted microbiota and opportunistic pathogen colonization in caesarean-section birth. Nature 2019;574(7776):117–21.

44. Pammi M, Lal CV, Wagner BD, et al. Airway microbiome and development of bronchopulmonary dysplasia in preterm infants: a systematic review. J Pediatr 2019;204:126–33.e2.

45. Pammi M, Cope J, Tarr PI, et al. Intestinal dysbiosis in preterm infants preceding necrotizing enterocolitis: a systematic review and meta-analysis. Microbiome 2017;5(1):31.

46. Vuong HE, Hsiao EY. Emerging roles for the gut microbiome in autism spectrum disorder. Biol Psychiatry 2017;81(5):411–23.

47. Luna RA, Oezguen N, Balderas M, et al. Distinct microbiome-neuroimmune signatures correlate with functional abdominal pain in children with autism spectrum disorder. Cell Mol Gastroenterol Hepatol 2017;3(2):218–30.

48. Mulligan CM, Friedman JE. Maternal modifiers of the infant gut microbiota: metabolic consequences. J Endocrinol 2017;235(1):R1–12.

49. Jennewein MF, Abu-Raya B, Jiang Y, et al. Transfer of maternal immunity and programming of the newborn immune system. Semin Immunopathol 2017;39(6): 605–13.

50. Gomez de Aguero M, Ganal-Vonarburg SC, Fuhrer T, et al. The maternal microbiota drives early postnatal innate immune development. Science 2016; 351(6279):1296–302.

51. Gopalakrishna KP, Macadangdang BR, Rogers MB, et al. Maternal IgA protects against the development of necrotizing enterocolitis in preterm infants. Nat Med 2019;25(7):1110–5.

52. Olszak T, An D, Zeissig S, et al. Microbial exposure during early life has persistent effects on natural killer T cell function. Science 2012;336(6080):489–93.

53. Zhang H, DiBaise JK, Zuccolo A, et al. Human gut microbiota in obesity and after gastric bypass. Proc Natl Acad Sci U S A 2009;106(7):2365–70.

54. Saulnier DM, Riehle K, Mistretta TA, et al. Gastrointestinal microbiome signatures of pediatric patients with irritable bowel syndrome. Gastroenterology 2011; 141(5):1782–91.

55. Torrazza RM, Neu J. The altered gut microbiome and necrotizing enterocolitis. Clin Perinatol 2013;40(1):93–108.

56. Warner BB, Deych E, Zhou Y, et al. Gut bacteria dysbiosis and necrotising enterocolitis in very low birthweight infants: a prospective case-control study. Lancet 2016;387(10031):1928–36.

57. Ward DV, Scholz M, Zolfo M, et al. Metagenomic sequencing with strain-level resolution implicates uropathogenic E. coli in necrotizing enterocolitis and mortality in preterm infants. Cell Rep 2016;14(12):2912–24.

58. Alenghat T, Artis D. Epigenomic regulation of host-microbiota interactions. Trends Immunol 2014;35(11):518–25.

59. Alenghat T. Epigenomics and the microbiota. Toxicol Pathol 2015;43(1):101–6.

60. Kabat AM, Srinivasan N, Maloy KJ. Modulation of immune development and function by intestinal microbiota. Trends Immunol 2014;35(11):507–17.

61. Smith PM, Howitt MR, Panikov N, et al. The microbial metabolites, short-chain fatty acids, regulate colonic Treg cell homeostasis. Science 2013;341(6145): 569–73.

62. Deshmukh HS, Liu Y, Menkiti OR, et al. The microbiota regulates neutrophil homeostasis and host resistance to Escherichia coli K1 sepsis in neonatal mice. Nat Med 2014;20(5):524–30.

63. Arrowsmith CH, Bountra C, Fish PV, et al. Epigenetic protein families: a new frontier for drug discovery. Nat Rev Drug Discov 2012;11(5):384–400.

64. Takahashi K, Sugi Y, Nakano K, et al. Epigenetic control of the host gene by commensal bacteria in large intestinal epithelial cells. J Biol Chem 2011; 286(41):35755–62.
65. Ganal SC, Sanos SL, Kallfass C, et al. Priming of natural killer cells by nonmucosal mononuclear phagocytes requires instructive signals from commensal microbiota. Immunity 2012;37(1):171–86.
66. Kumar H, Lund R, Laiho A, et al. Gut microbiota as an epigenetic regulator: pilot study based on whole-genome methylation analysis. mBio 2014;5(6):4271550.
67. Caesar R, Fak F, Backhed F. Effects of gut microbiota on obesity and atherosclerosis via modulation of inflammation and lipid metabolism. J Intern Med 2010; 268(4):320–8.
68. Arpaia N, Campbell C, Fan X, et al. Metabolites produced by commensal bacteria promote peripheral regulatory T-cell generation. Nature 2013;504(7480): 451–5.
69. Hoverstad T, Midtvedt T. Short-chain fatty acids in germfree mice and rats. J Nutr 1986;116(9):1772–6.
70. Macfarlane S, Macfarlane GT. Regulation of short-chain fatty acid production. Proc Nutr Soc 2003;62(1):67–72.
71. Waldecker M, Kautenburger T, Daumann H, et al. Inhibition of histone-deacetylase activity by short-chain fatty acids and some polyphenol metabolites formed in the colon. J Nutr Biochem 2008;19(9):587–93.
72. Furusawa Y, Obata Y, Fukuda S, et al. Commensal microbe-derived butyrate induces the differentiation of colonic regulatory T cells. Nature 2013;504(7480): 446–50.
73. Canani RB, Costanzo MD, Leone L, et al. Potential beneficial effects of butyrate in intestinal and extraintestinal diseases. World J Gastroenterol 2011;17(12): 1519–28.
74. Angrisano T, Pero R, Peluso S, et al. LPS-induced IL-8 activation in human intestinal epithelial cells is accompanied by specific histone H3 acetylation and methylation changes. BMC Microbiol 2010;10:172.
75. Walker WA. The importance of appropriate initial bacterial colonization of the intestine in newborn, child, and adult health. Pediatr Res 2017;82(3):387–95.
76. Fulde M, Hornef MW. Maturation of the enteric mucosal innate immune system during the postnatal period. Immunol Rev 2014;260(1):21–34.
77. Neu J, Pammi M. Pathogenesis of NEC: impact of an altered intestinal microbiome. Semin Perinatol 2017;41(1):29–35.
78. Schirmer M, Smeekens SP, Vlamakis H, et al. Linking the human gut microbiome to inflammatory cytokine production capacity. Cell 2016;167(4):1125–36.e8.
79. Mihi B, Good M. Impact of toll-like receptor 4 signaling in necrotizing enterocolitis: the state of the science. Clin Perinatol 2019;46(1):145–57.
80. Kawai T, Akira S. The roles of TLRs, RLRs and NLRs in pathogen recognition. Int Immunol 2009;21(4):317–37.
81. Nadatani Y, Watanabe T, Shimada S, et al. Microbiome and intestinal ischemia/reperfusion injury. J Clin Biochem Nutr 2018;63(1):26–32.
82. Souza DG, Vieira AT, Soares AC, et al. The essential role of the intestinal microbiota in facilitating acute inflammatory responses. J Immunol 2004;173(6): 4137–46.
83. Yoshiya K, Lapchak PH, Thai TH, et al. Depletion of gut commensal bacteria attenuates intestinal ischemia/reperfusion injury. Am J Physiol Gastrointest Liver Physiol 2011;301(6):G1020–30.

84. Pisano C, Besner GE. Potential role of stem cells in disease prevention based on a murine model of experimental necrotizing enterocolitis. J Pediatr Surg 2019; 54(3):413–6.
85. Wipf P, Eyer BR, Yamaguchi Y, et al. Synthesis of anti-inflammatory alpha-and beta-linked acetamidopyranosides as inhibitors of toll-like receptor 4 (TLR4). Tetrahedron Lett 2015;56(23):3097–100.
86. Neal MD, Jia H, Eyer B, et al. Discovery and validation of a new class of small molecule Toll-like receptor 4 (TLR4) inhibitors. PLoS One 2013;8(6):e65779.
87. Verstraelen H, Vilchez-Vargas R, Desimpel F, et al. Characterisation of the human uterine microbiome in non-pregnant women through deep sequencing of the V1-2 region of the 16S rRNA gene. PeerJ 2016;4:e1602.
88. Baker JM, Chase DM, Herbst-Kralovetz MM. Uterine microbiota: residents, tourists, or invaders? Front Immunol 2018;9:208.
89. Collado MC, Rautava S, Aakko J, et al. Human gut colonisation may be initiated in utero by distinct microbial communities in the placenta and amniotic fluid. Sci Rep 2016;6:23129.
90. Aagaard K, Ma J, Antony KM, et al. The placenta harbors a unique microbiome. Sci Transl Med 2014;6(237):237ra265.
91. Leiby JS, McCormick K, Sherrill-Mix S, et al. Lack of detection of a human placenta microbiome in samples from preterm and term deliveries. Microbiome 2018;6(1):196.
92. Leon LJ, Doyle R, Diez-Benavente E, et al. Enrichment of clinically relevant organisms in spontaneous preterm-delivered placentas and reagent contamination across all clinical groups in a large pregnancy cohort in the United Kingdom. Appl Environ Microbiol 2018;84(14) [pii:e00483-18].
93. de Goffau MC, Lager S, Sovio U, et al. Human placenta has no microbiome but can contain potential pathogens. Nature 2019;572(7769):329–34.

Recent Advances in Necrotizing Enterocolitis Research

Strategies for Implementation in Clinical Practice

Mohan Pammi, MD, PhD[a], Isabelle G. De Plaen, MD[b],
Akhil Maheshwari, MD[c],*

KEYWORDS

- Neonate • Preterm • Necrotizing enterocolitis • NEC • Research • Strategies

KEY POINTS

- Evaluation of microbiome optimization, immunomodulation, growth factors, and human milk glycans, and integration of multiomics data from various platforms as research strategies for prevention of necrotizing enterocolitis (NEC).
- Validation of novel biomarkers for early diagnosis of disease and monitoring in multicenter clinical trials.
- Evaluation of the gut microbiome, immunomodulation, growth factors, and human milk glycans, and integration of multiomics data from various platforms as research strategies for prevention of necrotizing enterocolitis (NEC).
- Validation of novel biomarkers for early diagnosis of NEC and monitoring in multicenter clinical trials.
- Evaluation of prophylactic strategies including maternal milk feeding, probiotics, antibiotic stewardship, and protective immunomodulators.

INTRODUCTION

Our Current Understanding of Necrotizing Enterocolitis as a Disease Entity

Necrotizing enterocolitis (NEC) is an idiopathic, inflammatory bowel necrosis of premature infants that involves the small and the large intestine (**Box 1**). Despite decades

Funding: NIH awards DK116568 (to I.G. De Plaen) and HL124078, HL133022 (to A. Maheshwari).
[a] Department of Pediatrics, Baylor College of Medicine, Texas Children's Hospital, Houston, TX, USA; [b] Department of Pediatrics, Ann & Robert H. Lurie Children's Hospital of Chicago, Northwestern University, Feinberg School of Medicine, Chicago, IL, USA; [c] Department of Pediatrics, Johns Hopkins School of Medicine, Baltimore, MD, USA
* Corresponding author. Charlotte R. Bloomberg Children's Center, 1800 Orleans Street, Room 8530, Baltimore, MD 21287.
E-mail address: akhil@jhmi.edu

Clin Perinatol 47 (2020) 383–397
https://doi.org/10.1016/j.clp.2020.02.011
0095-5108/20/© 2020 Elsevier Inc. All rights reserved.

> **Box 1**
> **Highlights**
>
> - Necrotizing enterocolitis (NEC) is an inflammatory necrosis of the bowel wall, and is a leading cause of morbidity and mortality of premature infants.
> - NEC is often preceded by bacterial overgrowth. Lesions are marked by necrosis, inflammation, hemorrhages, and pneumatosis.
> - Associations: prematurity, bacterial overgrowth, anemia/red blood cell transfusions, splanchnic compromise, and antibiotic use.
> - Biomarkers may be useful in early diagnosis of NEC and further monitoring.
> - Maternal milk feeding may be superior in various quantities to any other human milk substitute.
> - Probiotics are likely to be useful in prevention of NEC.
> - Antibiotic stewardship may protect against NEC through effects on bacterial flora.
> - Protective immunomodulators may include lactoferrin; Toll-like receptor antagonists; amniotic fluid; growth factors; and specific chemicals, such as oligosaccharide 2'-fucosyllactose and peptidoglycans.
> - Intestinal stem cells may have a role in prevention of NEC.

of research, the etiopathologic hypotheses remain incomplete and still focused on disparate elements such as immaturity of the gut mucosal barrier, mucosal injury, ischemia, inflammation, and microbial dysbiosis, which may eventually allow luminal bacteria to translocate into the bowel wall to cause cellular necrosis and unregulated inflammation. In the clinical setting, about half of all infants with NEC respond to bowel rest, antibiotics, and supportive medical measures, but others develop progressive bowel disease or require surgical intervention; a third of these patients eventually die.[1] There is an unmet need for novel research strategies for prevention, early diagnosis, clinical monitoring, and treatment of NEC.

Most patients with NEC show disease evolution over a period of 24 to 48 hours, although a third may progress rapidly over just a few hours. The onset of NEC at a postnatal age of 2 to 5 weeks typically shows an inverse relationship with the gestational age at birth. At presentation, the systemic clinical signs are usually nonspecific and may include tachycardia with increased lethargy, apnea, and temperature instability; gastrointestinal signs may include feeding intolerance, delayed gastric emptying, abdominal distention, tenderness, and ileus with decreased bowel sounds. Grossly bloody stools are seen in approximately 25%. The severity of illness is often staged by using the modified Bell criteria, which define disease progression with an early stage of nonspecific systemic/gastrointestinal inflammatory response, a more definite stage of gastrointestinal disease and localized peritonitis, and eventually an advanced stage with diffuse peritonitis and systemic inflammatory response syndrome.

On histology, NEC lesions in the bowel wall are characterized by coagulative necrosis; inflammatory changes; bacterial overgrowth; pneumatosis intestinalis (gaseous cysts in the bowel wall); and, depending on the time elapsed since disease onset, reparative changes in the bowel wall.[2,3] The leukocyte infiltrates in NEC lesions show numerous newly recruited blood monocytes and macrophages (12.8 ± 1.1 cells/high-power field [HPF] in control tissue vs 128.6 ± 9.4 cells/HPF in NEC lesions).[4] There is also a modest increase in neutrophils (7.7 ± 1.7 cells/HPF in control vs 37.9 ± 5.8 cells/HPF in NEC). The increase in lymphocytes is less promi-nent, although there may be important changes in lymphocyte subsets.[5] This article summarizes the research strategies currently underway and others on the horizon, hoping that a multipronged approach will eventually improve the outcomes of preterm infants at risk of NEC.

Hematological and Inflammatory Changes During Necrotizing Enterocolitis

Anemia and red blood cell (RBC) transfusions have been associated with NEC. Numerous retrospective clinical studies have shown that 25% to 40% of all patients with NEC develop intestinal injury within 48 hours of receiving an RBC transfusion.[6–12] Compared with patients who develop NEC and do not have a history of a recent RBC transfusion, neonates with transfusion-associated NEC are often born at an earlier gestation, have lower birth weights, and have a delayed NEC onset at 3 to 5 weeks of postnatal age. In a recent study, MohanKumar and colleagues[13] showed that mouse pups rendered anemic by timed phlebotomy on postnatal days 2 to 10 and then given RBC transfusions 24 hours later developed NEC-like intestinal injury within 12 to 24 hours. These mice showed prominent bowel necrosis, inflammation, and submuco-sal edema/separation of the lamina propria in the ileocecal region and colon. The anemic intestine showed extensive infiltration with inflammatory macrophages, which were activated by subsequent RBC transfusions via a lipopolysaccharide receptor (Toll-like receptor-4 [TLR4])–mediated mechanisms to cause bowel injury. TLR4 expression is known to be higher in the premature intestine than in term infants. Chela-tion of RBC degradation products with haptoglobin, absence of TLR4, macrophage depletion, and inhibition of macrophage activation were protective.[13] Intestinal injury worsened with increasing severity and duration of anemia before transfusion, indicating a need for reevaluation of the current transfusion guidelines for premature infants.

Patients with NEC are also usually thrombocytopenic and show platelet counts less than 150×10^9/L within 24 to 72 hours of onset of disease.[14–17] The severity of this thrombocytopenia usually correlates with the Bell clinical stage of NEC, and a rapid decrease in platelet counts to less than 100×10^9/L is a sensitive, although not spe-cific, predictor of bowel gangrene and/or the need for surgical intervention.[14,17] Although most patients with NEC and thrombocytopenia do not show signs of dissem-inated intravascular coagulation, the primary mechanism for thrombocytopenia is widely thought to be increased platelet destruction. In a recent study, Namachivayam and colleagues[18] used their murine model of NEC to investigate the role of platelets in the pathogenesis of NEC. Ten-day-old mouse pups develop thrombocytopenia at 12 to 15 hours and develop an acute necrotizing ileocolitis resembling human NEC within 24 hours. Neonatal intestinal macrophages released tissue factor as early as 3 hours after the initiation of mucosal injury, which led to the activation of circulating thrombin and then platelets, causing widespread activation of inflammatory cascades and gut mucosal injury. Consistent with the murine data, there were increased levels of circu-lating tissue factor and thrombin-antithrombin complexes in patients with NEC.

TLR4-mediated lymphocyte influx may also play an important role in the develop-ment of NEC. Egan and colleagues[5] showed that human and murine NEC is rich in lymphocytes that are required for NEC development. They showed that recombination activating gene 1–deficient (Rag1$^{-/-}$) mice were protected from NEC and the transfer of intestinal lymphocytes from NEC mice into naive mice induced intestinal inflamma-tion. Similar to the findings in anemia and RBC transfusion–related NEC, intestinal TLR4 expression was required for C-C chemokine receptor type 9 (CCR9)/C-C Motif Chemokine Ligand 25 (CCL25) signaling and consequent lymphocyte influx. TLR4 also mediated a signal transducer and activator of transcription-mediated lymphocyte polarization toward increased proinflammatory cluster of differentiation (CD) 3[+], CD4[+], interleukin (IL)-17[+], and reduced tolerogenic Foxp3[+] T-regulatory lymphocytes (Tregs). T-helper (Th)-17 lymphocytes were required for NEC development, because inhibition of STAT3 or IL-17 receptor signaling attenuated NEC in mice, whereas IL-17 release impaired enterocyte tight junctions, increased enterocyte apoptosis, and reduced enterocyte proliferation, leading to NEC.

Vascular Remodeling and Microcirculation

Development of intestinal vasculature and intestinal vasoregulation are prime targets for NEC research.[19–21] In premature infants, splanchnic blood flow limitations may arise from limited production of endogenous vasodilators such as nitric oxide (NO) from dysfunctional endothelial cells[22] or excessive production of vasoconstrictors such as catecholamines and endothelins.[23] Blood flow disruptions related to maternal preeclampsia and congenital heart disease are also recognized as risk factors for NEC.[24,25] Endothelial TLR4 activation can also contribute to NEC pathogenesis by diminishing endothelial NO synthase expression and NO production.[22] Clearly, optimizing splanchnic vasoregulation is a strategic area of research to decrease intestinal injury and inflammation.

Increasing evidence indicates a role of gut microvasculature maldevelopment in NEC pathogenesis.[21] In mice, the intestinal microvasculature rapidly expands within the perinatal period from a thin, rudimentary matrix into a much more complex and organized network of blood vessels.[26] In our murine NEC model, impaired postnatal development of the gut microvasculature may predispose to histologic intestinal injury.[27] Near term, the fetal intestine shows strong expression of proangiogenic vascular endothelial cell factor (VEGF) and its cognate receptor VEGFR2, but this maturational increase is impaired by prenatal inflammation. Murine pups treated with a VEGFR2 inhibitor before experimental NEC show increased intestinal injury and mortality,[27] whereas promotion of intestinal VEGF production may be protective.[20] These experimental findings are consistent with decreased VEGF expression in healthy margins of human intestinal tissue resected for NEC compared with controls.[28] Therapeutic approaches to preserve intestinal microvasculature development and local VEGF and VEGFR2 expression may help prevent NEC in high-risk premature infants.[27]

Microbiome and Biotics Research

Microbial dysbiosis preceding NEC is characterized by a proteobacterial bloom and decrease in other phyla, namely Firmicutes and Bacteroidetes.[29] Microbiome optimization to offset dysbiosis is a promising research strategy. Manipulating gut microbiota composition by administering targeted antibiotics; supplementing specific strains of beneficial bacteria (probiotics), microbial products, and paraprobiotics (inactivated probiotics); or by modulating the TLR4 response to dysbiosis are promising research strategies.

The traditional microbial optimization method has been the use of probiotics, both single species and combinations of species of bacteria such as bifidobacteria and lactobacilli, and nonpathogenic fungi such as *Saccharomyces*. The World Health Organization (WHO) defines probiotics as "live microorganisms which when administered in adequate amounts confer a health benefit on the host."[30] The mechanisms by which probiotics may induce beneficial effects include gut barrier enhancement, improved epithelial survival, immune response modulation (eg, reduced responses from the TLR4 receptor, modulation of the effects of inflammatory cytokines), and competitive inhibition of gut colonization by pathogens.[31–33] Systematic reviews on probiotics, including the Cochrane Review, show that probiotics decrease NEC, late-onset sepsis, and all-cause mortality.[34-38] However, questions regarding the ideal combination of probiotics, duration of use, and dosage remain. Probiotic-related sepsis remains rare, but reports of sepsis[39] caused by contamination of probiotic products call for continued clinical caution in the selection of recipients.[40-42] Novel probiotic delivery systems such as biofilms, which may be more efficacious, are also being researched.[43]

The term paraprobiotics is used to define nonviable microbial cells (intact or broken) or crude cell extracts (ie, with a complex chemical composition), which, when administered (orally or topically) in adequate amounts, confer a benefit on the human or animal recipient.[44] The live cells (probiotics) are inactivated by heat, chemicals (eg, formalin), gamma or ultraviolet rays, or sonication.[44,45] Each of these inactivation methods affects the cells differently and, therefore, induces variable effects on immunomodulation.

Prebiotics are indigestible substances that stay unabsorbed and serve as substrates for growth of probiotic organisms. In a meta-analysis of 7 trials (417 infants), prebiotics did not decrease late-onset sepsis, NEC, or feed tolerance but increased the growth of Bifidobacterium in the stools.[46] Synbiotics, a combination of prebiotics and probiotics, has been investigated in few trials with varying results, and more research is needed.[47]

Human Milk Oligosaccharides and Glycans

Human milk oligosaccharides (HMOs) have gained increased awareness because of their luminal effects as prebiotics, which enhanced growth of beneficial bacteria (such as bifidobacteria), and as decoys in preventing pathogen colonization, and intestinal effects via promotion of the gut epithelial barrier and through maturation and enhancement of the leukocyte barrier in the lamina propria.[48,49] There may be some inconsistency in the HMO content not only by gestation (preterm vs term human milk) but also among mothers because of their secretor or genetic status. Lower amounts of HMO in their mothers' milk may predispose some infants to late-onset sepsis or NEC. Supplementation of preterm formula with HMOs may have beneficial effects on intestinal injury and inflammation.[50] Although HMO supplementation has been reported to be beneficial in animal models of intestinal injury,[51-53] human trials are yet to be conducted.

Multiomic Strategies and Integration of Microbiome, Proteome, Metabolome, and Epigenome Data

Advancing technology, including next-generation sequencing, proteomics, metabolomics, transcriptomics, and epigenomics, has provided better and holistic understanding of perinatal pathophysiology.[54] There is an ever-increasing need for integrative analysis of the human microbiome, with increasing information on genomics and the proteome, metabolome, and the epigenome, with integrative analysis, and correlation of these to the clinical outcomes. The host genome provides the backdrop for additional and multiple system interactions. The host and these microbes also produce large quantities of metabolites, adding another layer of complexity. Metabolomics is the science of detecting small molecules, the result of metabolic pathways from biological specimens such as plasma, serum, urine, and tissues, and is the latest of the omics technologies.[55-58] This testing detects the products of the metabolic pathways in an organism, which may be useful in diagnosis, prediction, prognosis, or assigning disease status (biomarker detection). Metabolomics allows identification of distinct patterns of small molecules generated during both host and microbial cellular metabolism and may be useful in searching for biomarkers of microbiome patterns and dysbiosis. Metabolite patterns are dynamic, changing with gestational age, time, or disease process, and evaluation at a time point provides a snapshot of the metabolic milieu of the organism. The complexity and the numerous metabolites that need to be measured need sophisticated analytical techniques. Nuclear magnetic resonance spectroscopy and mass spectrometry are the most common techniques used. The metabolites produced by microbes and/or the host may also regulate transcriptional and translational events that can be evaluated using transcriptomics and proteomics.[59]

There is a need for integration, analysis, and interpretation of information collected from different platforms related to the microbiome, transcription, proteomics, metabolomics, and the immune function to have a comprehensive view of these biological processes. This need brings up a significant bioinformatics challenge given the complexity of biological systems, the technological limits, the large number of biological variables, and limitations in the number of biological samples. Many network-based and graphical models (bayesian and nonbayesian) are being used to integrate these data. Bioinformatic techniques and expertise in dealing with these multiomics data are often the key in multiomic studies.[60,61] Integration of multiomics data may give a holistic view of pathophysiologic processes that lead to perinatal diseases and may inform novel preventive and therapeutic approaches.

Liquid biopsy of stools
A novel method of assessing microbiome and host responses is to salvage intestinal cells from stools, which can then be tested for microbiome, gene expression, and epigenetic profiles all in the same stool specimen, which can be followed longitudinally.[62]

Immunomodulation

Intestinal injury and inflammation and necrosis are important features of NEC, and excessive inflammation has been proposed as a causal factor in NEC.[63] Hence the interest in immunomodulators, which can decrease inflammation and intestinal injury.

Lactoferrin
Lactoferrin is a multifunctional molecule that has iron binding and immunomodulatory properties. It is a component of the innate immune system and may decrease inflammation. A meta-analysis of 12 studies, including small trials done worldwide, found that enteral supplementation of lactoferrin decreases length of stay but not mortality or NEC.[64] Two large recent trials of lactoferrin (ELFIN [Enteral Lactoferrin Supplementation in Newborn Very Preterm Infants] trial in the United Kingdom and the LIFT trial [Lactoferrin Infant Feeding Trial] in Australia and New Zealand) failed to show a decrease in sepsis, mortality. or NEC.[65,66]

Toll-like receptor antagonists
TLR4 signaling is an important signaling pathway that enhances intestinal inflammation via the lipopolysaccharide of gram-negative bacteria.[67] Therefore, TLR4 antagonists may be helpful in decreasing intestinal inflammation and injury. A novel family of TLR4 inhibitors from the laboratory of David Hackam and his colleagues,[68,69] including a lead TLR4 antagonist, C34, which is available for clinical use. C34 is an oligosaccharide, binds to the synthetic lipid A analogue eritoran (E5564), and thus inhibits TLR4. C34 inhibits TLR4 in vitro in intestinal epithelial cells and macrophages, and reduces TLR4-mediated inflammation in mouse models of endotoxemia and NEC.[68,69] Phase 1 clinical trials of C34 are being planned.

Other natural products, such as amniotic fluid,[70,71] breast milk,[72] and human milk oligosaccharide 2'-fucosyllactose,[73] have been shown to attenuate TLR4 signaling. Reciprocal expression of TLR4 and TLR9 signaling is seen in NEC, and TLR9 attenuates inflammation by antagonizing TLR4 mechanisms.[74] Peptidoglycan of gram-positive organisms may trigger TLR2 signaling, which has an antiinflammatory (via IL-10) and mucosal protective effect.[75] Variants of TLR2 have been associated with more severe inflammation. Novel strategies that use TLR2 ligands may decrease inflammation and disease severity in NEC.[75] TLR9 (cytosine phosphate-guanosine [CpG]-DNA is a TLR9 ligand) inhibits TLR4 signaling and is one of the mechanisms of action of probiotics.[74]

Growth Factors in the Prevention of Necrotizing Enterocolitis: Role for Amniotic Fluid and Breast Milk

Growth factors are essential for development, growth, and health of the gastrointestinal tract, and understanding the ontogeny may help clinicians understand the timing of NEC onset.[76] The amniotic fluid that bathes the fetal intestines and breast milk that is given after birth contain growth factors for the optimum development and function of the intestine. It can be hypothesized that decreased or absent growth factors during critical stages during fetal or postnatal development may increase the risk of NEC. Growth factors mediate cellular activities, namely cellular proliferation, migration, differentiation, and survival. This research has focused on enterocyte growth and trophic factors such as the epidermal growth factor (EGF) and heparin binding– EGF, but similar beneficial roles have been identified for glucagonlike peptide 2, insulinlike growth factor 1, erythropoietin, growth hormone, hepatocyte growth factor, and even for inflammatory mediators such as CXC chemokines such as IL-8.

The role of amniotic fluid in the prevention of NEC, which contains growth and trophic factors, is being researched.[70] By urination and swallowing, the fetus contributes to the volume and composition of the amniotic fluid mostly in the second half of pregnancy. Interruption of amniotic fluid flow in the intestines causes mucosal and villus atrophy, which can be reversed by restoring flow of amniotic fluid but not by Ringer lactate.[77,78] This finding shows that trophic factors (insulinlike growth factors I and II, EGF, hepatocyte growth factor) in the amniotic fluid are more essential to fetal gut development and maturation than the volume of the fluid.[79] In addition, the amniotic fluid also contains cytokines and stem cells (SCs).[80] Animal studies have shown that amniotic fluid administration, postnatally in mice, decreases TLR4 signaling and inflammation, and enhances repair of the intestine.[71,81–83] However, questions remain regarding collection of amniotic fluid; when, how, what gestation, and when to administer to neonates; sterilization practices; donor amniotic fluid; and potential adverse effects of this intervention.

Human Stem Cells and Their Role in Prevention of Necrotizing Enterocolitis

The use of SCs, which have the potential to help in intestinal restitution from injury, is a promising avenue of research in NEC prevention. SCs produce an array of cytokines, growth factors, microRNAs, and extracellular vesicles that may decrease intestinal injury in animal models of NEC.[84] Research from the Besner laboratory has reported that different types of SC reduce the incidence and severity of NEC and preserve intestinal barrier function during NEC.[85,86] SCs from the amniotic fluid also protect the intestines from injury and facilitate repair, and hence amniotic fluid therapy holds great promise for prevention of NEC.[87] Once NEC has set in, rescue therapy is also possible with enteric neural SCs. Administered SCs engraft at low rates and do not explain the beneficial effects of SC administration, and, therefore, SC-secreted factors may be more important. SC-derived exosomes as a paracrine secretion that is responsible for the beneficial effects of SCs is currently being researched.[85,86]

BIOMARKER DISCOVERY FOR EARLY DIAGNOSIS AND MONITORING

The signs and symptoms in the early phases of NEC are nonspecific and can be confused with other diseases (spontaneous intestinal perforation [SIP]), ischemic bowel caused by cardiovascular diseases, or food protein–sensitive enteritis. Pneumoperitoneum on the radiograph may also be caused by SIP without intestinal necrosis, and pneumatosis intestinalis may be confused with air bubbles mixed with stool. Ultrasonography examination of the abdomen may be useful but can be subjective, needs expertise to perform and interpret, and becomes more specific in the later stages of the disease. Biomarkers that can diagnose NEC in the early stages of the disease are necessary to differentiate it from other diagnoses. None of the currently available biomarkers have adequate sensitivity or specificity for use in diagnostic tests. Development of a disease-specific screening tool may not only help in the early diagnosis of the disease but also improve the understanding of the pathogenesis and aid targeted treatment.

Biomarkers, end points, and other tools (BEST) defines a biomarker as "a defined characteristic that is, measured as an indicator of normal biological processes, pathogenic processes, or response to an exposure or intervention."[88] Molecular, histologic, radiographic, or physiologic characteristics are types of biomarkers. A biomarker would be highly useful in the following clinical scenarios[89]:

1. Risk assessment of likelihood or probability of NEC in all very low birth weight infants.
2. Early NEC diagnosis, before progression of disease to irreversible intestinal injury.
3. Excluding NEC in infants with symptoms suspicious for NEC (ie, high negative predictive value and specificity).
4. Early NEC prognostication, determining which newborns are likely to have disease progression.

CATEGORIES OF BIOMARKERS

1. Biomarkers associated with systemic inflammation: C-reactive protein (CRP), white cell count, thrombocytopenia, procalcitonin, and other cytokines. Increased CRP and procalcitonin levels have been reported to be highly specific for NEC diagnosis in some studies, although these studies do not include a control group of patients with sepsis alone without NEC, leading to misclassification bias.
2. Biomarkers specific for gut injury: calprotectin, intestinal fatty acid binding protein, claudins, and interalpha inhibitor protein.
3. Microbial metabolites including fecal volatile organic compounds (VOCs).
4. Composite of multiple biomarkers; for example, combination of inflammatory, gut injury specific and imaging.

Metabolomics allow identification of distinct patterns of small molecules generated during host and microbial cellular metabolism, which may detect microbiome and metabolomic signatures of dysbiosis.[90–94] Morrow and colleagues[95] evaluated urinary metabolome patterns in association with gut dysbiosis preceding NEC. Alanine was directly correlated with the relative abundance of Firmicutes, and inversely correlated with the relative abundance of both Proteobacteria and *Propionibacterium*.[95] Ratio of alanine to histidine was positively associated with overall NEC and inversely associated with the relative abundance of *Propionibacterium*. Other studies show differences in metabolites related to carbohydrate, steroid hormone biosynthesis, gluconic acid, leukotriene and prostaglandin metabolism, lineolate metabolism, lipid metabolism, and intracellular signaling between infants with NEC and control infants.[96-98] There is no unifying hypothesis related to altered metabolism in NEC (host or microbial) and integration of all omics platforms, including metabolomics, is necessary to understand the pathophysiology in NEC.

Fecal VOCs are considered to reflect not only gut microbiota composition but also their metabolic activity and concurrent interaction with the host.[99] A NEC-specific or a sepsis-specific microbial or metabolic signature has not yet been determined. Identification of disease-specific VOCs and microbiota composition may increase understanding on pathophysiologic mechanisms in NEC. To date, only 2 studies report on fecal VOCs in NEC.[99-101] Garner and colleagues[101] observed that the number of VOCs increases significantly with age in infants without NEC (n = 7), whereas a reduction was observed in infants with NEC (n = 6) days before diagnosis. The NEC cases did not show 4 specific esters: hexadecenoic acid ethyl ester, 2-ethylhexyl acetic ester, decanoic acid ethyl ester, and dodecanoic acid ethyl ester, which were present in control infants. de Meij and colleagues[100] reported that fecal VOC profiles allowed discrimination between cases (n = 13) and controls (n = 14) up to 3 days before clinical onset of NEC, with increasing accuracy closer to the day of diagnosis.

Currently available biomarkers lack utility[89] because they have not been rigorously assessed in appropriate samples of preterm infants. They lack validity testing with reproducibility of results; for example, IAIP, hydrogen excretion, VOCs, fecal microbiota analysis, and proteomics. There is an urgent need to evaluate these biomarkers in prospective multicenter studies to assess analytical validity (reproducibility), clinical validity (discrimination and calibration), and ability to generalize.

SUMMARY

This article summarizes the multipronged research being pursued in the domain of NEC. Advances in technology and multiomic platforms of the microbiome, transcriptomics, proteomics, and metabolomics have provided an opportunity to have a holistic view on biological processes in NEC, which can then be targeted to improve clinical outcomes. Multiomics can also provide host-related or microbiome-related biomarkers for early diagnosis and monitoring. However, most of this cutting-edge research needs further evaluation in experimental situations, and then for reproducibility and the ability to generalize in wider clinical applications.

REFERENCES

1. Moss RL, Kalish LA, Duggan C, et al. Clinical parameters do not adequately predict outcome in necrotizing enterocolitis: a multi-institutional study. J Perinatol 2008;28(10):665–74.
2. Ballance WA, Dahms BB, Shenker N, et al. Pathology of neonatal necrotizing enterocolitis: a ten-year experience. J Pediatr 1990;117(1 Pt 2):S6–13.
3. Santulli TV, Schullinger JN, Heird WC, et al. Acute necrotizing enterocolitis in infancy: a review of 64 cases. Pediatrics 1975;55(3):376–87.
4. Remon JI, Amin SC, Mehendale SR, et al. Depth of bacterial invasion in resected intestinal tissue predicts mortality in surgical necrotizing enterocolitis. J Perinatol 2015;35(9):755–62.

5. Egan CE, Sodhi CP, Good M, et al. Toll-like receptor 4-mediated lymphocyte influx induces neonatal necrotizing enterocolitis. J Clin Invest 2016;126(2): 495–508.
6. Teiserskas J, Bartasiene R, Tameliene R. Associations between red blood cell transfusions and necrotizing enterocolitis in very low birth weight infants: ten-year data of a tertiary neonatal unit. Medicina (Kaunas) 2019;55(1) [pii:E16].
7. Janjindamai W, Prapruettrong A, Thatrimontrichai A, et al. Risk of necrotizing enterocolitis following packed red blood cell transfusion in very low birth weight infants. Indian J Pediatr 2019;86(4):347–53.
8. Garg P, Pinotti R, Lal CV, et al. Transfusion-associated necrotizing enterocolitis in preterm infants: an updated meta-analysis of observational data. J Perinat Med 2018;46(6):677–85.
9. Maheshwari A, Patel RM, Christensen RD. Anemia, red blood cell transfusions, and necrotizing enterocolitis. Semin Pediatr Surg 2018;27(1):47–51.
10. Crabtree CS, Pakvasa M, Radmacher PG, et al. Retrospective case-control study of necrotizing enterocolitis and packed red blood cell transfusions in very low birth weight infants. J Neonatal Perinatal Med 2018;11(4):365–70.
11. Patel RM, Knezevic A, Shenvi N, et al. Association of red blood cell transfusion, anemia, and necrotizing enterocolitis in very low-birth-weight infants. JAMA 2016;315(9):889–97.
12. Wan-Huen P, Bateman D, Shapiro DM, et al. Packed red blood cell transfusion is an independent risk factor for necrotizing enterocolitis in premature infants. J Perinatol 2013;33(10):786–90.
13. MohanKumar K, Namachivayam K, Song T, et al. A murine neonatal model of necrotizing enterocolitis caused by anemia and red blood cell transfusions. Nat Commun 2019;10(1):3494.
14. O'Neill JA Jr. Neonatal necrotizing enterocolitis. Surg Clin North Am 1981;61(5): 1013–22.
15. Hutter JJ Jr, Hathaway WE, Wayne ER. Hematologic abnormalities in severe neonatal necrotizing enterocolitis. J Pediatr 1976;88(6):1026–31.
16. Patel CC. Hematologic abnormalities in acute necrotizing enterocolitis. Pediatr Clin North Am 1977;24(3):579–84.
17. Ververidis M, Kiely EM, Spitz L, et al. The clinical significance of thrombocytopenia in neonates with necrotizing enterocolitis. J Pediatr Surg 2001;36(5): 799–803.
18. Namachivayam K, MohanKumar K, Garg L, et al. Neonatal mice with necrotizing enterocolitis-like injury develop thrombocytopenia despite increased megakaryopoiesis. Pediatr Res 2017;81(5):817–24.
19. Nair J, Lakshminrusimha S. Role of NO and other vascular mediators in the etiopathogenesis of necrotizing enterocolitis. Front Biosci (Schol Ed) 2019;11:9–28.
20. Bowker RM, Yan X, Managlia E, et al. Dimethyloxalylglycine preserves the intestinal microvasculature and protects against intestinal injury in a neonatal mouse NEC model: role of VEGF signaling. Pediatr Res 2018;83(2):545–53.
21. Bowker RM, Yan X, De Plaen IG. Intestinal microcirculation and necrotizing enterocolitis: the vascular endothelial growth factor system. Semin Fetal Neonatal Med 2018;23(6):411–5.
22. Yazji I, Sodhi CP, Lee EK, et al. Endothelial TLR4 activation impairs intestinal microcirculatory perfusion in necrotizing enterocolitis via eNOS-NO-nitrite signaling. Proc Natl Acad Sci U S A 2013;110(23):9451–6.
23. Nowicki PT, Dunaway DJ, Nankervis CA, et al. Endothelin-1 in human intestine resected for necrotizing enterocolitis. J Pediatr 2005;146(6):805–10.

24. Giannone PJ, Luce WA, Nankervis CA, et al. Necrotizing enterocolitis in neonates with congenital heart disease. Life Sci 2008;82(7–8):341–7.
25. Perger L, Mukhopadhyay D, Komidar L, et al. Maternal pre-eclampsia as a risk factor for necrotizing enterocolitis. J Matern Fetal Neonatal Med 2016;29(13): 2098–103.
26. Hatch J, Mukouyama YS. Spatiotemporal mapping of vascularization and innervation in the fetal murine intestine. Dev Dyn 2015;244(1):56–68.
27. Yan X, Managlia E, Liu SX, et al. Lack of VEGFR2 signaling causes maldevelopment of the intestinal microvasculature and facilitates necrotizing enterocolitis in neonatal mice. Am J Physiol Gastrointest Liver Physiol 2016;310(9):G716–25.
28. Sabnis A, Carrasco R, Liu SX, et al. Intestinal vascular endothelial growth factor is decreased in necrotizing enterocolitis. Neonatology 2015;107(3):191–8.
29. Pammi M, Cope J, Tarr PI, et al. Intestinal dysbiosis in preterm infants preceding necrotizing enterocolitis: a systematic review and meta-analysis. Microbiome 2017;5(1):31.
30. Guidelines for the evaluation of probiotics in food: report of a joint FAO/WHO Working group on drafting guidelines for the evaluation of probiotics in food 2002. Available at: https://www.who.int/foodsafety/fs_management/en/probiotic_guidelines.pdf. Accessed December 27, 2019.
31. Rao RK, Samak G. Protection and restitution of gut barrier by probiotics: nutritional and clinical implications. Curr Nutr Food Sci 2013;9(2):99–107.
32. Walker A. Intestinal colonization and programming of the intestinal immune response. J Clin Gastroenterol 2014;48(Suppl 1):S8–11.
33. Good M, Sodhi CP, Ozolek JA, et al. Lactobacillus rhamnosus HN001 decreases the severity of necrotizing enterocolitis in neonatal mice and preterm piglets: evidence in mice for a role of TLR9. Am J Physiol Gastrointest Liver Physiol 2014; 306(11):G1021–32.
34. Underwood MA. Probiotics and the prevention of necrotizing enterocolitis. J Pediatr Surg 2019;54(3):405–12.
35. Alfaleh K, Anabrees J, Bassler D, et al. Probiotics for prevention of necrotizing enterocolitis in preterm infants. Cochrane Database Syst Rev 2011;(3):CD005496.
36. Deshpande G, Rao S, Patole S, et al. Updated meta-analysis of probiotics for preventing necrotizing enterocolitis in preterm neonates. Pediatrics 2010; 125(5):921–30.
37. Olsen R, Greisen G, Schroder M, et al. Prophylactic probiotics for preterm infants: a systematic review and meta-analysis of observational studies. Neonatology 2016;109(2):105–12.
38. Rao SC, Athalye-Jape GK, Deshpande GC, et al. Probiotic supplementation and late-onset sepsis in preterm infants: a meta-analysis. Pediatrics 2016;137(3): e20153684.
39. Salminen MK, Tynkkynen S, Rautelin H, et al. Lactobacillus bacteremia during a rapid increase in probiotic use of Lactobacillus rhamnosus GG in Finland. Clin Infect Dis 2002;35(10):1155–60.
40. Lewis ZT, Shani G, Masarweh CF, et al. Validating bifidobacterial species and subspecies identity in commercial probiotic products. Pediatr Res 2016;79(3): 445–52.
41. Vallabhaneni S, Walker TA, Lockhart SR, et al. Notes from the field: fatal gastrointestinal mucormycosis in a premature infant associated with a contaminated dietary supplement–Connecticut, 2014. MMWR Morb Mortal Wkly Rep 2015; 64(6):155–6.

42. Vermeulen MJ, Luijendijk A, van Toledo L, et al. Quality of probiotic products for preterm infants: contamination and missing strains. Acta Paediatr 2020;109(2): 276–9.
43. Olson JK, Rager TM, Navarro JB, et al. Harvesting the benefits of biofilms: a novel probiotic delivery system for the prevention of necrotizing enterocolitis. J Pediatr Surg 2016;51(6):936–41.
44. Taverniti V, Guglielmetti S. The immunomodulatory properties of probiotic microorganisms beyond their viability (ghost probiotics: proposal of paraprobiotic concept). Genes Nutr 2011;6(3):261–74.
45. Zorzela L, Ardestani SK, McFarland LV, et al. Is there a role for modified probiotics as beneficial microbes: a systematic review of the literature. Benef Microbes 2017;8(5):739–54.
46. Srinivasjois R, Rao S, Patole S. Prebiotic supplementation in preterm neonates: updated systematic review and meta-analysis of randomised controlled trials. Clin Nutr 2013;32(6):958–65.
47. Johnson-Henry KC, Abrahamsson TR, Wu RY, et al. Probiotics, prebiotics, and synbiotics for the prevention of necrotizing enterocolitis. Adv Nutr 2016;7(5): 928–37.
48. Plaza-Diaz J, Fontana L, Gil A. Human milk oligosaccharides and immune system development. Nutrients 2018;10(8) [pii:E1038].
49. Bering SB. Human milk oligosaccharides to prevent gut dysfunction and necrotizing enterocolitis in preterm neonates. Nutrients 2018;10(10) [pii:E1461].
50. Cilieborg MS, Bering SB, Ostergaard MV, et al. Minimal short-term effect of dietary 2'-fucosyllactose on bacterial colonisation, intestinal function and necrotising enterocolitis in preterm pigs. Br J Nutr 2016;116(5):834–41.
51. Autran CA, Schoterman MH, Jantscher-Krenn E, et al. Sialylated galacto-oligosaccharides and 2'-fucosyllactose reduce necrotising enterocolitis in neonatal rats. Br J Nutr 2016;116(2):294–9.
52. Jantscher-Krenn E, Zherebtsov M, Nissan C, et al. The human milk oligosaccharide disialyllacto-N-tetraose prevents necrotising enterocolitis in neonatal rats. Gut 2012;61(10):1417–25.
53. Yu H, Yan X, Autran CA, et al. Enzymatic and chemoenzymatic syntheses of disialyl glycans and their necrotizing enterocolitis preventing effects. J Org Chem 2017;82(24):13152–60.
54. Neu J. Multiomics-based strategies for taming intestinal inflammation in the neonate. Curr Opin Clin Nutr Metab Care 2019;22(3):217–22.
55. Kell DB, Oliver SG. The metabolome 18 years on: a concept comes of age. Metabolomics 2016;12(9):148.
56. Ursell LK, Haiser HJ, Van Treuren W, et al. The intestinal metabolome: an intersection between microbiota and host. Gastroenterology 2014;146(6):1470–6.
57. Fanos V, Van den Anker J, Noto A, et al. Metabolomics in neonatology: fact or fiction? Semin Fetal Neonatal Med 2013;18(1):3–12.
58. Antonucci R, Atzori L, Barberini L, et al. Metabolomics: the "new clinical chemistry" for personalized neonatal medicine. Minerva Pediatr 2010;62(3 Suppl 1): 145–8.
59. Howell KJ, Kraiczy J, Nayak KM, et al. DNA methylation and transcription patterns in intestinal epithelial cells from pediatric patients with inflammatory bowel diseases differentiate disease subtypes and associate with outcome. Gastroenterology 2018;154(3):585–98.
60. Chong J, Xia J. Computational approaches for integrative analysis of the metabolome and microbiome. Metabolites 2017;7(4) [pii:E62].

61. Hasin Y, Seldin M, Lusis A. Multi-omics approaches to disease. Genome Biol 2017;18(1):83.

62. Donovan SM, Wang M, Monaco MH, et al. Noninvasive molecular fingerprinting of host-microbiome interactions in neonates. FEBS Lett 2014;588(22):4112–9.

63. Nanthakumar N, Meng D, Goldstein AM, et al. The mechanism of excessive intestinal inflammation in necrotizing enterocolitis: an immature innate immune response. PLoS One 2011;6(3):e17776.

64. Pammi M, Suresh G. Enteral lactoferrin supplementation for prevention of sepsis and necrotizing enterocolitis in preterm infants. Cochrane database Syst Rev 2017;(6):CD007137.

65. Trial: Enteral LactoFerrin In Neonates. ISRCT registry N88261002. https://doi.org/10.1186/ISRCTN88261002. Accessed October 27, 2019.

66. Trial: Lactoferrin Infant Feeding Trial - LIFT_Canada. ClinicalTrials.gov Identifier: NCT03367013. Accessed October 27, 2019.

67. Hackam DJ, Sodhi CP, Good M. New insights into necrotizing enterocolitis: from laboratory observation to personalized prevention and treatment. J Pediatr Surg 2019;54(3):398–404.

68. Neal MD, Jia H, Eyer B, et al. Discovery and validation of a new class of small molecule Toll-like receptor 4 (TLR4) inhibitors. PLoS One 2013;8(6):e65779.

69. Wipf P, Eyer BR, Yamaguchi Y, et al. Synthesis of anti-inflammatory alpha-and beta-linked acetamidopyranosides as inhibitors of toll-like receptor 4 (TLR4). Tetrahedron Lett 2015;56(23):3097–100.

70. Dasgupta S, Jain SK. Protective effects of amniotic fluid in the setting of necrotizing enterocolitis. Pediatr Res 2017;82(4):584–95.

71. Good M, Siggers RH, Sodhi CP, et al. Amniotic fluid inhibits Toll-like receptor 4 signaling in the fetal and neonatal intestinal epithelium. Proc Natl Acad Sci U S A 2012;109(28):11330–5.

72. Good M, Sodhi CP, Egan CE, et al. Breast milk protects against the development of necrotizing enterocolitis through inhibition of Toll-like receptor 4 in the intestinal epithelium via activation of the epidermal growth factor receptor. Mucosal Immunol 2015;8(5):1166–79.

73. Good M, Sodhi CP, Yamaguchi Y, et al. The human milk oligosaccharide 2'-fucosyllactose attenuates the severity of experimental necrotising enterocolitis by enhancing mesenteric perfusion in the neonatal intestine. Br J Nutr 2016;116(7):1175–87.

74. Gribar SC, Sodhi CP, Richardson WM, et al. Reciprocal expression and signaling of TLR4 and TLR9 in the pathogenesis and treatment of necrotizing enterocolitis. J Immunol 2009;182(1):636–46.

75. Cario E. Barrier-protective function of intestinal epithelial Toll-like receptor 2. Mucosal Immunol 2008;1(Suppl 1):S62–6.

76. Shelby RD, Cromeens B, Rager TM, et al. Influence of growth factors on the development of necrotizing enterocolitis. Clin Perinatol 2019;46(1):51–64.

77. Trahair JF, Harding R. Restitution of swallowing in the fetal sheep restores intestinal growth after midgestation esophageal obstruction. J Pediatr Gastroenterol Nutr 1995;20(2):156–61.

78. Trahair JF, Harding R. Ultrastructural anomalies in the fetal small intestine indicate that fetal swallowing is important for normal development: an experimental study. Virchows Arch A Pathol Anat Histopathol 1992;420(4):305–12.

79. Drozdowski L, Thomson AB. Intestinal hormones and growth factors: effects on the small intestine. World J Gastroenterol 2009;15(4):385–406.

80. Maheshwari A. Role of cytokines in human intestinal villous development. Clin Perinatol 2004;31(1):143–55.

81. Zani A, Cananzi M, Lauriti G, et al. Amniotic fluid stem cells prevent development of ascites in a neonatal rat model of necrotizing enterocolitis. Eur J Pediatr Surg 2014;24(1):57–60.

82. Jain SK, Baggerman EW, Mohankumar K, et al. Amniotic fluid-borne hepatocyte growth factor protects rat pups against experimental necrotizing enterocolitis. Am J Physiol Gastrointest Liver Physiol 2014;306(5):G361–9.

83. Siggers J, Ostergaard MV, Siggers RH, et al. Postnatal amniotic fluid intake reduces gut inflammatory responses and necrotizing enterocolitis in preterm neonates. Am J Physiol Gastrointest Liver Physiol 2013;304(10):G864–75.

84. Pisano C, Besner GE. Potential role of stem cells in disease prevention based on a murine model of experimental necrotizing enterocolitis. J Pediatr Surg 2019; 54(3):413–6.

85. McCulloh CJ, Olson JK, Zhou Y, et al. Stem cells and necrotizing enterocolitis: a direct comparison of the efficacy of multiple types of stem cells. J Pediatr Surg 2017;52(6):999–1005.

86. McCulloh CJ, Olson JK, Wang Y, et al. Evaluating the efficacy of different types of stem cells in preserving gut barrier function in necrotizing enterocolitis. J Surg Res 2017;214:278–85.

87. Rager TM, Olson JK, Zhou Y, et al. Exosomes secreted from bone marrow-derived mesenchymal stem cells protect the intestines from experimental necrotizing enterocolitis. J Pediatr Surg 2016;51(6):942–7.

88. FDA-NIH Biomarker Working Group. BEST (Biomarkers, EndpointS, and other Tools). Food and Drug Administration, Silver Spring (MD), and National Institutes of Health, Bethesda (MD): 2016.

89. Goldstein GP, Sylvester KG. Biomarker discovery and utility in necrotizing enterocolitis. Clin Perinatol 2019;46(1):1–17.

90. Tuohy KM, Gougoulias C, Shen Q, et al. Studying the human gut microbiota in the trans-omics era–focus on metagenomics and metabonomics. Curr Pharm Des 2009;15(13):1415–27.

91. Swann JR, Tuohy KM, Lindfors P, et al. Variation in antibiotic-induced microbial recolonization impacts on the host metabolic phenotypes of rats. J Proteome Res 2011;10(8):3590–603.

92. Ponnusamy K, Choi JN, Kim J, et al. Microbial community and metabolomic comparison of irritable bowel syndrome faeces. J Med Microbiol 2011;60(Pt 6):817–27, 3167923.

93. Dai ZL, Zhang J, Wu G, et al. Utilization of amino acids by bacteria from the pig small intestine. Amino acids 2010;39(5):1201–15.

94. Cevallos-Cevallos JM, Danyluk MD, Reyes-De-Corcuera JI. GC-MS based metabolomics for rapid simultaneous detection of Escherichia coli O157:H7, Salmonella Typhimurium, Salmonella Muenchen, and Salmonella Hartford in ground beef and chicken. J Food Sci 2011;76(4):M238–46.

95. Morrow AL, Lagomarcino AJ, Schibler KR, et al. Early microbial and metabolomic signatures predict later onset of necrotizing enterocolitis in preterm infants. Microbiome 2013;1(1):13, 3971624.

96. Wilcock A, Begley P, Stevens A, et al. The metabolomics of necrotising enterocolitis in preterm babies: an exploratory study. J Matern Fetal Neonatal Med 2016;29(5):758–62.

97. Stewart CJ, Embleton ND, Marrs EC, et al. Temporal bacterial and metabolic development of the preterm gut reveals specific signatures in health and disease. Microbiome 2016;4(1):67.

98. De Magistris A, Corbu S, Cesare Marincola F. NMR-based metabolomics analysis of urinary changes in neonatal necrotizing enterocolitis. Jpnim 2015;37–8.

99. Berkhout DJC, Niemarkt HJ, de Boer NKH, et al. The potential of gut microbiota and fecal volatile organic compounds analysis as early diagnostic biomarker for necrotizing enterocolitis and sepsis in preterm infants. Expert Rev Gastroenterol Hepatol 2018;12(5):457–70.

100. de Meij TG, van der Schee MP, Berkhout DJ, et al. Early detection of necrotizing enterocolitis by fecal volatile organic compounds analysis. J Pediatr 2015; 167(3):562–7.e1.

101. Garner CE, Ewer AK, Elasouad K, et al. Analysis of faecal volatile organic compounds in preterm infants who develop necrotising enterocolitis: a pilot study. J Pediatr Gastroenterol Nutr 2009;49(5):559–65.

Transfusion-related Gut Injury and Necrotizing Enterocolitis

Allison Thomas Rose, MD, Vivek Saroha, MD, PhD,
Ravi Mangal Patel, MD, MSc*

KEYWORDS

• Preterm • Transfusion • Anemia • Feeding • Morbidity

KEY POINTS

- Preclinical studies have identified plausible biological mechanisms of gut injury from red blood cell (RBC) transfusion in the setting of anemia. These studies may explain the epidemiologic associations observed in studies of preterm infants between severe anemia, RBC transfusion, and necrotizing enterocolitis (NEC).
- The optimal hemoglobin transfusion thresholds to reduce the risk of NEC and other important adverse outcomes in preterm infants are uncertain. Ongoing randomized trials, coupled with advanced monitoring techniques such as near-infrared spectroscopy, may provide new information to guide approaches to red cell transfusion in preterm infants.
- The implementation of standardized feeding protocols is associated with a reduction in the risk of NEC; however, the effects of withholding enteral feeds during RBC transfusion on NEC and other important outcomes is uncertain.
- Additional studies are needed to further understand the effects of RBC product characteristics on transfusion-related outcomes in preterm infants.

INTRODUCTION

Necrotizing enterocolitis (NEC) causes significant morbidity and mortality in infants, accounting for 10% of deaths in neonatal intensive care units.[1] Multiple randomized trials and observational studies have identified a variety of factors associated with NEC, although the causal effects of many of these factors are unclear.[2] Because NEC is a multifactorial disease, there are likely several distinct causal mechanisms leading to an eventual common disease phenotype, with intestinal inflammation a central theme in the pathogenesis of NEC. The association between NEC, red blood cell

Division of Neonatology, Department of Pediatrics, Emory University School of Medicine, Children's Healthcare of Atlanta, 2015 Uppergate Drive Northeast, Atlanta, GA 30322, USA
* Corresponding author.
E-mail address: rmpatel@emory.edu
Twitter: @404Rose (A.T.R.); @vsaroha (V.S.); @ravimpatelmd (R.M.P.)

Clin Perinatol 47 (2020) 399–412
https://doi.org/10.1016/j.clp.2020.02.002

(RBC) transfusion, and anemia has been investigated in multiple observational studies. Meta-analyses of these studies have found conflicting results, with a 2012 analysis suggesting an increased odds of NEC after RBC transfusion (odds ratio [OR], 2.01; 95% confidence interval [CI], 1.61–2.5)[3] and a more recent analysis suggesting no association (OR, 0.96; 95% CI, 0.53–1.71).[4] Although up to one-third of NEC cases occur in the setting of antecedent RBC transfusion exposure,[5] few cases of NEC occur within 48 hours of RBC transfusion (0.5%–1.4%).[6,7] Two recent animal studies may help illuminate the biological mechanisms underlying the associations between anemia, RBC transfusion, and gut injury.[8,9] This article summarizes the most recent data on NEC following RBC transfusion, which some groups have termed transfusion-related acute gut injury (TRAGI) or transfusion-associated NEC (TANEC). It also highlights the potential mechanisms in preclinical and human physiologic studies. Because enteral feeding, including the type of feeding, may influence the risk of NEC, this article reviews what is known about the role of feeding during RBC transfusion and the risk of NEC. Although publications on TRAGI extend back to its first description in 1987 by McGrady and colleagues,[10] this article is limited to the most recent publications as well as discussions of ongoing trials. Although studies use different terminology to define NEC in relation to an antecedent RBC transfusion, this article consistently uses TRAGI to refer to NEC that occurs within 48 hours of RBC transfusion and notes when studies consider NEC occurring at different time points following RBC transfusion. This is partially because the 48 hour cutoff of NEC occurring following RBC transfusion is arbitrary.

META-ANALYSIS OF OBSERVATIONAL STUDIES OF RED BLOOD CELL TRANSFUSION AND NECROTIZING ENTEROCOLITIS

Five meta-analyses over the past 7 years have collected data from 28 unique observational studies to determine the association between RBC transfusion and NEC. A systematic review and meta-analysis from 2012 reported on 12 trials (publication years 2006–2011) assessing the association of transfusion and NEC. In 5 of 12 studies reporting unadjusted outcomes, the analysis found an association between RBC transfusion and NEC (OR, 3.91; 95% CI, 2.97–5.14). This point estimate was attenuated when examining 4 of the 12 studies that reported adjusted outcomes (OR, 2.01; 95% CI, 1.61–2.50).[3] Also published in 2012, a second review examined data from randomized controlled trials (RCTs) of transfusion thresholds (discussed later) as well as observational data from 6 cohort studies and 4 case-control studies. Although the pooled OR and CI for RCT data remained nonsignificant (OR, 1.67; 95% CI, 0.82–3.38), the study noted the pooled point estimate was in the direction toward more NEC in the restrictive transfusion group, suggesting the opposite of what would be expected if RBC transfusions alone were causative for NEC.[11] The pooled estimate from randomized trials in this review were in the opposite direction of the pooled estimates from observational cohort studies (OR, 7.48; 95% CI, 5.87-9.53) and case-control studies (OR, 2.19; 95% CI, 1.52-3.17).[11] Thus, the investigators concluded that the observational data are hypothesis generating in that they identify a potential cause of NEC that deserves further study, but they are not conclusive of a causal relationship between RBC transfusion and NEC.

Three additional meta-analyses published 6 years on from these first two suggest there is continued uncertainty regarding the causal relationship between RBC transfusion and NEC. In 2017, a Grading of Recommendations Assessment, Development and Evaluation (GRADE) analysis of clinical data on transfusions and NEC suggested that the overall quality of evidence was low to very low in the association between RBC transfusion and NEC.[12] This study found no increased odds of TRAGI based on 13 observational studies (OR, 1.13; 95% CI, 0.99-1.29), but increased odds for NEC any time after transfusion (OR, 1.95; 95% CI, 1.60-2.38; 9 studies). Two additional meta-analyses noted 2 different conclusions: a meta-analysis of 17 observational studies found no association between RBC transfusion and NEC (OR, 0.96; 95 CI, 0.53–1.17)[4] and a meta-analysis of 10 studies found RBC transfusion was associated with a lower risk of NEC (OR, 0.55; 95% CI, 0.31–0.98).[13] Although attempts to summarize the evidence through systematic reviews and meta-analyses have led to different estimates of the association between RBC transfusion and NEC, all meta-analyses note the inherent limitations of observational data, with bias and confounding by indication that limit causal inference. As such, data from large, ongoing RCTs will provide important information, as discussed later.

DATA FROM RED BLOOD CELL TRANSFUSION TRIALS

RCT data on restrictive versus liberal transfusion thresholds have not indicated that more liberal RBC transfusion approaches increase the risk of NEC. The Premature Infants in Need of Transfusion (PINT) trial[14] randomized 451 infants less than 1000 g and less than 31 weeks' gestational age to either restrictive or liberal transfusion thresholds. In the PINT trial,[15] the mean hemoglobin difference between the 2 study arms was approximately 1 g/dL, with a mean hemoglobin level of 10.1 mg/dL in the restrictive arm at 4 weeks compared with 11.2 mg/dL in the liberal arm. The differences in transfusion thresholds resulted in a mean difference in number of transfusions of −0.83 (95% CI, −1.68–0.02; $P = .07$). There was no statistically significant difference in the risk of NEC between the 2 study arms. The Iowa trial randomized 100 infants to restrictive or liberal transfusions and achieved a mean difference in hemoglobin of 2.7 g/dL between study arms.[16] A single episode of NEC occurred in each study arm.[17] A 2011 Cochrane Review pooled analysis from 3 RCTs of restrictive versus liberal transfusion practices, including the PINT and Iowa trials, and found no difference in the risk of NEC (relative risk [RR], 1.62; 95% CI, 0.82–3.13); the PINT trial accounted for 90% of the weighted result.[17] NEC was not the primary outcome in any of the randomized trials, and none reported on a temporal relationship between RBC transfusion and NEC. Two future RCTs comparing restrictive versus liberal transfusion thresholds will report on survival and ~2-year neurodevelopmental outcomes with NEC as a secondary outcome. In the United States, the Transfusion of Prematures (TOP) trial from the National Institute of Child Health and Human Development Neonatal Research Network has completed enrollment of 1824 infants randomized to restrictive versus liberal transfusion thresholds based on postnatal age and respiratory support.[18] In Germany, The Effects of Transfusion Thresholds on Neurocognitive Outcome of Extremely Low Birth Weight Infants (ETTNO) trial has enrolled 920 infants with similar design to TOP.[19] Together, these studies may contribute information from approximately 2700 infants to update current evidence from past trials that will be important in guiding transfusion decisions and how such decisions may influence the risk of NEC as well as other important outcomes, such as death or long-term neurodevelopmental impairment.

ROLE OF UNDERLYING SEVERITY OF ANEMIA

Premature infants are at risk for severe anemia because of several endogenous factors (ie, decreased erythropoietin production and increased erythropoietin catabolism)[20] as well as exogenous factors (ie, iatrogenic blood loss, nutritional deficiencies, infection, chronic illness). Recent trends in clinical practice have moved away from frequent

RBC transfusions to treat anemia of prematurity[21]; however, it has been proposed that anemia leading to decreased oxygen delivery and tissue hypoxia may cause intestinal injury in premature infants, thus setting up the potential for the development of NEC. A 2011 case-control study of 333 premature infants (111 with NEC and 222 matched controls without) found a 10% increase risk of NEC for every 1-g/dL decrease in hemoglobin nadir in multivariate modeling (OR, 1.10; 95% CI, 1.02–1.18).[22] In a prospective study of 598 very low birth weight (VLBW) infants, infants with severe anemia (≤8 g/dL) had a significantly increased rate of NEC compared with those without severe anemia (adjusted cause-specific hazard ratio [CSHR], 6.0; 95% CI, 2.00–18.0).[7] In the same study, an analysis of 319 VLBW infants who received at least 1 RBC transfusion found no association between RBC transfusion and NEC; however, severe anemia continued to be a risk factor after adjustment for other confounding variables (CSHR, 6.32; 95% CI, 1.94-20.06).

Untangling the relationship between RBC transfusion, anemia, and NEC is challenging because RBC transfusion is often a treatment of anemia. In observational studies, it may be difficult to distinguish whether anemia and the resulting RBC transfusion preceded the onset of NEC or was in response to the development of symptoms associated with NEC. In addition, assessing the statistical interaction between RBC transfusion and anemia on the risk of NEC requires a much larger sample size than examining each exposure alone.[23] Although larger RCTs are ongoing (see prior discussion of TOP, ETTNO and, later, for WHEAT [Withholding Enteral Feeds Around Packed RBC Transfusion]), preclinical animal studies may give insight into the interaction of RBC transfusion and anemia, and the mechanisms by which such exposures might result in intestinal injury. Although animal studies may not perfectly model the human preterm gut or the development of NEC, they offer information on plausible biological mechanisms through which anemia or RBC transfusion may influence intestinal injury that could predispose to NEC. Two recent studies focus specifically on anemia and the combination of anemia and RBC transfusion, as discussed later.[8,9]

PRECLINICAL STUDIES OF ANEMIA AND RED BLOOD CELL TRANSFUSION

Development of NEC is the outcome of multiple causal factors, the combination of which leads to the development of signs, symptoms, and intestinal pathology consistent with the diagnosis. Progressive tissue inflammation and disruption of intestinal mucosal integrity are considered important mechanisms for the development of intestinal injury that may predispose an infant to NEC. Changes to intestinal circulation in response to anemia and blood transfusion have the potential to cause tissue hypoxia and reoxygenation, which are possible stimulants for gut inflammation and mucosal barrier damage[24,25] (Fig. 1).

Effect of Anemia and Transfusion on Gut Vasculature

Following birth, the intestines increase metabolic activity from feeding, which may influence susceptibility to perturbations in oxygen delivery.[26] Oxygen delivery to tissues depends on hemoglobin, cardiac output, vascular tone, and tissue demand. Decreasing blood hemoglobin concentrations leads to circulatory adjustments, such as increases in cardiac output, capillary perfusion, and increased oxygen extraction by tissues.[27] Progressive anemia in newborn lambs has been shown to be associated with compensatory mechanisms, including increase in oxygen extraction to maintain tissue oxygen consumption.[28,29] However, profound anemia may overwhelm the body's compensatory mechanisms, and resulting decreases in oxygen delivery may induce direct tissue hypoxia and ischemia when oxygen supply does not meet

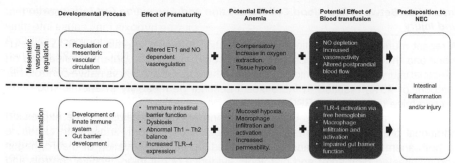

Fig. 1. Potential mechanisms that may explain the intestinal inflammation or injury resulting from anemia and RBC transfusion. ET1, endothelin 1; NO, nitric oxide; Th, T helper cell; TLR, toll-like receptor. (*Adapted from* Saroha V, Josephson CD, Patel RM. Epidemiology of Necrotizing Enterocolitis: New Considerations Regarding the Influence of Red Cell Transfusions and Anemia. *Clin Perinatol.* 2019 Mar;46(1):101-117; with permission.)

demand.[30,31] On histology, such hypoxic changes have been shown in the intestinal lamina propria of anemic murine pups.[8] The presence of systemic changes such as hypotension, hypoxemia, and lower oxygen saturation targeting may further compound the effect of anemia on tissue oxygen delivery.[30,32,33]

Intestinal circulation is governed by a dynamic balance between vasoconstrictive (catecholamine and endothelin) and vasodilatory mediators (nitric oxide [NO]).[34] Neonatal intestinal circulation is predominantly regulated by endothelium-derived NO (eNO),[35] which is present in increased concentration compared with mature infants. Furthermore, NO inhibition in neonates is associated with a greater increase in vascular resistance compared with mature infants. RBC transfusion has the potential to disrupt the balance of vascular tone, as shown in a model of preterm lambs where, compared with controls, mesenteric arterial rings isolated from lambs following transfusion with RBCs showed increased vasoreactivity associated with decreased expression of mesenteric arterial eNOS protein.[36] Stored RBCs are known to have declining amounts of constitutive vasodilator components such as S-nitrosothiol[37]; release of intracellular arginase, which depletes the NO precursor arginine[38]; and increased free hemoglobin, which binds to free NO,[39] all potentially contributing to increased vasoreactivity following blood transfusion. Studies using near-infrared spectroscopy (NIRS) to measure regional tissue oxygen saturation (rSo_2) have shown greater fluctuation and decreases in mesenteric oxygen patterns in infants who developed NEC posttransfusion compared with infants who were transfused and did not develop NEC.[40]

Effect of Anemia on Gut Inflammation and Barrier Function

In a murine model examining the effects of anemia on the neonatal gut, phlebotomy induced anemia (PIA) in P8 murine pups (term-equivalent structural and functional gut maturity by P18–21[41]) to a mean hematocrit of less than 25% compared with mean hematocrit of 45% in controls. It did not lead to increased hypoxia at the villous level (measured by hydroxyprobe, a marker of tissue hypoxia) or increased expression of multiple proinflammatory cytokines in the macrophages isolated from intestinal lamina propria, including tumor necrosis factor-alpha and interferon-gamma.[8] This finding was associated with increased intestinal barrier permeability and decreased tight junction protein expression, with reduction in abnormalities following macrophage depletion. This study suggests intestinal macrophages play an important role in anemia-induced inflammation, with findings confirmed by another recent study, as described later.[9]

Interaction Between Red Blood Cell Transfusion and Anemia on Gut Inflammation and Injury

A recent murine study examined the interaction between anemia and RBC transfusions and the underlying mechanisms that could explain the potential influences on intestinal injury.[9] PIA in P13 mice pups (mean hematocrit, 22.5% vs native controls hematocrit of 45%) resulted in increased intestinal permeability in anemic mice and anemic mice that received RBC transfusion compared with nonanemic controls and nonanemic transfused mice. Both anemic and anemic transfused mice expressed additional proinflammatory macrophage populations but only those with exposure to both anemia and RBC transfusion showed increased activation of macrophages and manifested biomarker and histologic evidence of gut injury. Native controls and nonanemic RBC transfused mice did not show such macrophage infiltration, activation, or associated gut injury. In addition, protection against the development of gut injury in this model was shown following chelation of RBC degradation products with haptoglobin, absence of Toll-like receptor-4 (TLR-4), and macrophage depletion, suggesting these may be obligatory in the pathway of gut injury in this model. A dose-response to the severity and duration of anemia was noted, with increasing severity of bowel injury in the setting of more severe and prolonged anemia.

Worsening gut injury following RBC transfusion in the presence of severe anemia or prolonged anemia in this model indicates progressive susceptibility caused by a priming step (anemia) and activation step (RBC transfusion) to induce bowel injury.[9] It is plausible that other factors, such as an altered microbiome[42] secondary to antibiotics use, formula feeds, or mucosal exposure to substrates and hypoxia,[25] may in combination, or independently, provoke immunologic shifts[43] and increase the susceptibility of the gut to injury and, potentially, NEC, that is similar to the effects of anemia. Additional preclinical models that investigate combinations of such factors, in addition to varying levels of oxygenation, may help better understand how anemia and/or RBC transfusion interact with other mediators to influence gut injury in preterm infants.

INFLUENCE OF FEEDING DURING RED BLOOD CELL TRANSFUSION

Given the potential increased risk of NEC following RBC transfusion, several observational studies and a small RCT have investigated the effect of feeding during RBC transfusion on the risk of NEC. In a retrospective case-control study of 100 infants less than or equal to 34 weeks' gestational age with NEC (Bell stage 2A or greater), infants who developed TRAGI were more likely to be nil by mouth compared with infants that developed NEC remote from transfusions (84.6% vs 36.8%; P<.001); however, there was no standard feeding protocol or approach to feeding during transfusions during the 9-year study period.[44] Another study evaluated the impact of a peritransfusion feeding protocol, comparing infants less than or equal to 1500 g who were nil by mouth during all RBC transfusions with those who were fed at least once during any transfusion.[45] They found no difference in the risk of NEC between the 2 groups (5 out of 64 vs 16 out of 116; adjusted OR, 0.54; 95% CI, 0.16–1.51). Of the 21 infants in the study who developed NEC, 11 did so within 48 hours of a transfusion; 6 infants were fed during the prediagnosis transfusion and 5 were nil by mouth for a prolonged period. When infants with TRAGI were compared with a control group of transfused infants who did not develop NEC, there was no difference in the rate of nil by mouth during transfusions or in the feeding rate (mL/kg/d) just before diagnosis.[46]

The implementation of standardized feeding protocols has been associated with a decrease in the risk of NEC.[47] Several studies have reported NEC outcomes after standardization of feedings around RBC transfusions. The results, primarily from single centers, report some conflicting data. An early 2011 study from a single institution reported a decrease in overall NEC incidence from 18 months before to 18 months after implementation of a feeding protocol holding feeds before and during RBC transfusions (NEC incidence, 5.3% [before] vs 1.3% [after]; P = .047).[48] The investigators recognize that their observation period may not have been long enough to identify a true trend. A quality improvement (QI) initiative that involved conservative feeding during RBC transfusion and indomethacin administration reported an overall decrease in NEC from 8.0% to less than 4.0%.[49] However, transfusion feeding guidelines were only a portion of the QI interventions, and they were implemented at the same time as an initiative to feed mother's own milk or donor milk early in a standardized fashion. The investigators succeeded in increasing the percentage of discharged infants fed mother's milk before day of life 3 from 0% to 50% over the course of the project. This improvement alone could have a major effect on declines in NEC incidence, and, thus, it is not possible from the data presented to determine the independent effect of the peritransfusion feeding guideline on overall reductions in NEC incidence. In another study of prefeeding/postfeeding protocol implementation, breast milk feedings increased but there was no change in rates of NEC or TRAGI despite the emphasis on early breast milk feeds and holding feeds for 12 to 24 hours during RBC transfusion[50]; the study did find a trend toward more bloodstream infection during the epoch in which feeds were held for transfusion (3 out of 189 prefeeding protocol vs 11 out of 192 postfeeding protocol with feeds held; P = .053). Another single-institution prefeeding/postfeeding protocol study showed a decrease in the rate of TRAGI, although the protocol did not address feeding practices during transfusions but emphasized prolonged nil-by-mouth times up to 14 days of life, trophic feeds for up to 7 days of life, and slow advancement of enteral feeds with full feeds (150 mL/kg/d) not established until 44 to 52 days of life.[51] A regional case-crossover trial found no association between feed fortification (OR, 1.67; 95% CI, 0.61-4.59), feed volume increase (OR, 0.63; 95% CI, 0.28-1.38), or RBC transfusion (OR, 1.8; 95% CI, 0.60-5.37) on the odds of developing NEC.[52] Infants served as their own controls, with the 48 hours before NEC onset defined as the hazard period and the 48 hours before the hazard period defined as the control period. Institutional practice was to hold feeds during transfusions and not to advance volume or calories on the day of transfusion. Thus, conservative feeding practices were already adopted as standard practice. A 2017 systematic review and meta-analysis examined a combination of abstracts and published articles reporting the effects of before-and-after results of peritransfusion feeding policies.[53] Although the review concludes that withholding feeds around the time of transfusion reduced the incidence of TRAGI (RR, 0.47; 95% CI, 0.28-0.80), the study's dependence on unadjusted, observational data limits the certainty with which its conclusion can be accepted because of the possibility of residual confounding by other changes over the study periods.

The studies discussed earlier, with their wide variation in protocols as well as differing outcomes on overall NEC and TRAGI rates, make it difficult to determine the best feeding practice around RBC transfusions. This difficulty is particularly relevant because few cases of NEC occur within 48 hours of RBC transfusion (0.5%–1.4%).[6,7] At this time, there is 1 small RCT that examined whether withholding feeding during RBC transfusion decreases the risk of TRAGI.[54] The study population constituted hemodynamically stable preterm infants less than or equal to 32 weeks' gestation and less than or equal to 1500 g at birth who were tolerating 130 to 180 mL/kg/d of enteral feeds. In addition, infants with anomalies, severe hypoxia, asphyxia, and those who received RBC transfusion in the first 7 days of life were excluded. RBC transfusions were given per an established unit protocol. Infants were randomized to a nil-by-mouth group (1–2 feeds held before, during, and after transfusion, resulting in 8–12 hours of nil-by-mouth time) or a FED (feeds continued as per established unit feeding protocol) group. The study's primary outcomes were an increase in abdominal circumference and NEC development in the first 72 hours after transfusion. One-hundred and twelve infants were randomized, 52 in the nil-by-mouth group and 58 in the FED group, at which point no further randomization occurred because of low NEC rates and futility. There was no difference between the 2 groups in abdominal circumference, feeding intolerance, or NEC. The combined outcome of feeding intolerance and/or NEC and mortality was significantly higher in the FED group (17.2% vs 1.9%; $P = .009$) with a trend to increase mortality in the FED group (0 vs 6.8%; $P = .06$). However, these results should be interpreted with caution because the study was stopped early and was underpowered to detect such differences in mortality. A pilot point-of-care RCT, WHEAT, has finished initial enrollment in the United Kingdom (https://www.npeu.ox.ac.uk/wheat) and may expand to a larger, multicenter trial in the United Kingdom or elsewhere. This trial randomizes infants born at less than 30 weeks' gestation to either continue enteral feedings during RBC transfusion or to withhold feeds for 4 hours before, during, and 4 hours after the transfusion. This trial should provide further information to guide feeding practices during RBC transfusions, including effects on NEC as well as other important outcomes, such as late-onset infection.

USE OF NEAR-INFRARED SPECTROSCOPY MONITORING

As approaches to RBC transfusion and feeding during RBC transfusion in the aforementioned studies are applied broadly to preterm infants, tools such as NIRS may provide some insight into the effect of anemia, RBC transfusion, and feeding on intestinal oxygenation for individual infants. The use of NIRS monitoring of splanchnic rSo_2 during feeding has been reported in several studies. Infants with feeding intolerance were noted to have lower splanchnic rSo_2 or splanchnic to cerebral oxygenation ratio (SCOR), a measure of relative intestinal oxygenation.[26,55] In addition, bolus feeds seem to result in increased superior mesenteric artery velocity as measured by Doppler and rSo_2 as measured by NIRS that is not seen in the setting of continuous feeds.[56–58] In a study of 50 anemic preterm infants (hematocrit $\leq$ 28%), the SCOR decreased from baseline during feedings and splanchnic rSo_2 trended toward decreased levels during feedings. In addition, after feeding there was not an increase in splanchnic rSo_2 as shown in other feeding studies.[31] These findings suggest that anemic infants may have less ability to meet the metabolic demand of feeding and digestion, potential making them more vulnerable to the consequences of imbalanced oxygen demand and supply. However, there is currently insufficient evidence to support the use of NIRS to guide RBC transfusion or approaches to feeding during RBC transfusion.

CHARACTERISTICS OF TRANSFUSED RED BLOOD CELL PRODUCTS

If the transfusion of blood products has the ability to alter intestinal circulation and incite inflammatory responses based on data from preclinical studies, then blood banking practices, donor characteristics, and RBC characteristics may influence recipient responses to transfusion. Transfusion practices for neonates vary between blood banks in terms of preservation solution used, timing of irradiating of RBCs, and age of RBCs transfused.[59] Little is known about whether these practices influence neonatal outcomes, including NEC. Preclinical data suggest transfused RBCs can introduce exogenous biological response modifiers that may play a role in gut inflammation and intestinal injury.[23] In the anemic transfused mice model developed by MohanKumar and colleagues,[9] the inflammatory effects of RBC transfusion were isolated to factors released by stored RBCs. Increased inflammatory signaling was seen only in the setting of exposure to stored RBC product (7-day RBC or 7-day plasma with fresh RBCs), and minimal inflammation was seen with fresh RBC transfusion, fresh plasma transfusion, or 7-day plasma supernatant without exposure to RBCs.[9] However, 7-day-old stored murine RBCs may not reflect what is transfused to human neonates. In the multicenter Age of Red Blood Cells in Premature Infants (ARIPI) trial, low birth weight infants were randomized at Canadian centers to receive transfusion of RBCs stored for 7 days or less (188 infants) versus standard blood banking practice (189 infants). The study's primary outcome was a composite of major neonatal morbidities, including NEC. The mean age of transfused blood in the intervention group was 5.1 days (standard deviation [SD], 2.0 days) and 14.6 days (SD, 8.3 days) in the standard practice group. There was no difference in the primary outcome between the 2 groups (RR, 1.00; 95% CI, 0.82-1.2) or in NEC alone (RR, 1.00; 95% CI, 0.48-2.12).[60] Therefore, there are currently no data from clinical trials that would support transfusion of only fresh RBCs into neonates. Beyond chronologic storage age, the storage duration after RBC product irradiation has been shown to be negatively correlated with the magnitude of regional cerebral oxygen saturation response to RBC transfusion, suggesting the time from irradiation to RBC transfusion may influence the effect of transfused RBCs on changes in oxygen delivery.[61] The impact of irradiation is currently being studied in a prospective cohort study that will examine the relationship between prolonged irradiation storage time, RBC metabolomics profiles, and anemia on intestinal oxygenation and the development of NEC in premature infants.[62]

Outside of RBC product transfusion, the role of platelet transfusions in the pathogenesis or propagation of NEC is unclear.[63,64] Neuropeptide Y, a molecule that can play a role in splanchnic vasoconstriction as well as macrophage adhesion, was found in increasing levels in stored platelets, suggesting platelet-derived active substances present in stored platelets may contribute to NEC injury.[64] One retrospective study found increased morbidity in preterm neonates with NEC who received greater number and volume of platelet transfusion,[63] although another found no difference in platelet transfusion rate and death from NEC.[64] In the Platelets for Neonatal Transfusion Study 2 (PlaNeT-2), in which infants were randomized to high (50,000/mm3) versus low (25,000/mm3) platelets transfusion threshold, 16% of infants randomized had NEC at the time of randomization, and there was no difference in additional NEC cases between the 2 groups.[65]

SUMMARY

The impact of NEC on neonatal morbidity and mortality, as well as the concern that a common neonatal physiologic state (anemia) and intervention (RBC transfusion) may predispose premature infants to NEC, make understanding the causal effects of anemia and RBC transfusion and underlying mechanisms important to researchers and clinicians. Recently developed preclinical murine models that investigate the impact of anemia and RBC transfusion on gut injury are providing some insight into the observed clinical phenomenon of TRAGI. The effect of anemia and transfusion on gut barrier integrity, inflammation, and tissue hypoxia may be related to alterations in endogenous vasoactive mediators, upregulation of TLR-4, and activation of proinflammatory macrophages. Other factors, such as transfusion product and donor characteristics, need additional studies to determine whether they influence outcomes such as NEC. In addition, ongoing trials comparing RBC transfusion thresholds and the effect of withholding of feeding during RBC transfusion will provide important information regarding how these common interventions may influence the risk of NEC and other important outcomes in preterm infants.

DISCLOSURE

Dr R.M. Patel reports receiving grant support from the National Institutes of Health (K23 HL128942). The authors have no other relevant conflicts of interest to disclose.

Best Practices

What is the current practice?

At present, there is uncertainty about the optimal hemoglobin thresholds for RBC transfusion, the safest RBC product characteristics for preterm infants, and the best approach to enteral feeding during RBC transfusions.

What changes in current practice are likely to improve outcomes?

1. The implementation of standardized feeding protocols that include the use of human milk feedings has been associated with a reduction in the risk of NEC. Implementation of such protocols may be helpful to reduce the risk of NEC until further data from RCTs about feeding practices during RBC transfusions are available.

2. Preclinical and clinical data suggest severe anemia may influence the risk of gut injury. Strategies to reduce severe anemia, such as minimizing unnecessary phlebotomy-related blood loss, provision of delayed cord clamping, and avoidance of transfusion thresholds lower than those studied in trials to date, are suggested care approaches, although additional studies will provide better data on the safety of tolerating neonatal anemia.

Summary Statement

Anemia (priming step) and RBC transfusion (activating step) may play a role in gut injury. Results from ongoing RCTs of transfusion thresholds as well as feeding practices during RBC transfusion should inform important clinical decisions surrounding approaches to RBC transfusions and enteral feedings during transfusion.

REFERENCES

1. Jacob J, Kamitsuka M, Clark RH, et al. Etiologies of NICU deaths. Pediatrics 2015;135(1):e59–65.

2. Rose AT, Patel RM. A critical analysis of risk factors for necrotizing enterocolitis. Semin Fetal Neonatal Med 2018;23(6):374–9.

3. Mohamed A, Shah PS. Transfusion associated necrotizing enterocolitis: a meta-analysis of observational data. Pediatrics 2012;129(3):529–40.

4. Garg P, Pinotti R, Lal CV, et al. Transfusion-associated necrotizing enterocolitis in preterm infants: an updated meta-analysis of observational data. J Perinat Med 2018;46(6):677–85.

5. Maheshwari A, Patel RM, Christensen RD. Anemia, red blood cell transfusions, and necrotizing enterocolitis. Semin Pediatr Surg 2018;27(1):47–51.

6. Paul DA, Mackley A, Novitsky A, et al. Increased odds of necrotizing enterocolitis after transfusion of red blood cells in premature infants. Pediatrics 2011;127(4): 635–41.

7. Patel RM, Knezevic A, Shenvi N, et al. Association of red blood cell transfusion, anemia, and necrotizing enterocolitis in very low-birth-weight infants. JAMA 2016; 315(9):889–97.
8. Arthur CM, Nalbant D, Feldman HA, et al. Anemia induces gut inflammation and injury in an animal model of preterm infants. Transfusion 2019;59(4):1233–45.
9. MohanKumar K, Namachivayam K, Song T, et al. A murine neonatal model of necrotizing enterocolitis caused by anemia and red blood cell transfusions. Nat Commun 2019;10(1):3494.
10. McGrady GA, Rettig PJ, Istre GR, et al. An outbreak of necrotizing enterocolitis. Association with transfusions of packed red blood cells. Am J Epidemiol 1987; 126(6):1165–72.
11. Kirpalani H, Zupancic JAF. Do transfusions cause necrotizing enterocolitis? The complementary role of randomized trials and observational studies. Semin Perinatol 2012;36(4):269–76.
12. Hay S, Zupancic JAF, Flannery DD, et al. Should we believe in transfusion-associated enterocolitis? Applying a GRADE to the literature. Semin Perinatol 2017;41(1):80–91.
13. Rai SE, Sidhu AK, Krishnan RJ. Transfusion-associated necrotizing enterocolitis re-evaluated: a systematic review and meta-analysis. J Perinat Med 2017. https://doi.org/10.1515/jpm-2017-0048.
14. Kirpalani H, Whyte RK, Andersen C, et al. The premature infants in need of transfusion (pint) study: a randomized, controlled trial of a restrictive (LOW) versus liberal (HIGH) transfusion threshold for extremely low birth weight infants. J Pediatr 2006;149(3):301–7.e3.
15. Bell EF. Transfusion thresholds for preterm infants: how low should we go? J Pediatr 2006;149(3):287–9.
16. Bell EF. Randomized trial of liberal versus restrictive guidelines for red blood cell transfusion in preterm infants. Pediatrics 2005;115(6):1685–91.
17. Whyte R, Kirpalani H. Low versus high haemoglobin concentration threshold for blood transfusion for preventing morbidity and mortality in very low birth weight infants. Cochrane Database Syst Rev 2011;(11):CD000512.
18. Transfusion of prematures trial (TOP). Available at: https://clinicaltrials.gov/ct2/show/NCT01702805. Accessed October 9, 2019.
19. ETTNO Investigators. The 'Effects of transfusion thresholds on neurocognitive outcome of extremely low birth-weight infants (ETTNO)' study: background, aims, and study protocol. Neonatology 2012;101(4):301–5.
20. Colombatti R, Sainati L, Trevisanuto D. Anemia and transfusion in the neonate. Semin Fetal Neonatal Med 2016;21(1):2–9.
21. Keir AK, Yang J, Harrison A, et al, Canadian Neonatal Network. Temporal changes in blood product usage in preterm neonates born at less than 30 weeks' gestation in Canada. Transfusion 2015;55(6):1340–6.
22. Singh R, Visintainer PF, Frantz ID, et al. Association of necrotizing enterocolitis with anemia and packed red blood cell transfusions in preterm infants. J Perinatol 2011;31(3):176–82.
23. Saroha V, Josephson CD, Patel RM. Epidemiology of necrotizing enterocolitis. Clin Perinatol 2019;46(1):101–17.
24. Li C, Jackson RM. Reactive species mechanisms of cellular hypoxia-reoxygenation injury. Am J Physiol Cell Physiol 2002;282(2):C227–41.
25. Chen Y, Koike Y, Miyake H, et al. Formula feeding and systemic hypoxia synergistically induce intestinal hypoxia in experimental necrotizing enterocolitis. Pediatr Surg Int 2016;32(12):1115–9.

26. Cortez J, Gupta M, Amaram A, et al. Noninvasive evaluation of splanchnic tissue oxygenation using near-infrared spectroscopy in preterm neonates. J Matern Fetal Neonatal Med 2011;24(4):574–82.
27. Alkalay AL, Galvis S, Ferry DA, et al. Hemodynamic changes in anemic premature infants: are we allowing the hematocrits to fall too low? Pediatrics 2003; 112(4):838–45.
28. Nowicki PT, Hansen NB, Oh W, et al. Gastrointestinal blood flow and oxygen consumption in the newborn lamb: effect of chronic anemia and acute hypoxia. Pediatr Res 1984;18(5):420–5.
29. Holzman IR, Tabata B, Edelstone DI. Effects of varying hematocrit on intestinal oxygen uptake in neonatal lambs. Am J Physiol 1985;248(4 Pt 1):G432–6.
30. Szabo JS, Mayfield SR, Oh W, et al. Postprandial gastrointestinal blood flow and oxygen consumption: effects of hypoxemia in neonatal piglets. Pediatr Res 1987; 21(1):93–8.
31. Braski K, Weaver-Lewis K, Loertscher M, et al. Splanchnic-cerebral oxygenation ratio decreases during enteral feedings in anemic preterm infants: observations under near-infrared spectroscopy. Neonatology 2018;113(1):75–80.
32. Reber KM, Nankervis CA, Nowicki PT. Newborn intestinal circulation. Physiology and pathophysiology. Clin Perinatol 2002;29(1):23–39. Available at: http://www.ncbi.nlm.nih.gov/pubmed/11917738.
33. Askie LM, Darlow BA, Finer N, et al. Association between oxygen saturation targeting and death or disability in extremely preterm infants in the neonatal oxygenation prospective meta-analysis collaboration. JAMA 2018;319(21):2190–201.
34. Bowker RM, Yan X, De Plaen IG. Intestinal microcirculation and necrotizing enterocolitis: the vascular endothelial growth factor system. Semin Fetal Neonatal Med 2018;23(6):411–5.
35. Watkins DJ, Besner GE. The role of the intestinal microcirculation in necrotizing enterocolitis. Semin Pediatr Surg 2013;22(2):83–7.
36. Nair J, Gugino SF, Nielsen LC, et al. Packed red cell transfusions alter mesenteric arterial reactivity and nitric oxide pathway in preterm lambs. Pediatr Res 2013; 74(6):652–7.
37. Bennett-Guerrero E, Veldman TH, Doctor A, et al. Evolution of adverse changes in stored RBCs. Proc Natl Acad Sci U S A 2007;104(43):17063–8.
38. Sanchez CMP, Palomero-Rodriguez MA, Garcia NR, et al. Relationship between packed red blood cell storage time and arginase concentration: 6AP5-6. Eur J Anaesthesiol 2011;28. p. 92, Available at: https://journals.lww.com/ejanaesthesiology/Fulltext/2011/06001/Relationship_between_packed_red_blood_cell_storage.293.aspx.
39. Nagababu E, Scott AV, Johnson DJ, et al. The impact of surgery and stored red blood cell transfusions on nitric oxide homeostasis. Anesth Analg 2016;123(2): 274–82.
40. Marin T, Moore J, Kosmetatos N, et al. Red blood cell transfusion-related necrotizing enterocolitis in very-low-birthweight infants: a near-infrared spectroscopy investigation. Transfusion 2013;53(11):2650–8.
41. Walthall K, Cappon GD, Hurtt ME, et al. Postnatal development of the gastrointestinal system: a species comparison. Birth Defects Res B Dev Reprod Toxicol 2005;74(2):132–56.
42. Pammi M, Cope J, Tarr PI, et al. Intestinal dysbiosis in preterm infants preceding necrotizing enterocolitis: a systematic review and meta-analysis. Microbiome 2017;5(1):31.

43. Zhang B, Ohtsuka Y, Fujii T, et al. Immunological development of preterm infants in early infancy. Clin Exp Immunol 2005;140(1):92–6.
44. Garg PM, Ravisankar S, Bian H, et al. Relationship between packed red blood cell transfusion and severe form of necrotizing enterocolitis: a case control study. Indian Pediatr 2015;52(12):1041–5. Available at: http://www.ncbi.nlm.nih.gov/pubmed/26713988.
45. Doty M, Wade C, Farr J, et al. Feeding during blood transfusions and the association with necrotizing enterocolitis. Am J Perinatol 2016;33(09):882–6.
46. Crabtree CS, Pakvasa M, Radmacher PG, et al. Retrospective case-control study of necrotizing enterocolitis and packed red blood cell transfusions in very low birth weight infants. J Neonatal Perinatal Med 2018;11(4):365–70.
47. Jasani B, Patole S. Standardized feeding regimen for reducing necrotizing enterocolitis in preterm infants: an updated systematic review. J Perinatol 2017; 37(7):827–33.
48. El-Dib M, Narang S, Lee E, et al. Red blood cell transfusion, feeding and necrotizing enterocolitis in preterm infants. J Perinatol 2011;31(3):183–7.
49. Talavera MM, Bixler G, Cozzi C, et al. Quality improvement initiative to reduce the necrotizing enterocolitis rate in premature infants. Pediatrics 2016;137(5): e20151119.
50. Bajaj M, Lulic-Botica M, Hanson A, et al. Feeding during transfusion and the risk of necrotizing enterocolitis in preterm infants. J Perinatol 2019;39(4):540–6.
51. Dako J, Buzzard J, Jain M, et al. Slow enteral feeding decreases risk of transfusion associated necrotizing enterocolitis. J Neonatal Perinatal Med 2018;11(3): 231–9.
52. Le VT, Klebanoff MA, Talavera MM, et al. Transient effects of transfusion and feeding advances (volumetric and caloric) on necrotizing enterocolitis development: a case-crossover study. PLoS One 2017;12(6):e0179724.
53. Jasani B, Rao S, Patole S. Withholding feeds and transfusion-associated necrotizing enterocolitis in preterm infants: a systematic review. Adv Nutr 2017;8(5): 764–9.
54. Sahin S, Gozde Kanmaz Kutman H, Bozkurt O, et al. Effect of withholding feeds on transfusion-related acute gut injury in preterm infants: a pilot randomized controlled trial. J Matern Fetal Neonatal Med 2019;1–6. https://doi.org/10.1080/14767058.2019.1597844.
55. Corvaglia L, Martini S, Battistini B, et al. Splanchnic oxygenation at first enteral feeding in preterm infants: correlation with feeding intolerance. J Pediatr Gastroenterol Nutr 2017;64(4):550–4.
56. Bozzetti V, Paterlini G, De Lorenzo P, et al. Impact of continuous vs bolus feeding on splanchnic perfusion in very low birth weight infants: a randomized trial. J Pediatr 2016;176:86–92.e2.
57. Dani C, Pratesi S, Barp J, et al. Near-infrared spectroscopy measurements of splanchnic tissue oxygenation during continuous versus intermittent feeding method in preterm infants. J Pediatr Gastroenterol Nutr 2013;56(6):652–6.
58. Corvaglia L, Martini S, Battistini B, et al. Bolus vs. continuous feeding: effects on splanchnic and cerebral tissue oxygenation in healthy preterm infants. Pediatr Res 2014;76(1):81–5.
59. Patel RM, Meyer EK, Widness JA. Research opportunities to improve neonatal red blood cell transfusion. Transfus Med Rev 2016;30(4):165–73.
60. Fergusson DA, Hébert P, Hogan DL, et al. Effect of Fresh red blood cell transfusions on clinical outcomes in premature, very low-birth-weight infants. JAMA 2012;308(14):1443.

61. Saito-Benz M, Murphy WG, Tzeng Y-C, et al. Storage after gamma irradiation affects in vivo oxygen delivery capacity of transfused red blood cells in preterm infants. Transfusion 2018;58(9):2108–12.
62. Marin T, Patel RM, Roback JD, et al. Does red blood cell irradiation and/or anemia trigger intestinal injury in premature infants with birth weight ≤ 1250 g? an observational birth cohort study. BMC Pediatr 2018;18(1):270.
63. Kenton AB, Hegemier S, Smith EO, et al. Platelet transfusions in infants with necrotizing enterocolitis do not lower mortality but may increase morbidity. J Perinatol 2005;25(3):173–7.
64. Patel RM, Josephson CD, Shenvi N, et al. Platelet transfusions and mortality in necrotizing enterocolitis. Transfusion 2019;59(3):981–8.
65. Curley A, Stanworth SJ, Willoughby K, et al. Randomized trial of platelet-transfusion thresholds in neonates. N Engl J Med 2019;380(3):242–51.

Gastrointestinal Endoscopy in the Neonate

Ethan A. Mezoff, MD[a,b,*], Kent C. Williams, MD[b], Steven H. Erdman, MD[b]

KEYWORDS

- Neonatal endoscopy • Bleeding • Gastrostomy tube
- Percutaneous endoscopic gastrostomy • Bedside

KEY POINTS

- Endoscopes of approximately 15 French/4.9 mm diameter are now available for inspection of the neonatal gastrointestinal tract.
- When considering neonatal endoscopic evaluation, a paucity of neonatal data underscores the need to apply a personalized risk and benefit assessment based on experience and relevant pediatric data
- Bedside endoscopic gastrostomy tube placement, evaluation and control of upper gastrointestinal bleeding, and dilation of fibromuscular congenital esophageal stenosis are examples of therapeutic endoscopic maneuvers possible in the neonate.

INTRODUCTION

Pediatric gastrointestinal endoscopy began in the mid-1980s with flexible fiberoptic endoscopes. These instruments allowed direct observation of the surface of the alimentary tract and later an array of functional adaptations, including tissue biopsy, fluid sampling, targeted ultrasonography, injections of drugs, electrocautery, application of various devices such as metal clips or elastic bands, and polypectomy. Although the development of smaller diameter endoscopes has safely opened many of these diagnostic and therapeutic possibilities to the neonatal population, endoscopy in neonates is governed by anecdote and extrapolation of techniques developed in larger patients. Endoscopic studies in the neonatal population are rare. We review the endoscopic techniques relevant to the neonatal population including approach, possible complications, and safety concerns. As strict indications and contraindications are relatively few, general diagnostic and therapeutic interventions are

[a] Center for Intestinal Rehabilitation and Nutrition Support, Nationwide Children's Hospital, The Ohio State University College of Medicine, 700 Children's Drive, Columbus, OH 43205, USA; [b] Division of Gastroenterology, Hepatology and Nutrition, Nationwide Children's Hospital, The Ohio State University College of Medicine, 700 Children's Drive, Columbus, OH 43205, USA
* Corresponding author.
E-mail address: Ethan.Mezoff@nationwidechildrens.org

Clin Perinatol 47 (2020) 413–422
https://doi.org/10.1016/j.clp.2020.02.012
0095-5108/20/© 2020 Elsevier Inc. All rights reserved.
perinatology.theclinics.com

discussed. Finally, where evidence or sufficient experience exists, we discuss specific indications and related technique.

OVERVIEW OF ENDOSCOPES

The basic design of flexible pediatric gastrointestinal endoscopes, henceforth referred to as "endoscopes," is similar across all manufacturers. The insertion tube, which enters the patient, is a flexible shaft of steel mesh and bands covered by a soft polymer containing the image senor or camera, fiberoptic light bundles, channel for water/insufflation and a "working channel" for suction and passage of instruments. Insertion tube diameter is an important consideration in neonatal endoscopy given limitations of esophageal diameter and potential compression of nearby structures. The typical pediatric gastroscope ranges in external diameter from 8 to 10 mm, with a working channel diameter of 2.8 mm. Most therapeutic accessories are designed to use in a ≥2.8-mm working channel. Ultrathin gastrointestinal endoscopes are available with an insertion tube diameter between 4.9 mm and 6.0 mm (approximately 15–18 French), permitting safer endoscopy in smaller infants even reportedly weighing as low as 0.9 kg (**Table 1**).[1–3] However, the smaller instruments come with a reduced field of vision and smaller working channel of 2.0 mm, restricting some therapeutic options. The diagnostic and therapeutic objective(s) of the procedure should be considered in instrument selection while planning endoscopy in the neonatal setting. Fortunately, there has been a recent expansion in accessory instruments offered that can pass through a 2.0-mm working channel (**Box 1**).

CONSIDERATIONS FOR PROCEDURE LOCATIONS

The choice of setting or venue for the procedure should be made on a case-by-case basis, with options including a well-equipped endoscopy unit, surgical operating

Table 1			
Common gastroscopes for neonatal endoscopy			
Manufacturer	Gastroscope Name	Insertion Tube Diameter, mm/ French[a]	Working Channel Diameter, mm
Olympus	GIF-N180	4.9/15	2.0
	GIF-XP180N	5.5/16 ½	2.0
	GIF-Q180	8.8/26 ½	2.8
	GIF-H180	9.8/29 ½	2.8
Fujinon	EG530N	5.9/18	2.0
	EG530NP	4.9/15	2.0
	EG-450PE5	8.1/24 ½	2.2
	EG-530WR	9.3/28	2.8
Pentax	EG1690K	5.4/16 ½	2.0
	EG1870K	6.0/18	2.0
	EG-2790i	9.0/27	2.8

[a] Approximation.

Adapted from Committee AT, Barth BA, Banerjee S, et al. Equipment for pediatric endoscopy. Gastrointest Endosc. 2012;76(1):8-17; with permission. And *Adapted from* Committee AT, Varadarajulu S, Banerjee S, et al. GI endoscopes. Gastrointest Endosc. 2011;74(1):1-6 e; with permission. Epub 2011/06/28.

Box 1

Accessories available for neonatal endoscopy with 2.0-mm working channel

Equipment compatible with 2.0-mm working channel
  Small biopsy forceps
  Small polyp snare
  Pediatric Roth net
  Small alligator forceps
  Small rat-tooth forceps
  Small injection needle
  Small argon plasma coagulation probe
  2-prong grasper

Adapted from Committee ASoP, Lightdale JR, Acosta R, et al. Modifications in endoscopic practice for pediatric patients. Gastrointest Endosc. 2014;79(5):699-710; with permission. Epub 2014/03/07.

---

room, or the neonatal intensive care unit bedside. When bedside procedures are a consideration, particularly with premature or unstable infants, a sober assessment of bedside space constraints for placement of endoscopists, technician, and endoscopic equipment should be made. Although endoscopy can be performed without sedation in infants, sedation or general anesthesia is commonly performed.[3] When sedation is indicated, American Academy of Pediatrics guidelines for pre-procedure fasting should be followed, at minimum.[4] Attention should be given to positioning of the sedating, credentialed clinician who requires ready access to the patient's airway.

SAFETY CONCERNS AND GENERAL COMPLICATIONS

Although a robust multisite description of endoscopy complications among neonates is not available, retrospective reports from comprehensive pediatric studies are informative. An overall complication rate of 2.3% for upper endoscopy and 1.1% for lower endoscopy were reported in the past decade.[5,6] Sedation-related cardiopulmonary compromise is considered responsible for most adverse events related to an endoscopic procedure.[6,7] Particularly relevant to the neonate with a small caliber and collapsible airway, vagal stimulation or airway compression can lead to patient deterioration and the need for termination of the procedure.[8] Neonates may also be at risk for hypothermia, warranting proactive use of warmers and frequent thermal monitoring. Additional adverse event categories are bleeding, infection, and perforation.[9,10]

Although clinically significant procedure-associated bleeding is rare, mild oozing accompanies tissue biopsy and therapeutic maneuvers disrupting the mucosal surface.[11] Clinically significant bleeding may arise from therapeutic maneuvers, such as when significant sheering or tearing forces occur with advancement of an endoscope around a tight turn or taking biopsies in the setting of a primary or secondary coagulation or platelet disorder. Platelet function is not routinely assessed but a platelet count of greater than 50×10^3 μL is suggested if obtaining mucosal biopsies and greater than 20×10^3 μL for endoscopic mucosal inspection based on recent adult recommendations.[10] Reported rates of postprocedure bleeding among children range from 0.11% to 0.3%.[6,12] A bleeding complication commonly reported among children following bone marrow transplantation but possible in others, intramural duodenal hematoma is particularly worrisome as a partial or complete but transient bowel obstruction may occur without overt signs of bleeding during the procedure.[11,13] Signs of vomiting or abdominal distension following an endoscopic procedure should alert the astute clinician to this possibility.

Endogenous infections from bowel flora after routine biopsies are infrequent among immunocompetent patients. Transient bacteremia, although reported, is rare.[14] Guidance regarding antibiotic prophylaxis among "high-risk" neonates subjected to endoscopy do not exist, justifying a case-by-case evaluation of risk and benefit among neonates with complex congenital heart disease, congenital or acquired immune deficiency, or liver disease.[9] In adults, the most common postprocedural complication following percutaneous endoscopic gastrostomy (PEG) placement is peristomal wound infection, warranting perioperative antibiotic prophylaxis.[15] Exogenous infection, that occurring in association with contaminated equipment, is considered extremely rare with present-day cleaning techniques; however, recent reports of contaminated side-viewing duodenoscopes related to difficulty cleaning this specific design have returned the issue to the fore.[16,17] With appropriate, high-level disinfection, and as few situations require use of a side-viewing duodenoscope in the neonate, exogenous infection remains an exceedingly rare event.

Perforation, defined as injury to bowel resulting in extragastrointestinal leakage of air or other luminal contents, has been reported and relates to both patient comorbidity (eg, presence of intestinal stricture, bowel dilation, spinal muscular atrophy) and technique (eg, intracolonic loop formation, excessive air insufflation, sharp angulation, patient: endoscope size discrepancy).[9] Perforation should be suspected with abdominal distension, vomiting, vital sign instability, or other nonspecific but concerning findings. Abdominal radiographs in 2 views, computerized tomography, or fluoroscopy with a water-soluble contrast agent are diagnostic tests of choice.

GENERAL USE, INDICATIONS, AND CONTRAINDICATIONS

It is important to appreciate the breadth and limits of endoscopic diagnostic and treatment modalities when evaluating the appropriateness for a patient. Endoscopy permits visual inspection of the gastrointestinal mucosa, typically to the depth of the mid-duodenum during esophagogastroduodenoscopy (EGD). Colonoscopy in the neonate is generally performed with ultrathin devices designed for upper gastrointestinal endoscopy and is generally limited to the distal colon though intubation of the terminal ileum is desirable in older infants and children.[18] Tissue biopsy is often performed, as risks of occult microscopic pathology, repeat endoscopy, and sedation outweigh risks of biopsy.[19,20] In addition to standard hematoxylin and eosin or specialized staining, other tests can be performed, such as disaccharidase analysis or electron microscopy, to evaluate for entities such as disaccharidase deficiency or microvillous inclusion disorder, respectively. Therapeutic options are largely dependent on institutional expertise and appropriately sized instrument availability. Smaller-sized biopsy forceps, snares, injection needles, bipolar electrocautery probes, and argon plasma coagulation are available. However, a clipping device and through-the-scope balloon dilation catheters are presently not available for the 2.0-mm working channel of smaller neonatal compatible endoscopes.

Indications for neonatal endoscopy are based on the coherent application of diagnostic or therapeutic treatment modalities to a problem when absolute and relative contraindications have been addressed. Indications for diagnostic endoscopy may include dysphagia, odynophagia, feeding difficulty or intolerance, recurrent vomiting, hematemesis, melena, hematochezia, chronic diarrhea/malabsorption, and a brief resolved unexplained event.[18] Further, nonspecific complaints of persistent fussiness, colic, poor growth, and unexplained iron deficiency are reasons to consider neonatal endoscopy.[18] A review of 1024 endoscopy cases spanning 2 decades and among patients less than 1 year of age found diarrhea and failure to thrive were the most frequent indications for endoscopy.[20] This series found a diagnostic yield (histologic abnormalities) in 63.8% of cases, with the highest yield among small bowel and colon biopsies.[20]

As standard diagnostic endoscopy is thought to be low risk, there are relatively few absolute contraindications, although prudence in case selection is highly encouraged in this vulnerable neonatal population. As an elective procedure, endoscopy is performed on medically stable patients with no features of airway instability, cardiovascular collapse, intestinal perforation, and peritonitis.[21] Inferred by this list, concern for necrotizing enterocolitis should preclude endoscopic evaluation. Relative contraindications include unstable cardiopulmonary disease, bowel obstruction, recent gastrointestinal operation, severe thrombocytopenia, coagulopathy, and neutropenia.[21] No weight "floor" has been established, and endoscopy using an ultrathin endoscope has been safely performed in neonates weighing 1.5 kg or less.[3,22]

NEONATAL GASTROINTESTINAL BLEEDING

Although often used as a diagnostic or therapeutic intervention for gastrointestinal bleeding in the older pediatric population, endoscopy has limited applications and is used infrequently to treat gastrointestinal bleeds in preterm and term infants due to both the causes of gastrointestinal bleeding and the size of neonates (Table 2).[23–25] Most of the common causes of gastrointestinal bleeding in neonates are due to conditions that therapeutic endoscopy cannot remedy, such as swallowed maternal blood, milk protein allergy, or necrotizing colitis. Even stress ulcers, for which therapeutic endoscopy is a common treatment modality in older pediatric populations, responds well to conservative medical management of acid suppression and supportive care, and rarely requires invasive or aggressive interventions.[26] In addition to differences in causes of gastrointestinal bleeding, the size of neonatal patients limits use of endoscopy to address gastrointestinal bleeding. The diameter of the endoscope used for therapeutic endoscopy is often larger than a neonate's esophageal lumen, therefore preventing the use of this treatment modality.[1,2] However, as previously mentioned, the recent expansion of accessory instruments for scopes with the smaller working channel may provide opportunity to use some therapeutic interventions for controlling gastrointestinal bleeding in neonates.[27,28] Although feasibility of therapeutic interventions are limited, there are times when direct observation and biopsy of gastrointestinal mucosa are helpful in assessing or differentiating between potential causes of gastrointestinal bleeding.[3] For instance, mucosal biopsies performed

Table 2	
Common causes of gastrointestinal bleeding in neonates	
Upper	**Lower**
1. Swallowed maternal blood	1. Necrotizing enterocolitis
2. Vitamin K deficiency	2. Malrotation with volvulus
3. Stress gastritis/ulcer	3. Milk protein/allergic colitis
4. Acid-peptic disease	4. Hirschsprung
5. Vascular anomalies	5. Vitamin K deficiency
6. Coagulopathy	6. Coagulopathy
7. Milk protein sensitivity	7. Infectious colitis

during upper or lower endoscopy showing increased eosinophils in the gastrointestinal mucosa can help determine whether persistent blood in recurring emesis or loose stools is due to milk protein allergy versus a discreet ulcer or infection. To help determine the value and feasibility of an endoscopic intervention are best made from the input of a multidisciplinary team of neonatologist, gastroenterologists, and pediatric surgeons.

STENOSIS OF THE UPPER GASTROINTESTINAL TRACT

Unlike gastrointestinal atresia with complete obstruction, congenital stenosis of the upper gastrointestinal tract can have a subtle presentation that at times can be seen in the neonatal period. Congenital esophageal stenosis can present with recurrent choking or vomiting during feeding or with the introduction of solids and poor weight gain later in infancy.[29] Congenital esophageal stenosis is typically located in the bottom half of the esophagus and can be attributed to 1 of 3 subtypes: fibromuscular (54%), tracheal cartilaginous remnants (30%), or a membranous web (~15%), with approximately 10% being associated with esophageal atresia as a second lesion.[30,31] Differentiating between stenosis subtypes was previously done by histologic examination of the resected stricture.[32–34] Strictures of the fibromuscular form show thickening and fibrosis of predominant layers of the esophagus (submucosa, muscularis mucosae, and muscularis propria), whereas those with tracheal remnants show muscle-layer proliferation/disarrangement, cartilaginous elements, and respiratory glands.[33] Recent guidelines suggest the preoperative use of radial endoscopic ultrasound with a miniprobe can help with delineation.[35] The importance of this technique as a diagnostic tool in differentiating congenital esophageal stenosis subtypes was highlighted in a recent review.[30] Through-the-scope balloon dilatation is possible with the fibromuscular forms but attempts at dilatation of strictures with cartilaginous remnants have a higher association of perforation.[30,36] For this reason, most studies suggest surgical resection of the stenosis with primary anastomosis for congenital strictures with tracheal remnants or endoscopic dilation failure to minimize the risk of postdilation esophageal perforation.[31]

Congenital pyloric stenosis is another disorder that can be seen during the newborn period. These infants typically have postprandial nonbilious emesis of breast milk or formula and, with time, will show poor weight gain and electrolyte abnormalities of alkalosis and hyperchloremia. The diagnosis is commonly made by abdominal ultrasound documenting an elongated and thickened pylorus. Pyloromyotomy remains the standard of care for this disorder, which usually addresses growth and electrolyte problems. However, like all surgical procedures, pyloromyotomy can be associated with complications such as insufficient release of the obstruction or mucosal perforation.[37] Recent interest in through-the-scope balloon dilatation of pyloric stenosis has developed. Further studies are needed to determine which method of treatment would be best in each clinical situation.

LACTOBEZOARS

Precipitated protein associated with both cow's milk formula and breast milk can be associated with the development of gastric lactobezoars, typically in small premature infants, although they have also been found in term infants. The exact incidence of this disorder is not clear; however, an increase in incidence was noted with the introduction of cow's milk formulas in the 1970s. Multiple factors are associated with the development of lactobezoars including prematurity, hyperosmolar formula, dehydration, altered gastrointestinal emptying, and secretion. Smaller lactobezoars can be asymptomatic; however, typically they lead to gastric outlet obstruction with abdominal distension and vomiting. As noted, prematurity is an associated factor with findings that overlap necrotizing enterocolitis. Recent case reports have associated gastric pneumatosis and rupture with lactobezoars.[38] Upper endoscopy can confirm the diagnosis and allow for mechanical disruption of the lactobezoar aiding passage into the intestinal tract.

PERCUTANEOUS ENDOSCOPIC GASTROSTOMY TUBE PLACEMENT

Nutrition support is a cornerstone of neonatal care that is often limited by delayed oral feeding skills that prevent adequate calorie intake for the sick or premature infant. Orogastric (OG) or nasogastric (NG) feeding tubes can help to meet nutrition goals. However, over time, chronic indwelling NG or OG tubes can interfere with the development of appropriate feeding skills and dislodgement is common. Reinsertion of NG tubes by parents at home has been a controversial issue in many institutions. Direct access to the stomach through the abdominal wall by way of gastrostomy tube placement can be accomplished by several methods and techniques. Percutaneous placement using an endoscope (PEG) is a common procedure in both pediatric and adult medicine. This same technique can be used in infants down to a weight of 1.8 kg (authors' note) using either general anesthesia or bedside intravenous sedation. This latter method avoids reintubation with further airway manipulation/injury.

The basic "pull" technique uses a looped guidewire that is inserted through the abdominal wall into the stomach. The wire is secured by the endoscope and pulled through the stomach, up the esophagus, and out the mouth where the PEG tube is attached to the wire. The wire extending from the abdominal incision is pulled bringing the tube down the esophagus, through the stomach and out through the abdominal wall incision. A gastric bumper on the end of the tube secures the tube in the stomach while an external bumper is attached to the tube to stabilize the tube and site. Over time, a durable resilient scar or adhesion develops between the gastric wall and anterior abdominal wall, creating a stable and fully sealed tract. When gastric access by way of the esophagus is not an option, a "push" method can be used to advance the gastrostomy tube directly into the stomach. This technique also can be used for initial placement of a gastrojejunal feeding tube and is typically done under general anesthesia.

SUMMARY

Neonatal endoscopy is a highly specialized procedure. Few data directly guide neonatal use; however, anecdote and extrapolation from pediatric and adult care is informative. With careful consideration of risks and benefits of endoscopy and thoughtful anticipation of intraprocedural concerns, the neonatal team and gastroenterological consultant can formulate a patient-specific plan to address complaints while minimizing risk. The small working channel diameter of endoscopes for neonatal use has historically limited some therapeutic maneuvers. However, growing experience and expansion of tools compatible with the 2.0-mm working channel have opened new possibilities to diagnose and treat gastrointestinal disease in this vulnerable population.

DISCLOSURE

The authors have no disclosures relevant to this work.

Best Practices

What is the current practice?

Neonatal gastrointestinal bleeding (upper and lower)

Percutaneous endoscopic gastrostomy

Best practice/guideline/care path objectives
- Stabilization, assessment, and initiation of medical treatment
- Prompt initial assessment of hemodynamic stability or blood loss assessment
- Consultation with Pediatric Gastroenterology and Pediatric surgery
- Early initiation of intravenous acid suppression therapy
- Appropriate assessment of the infant with persistent feeding skills insufficiency for gastrostomy tube placement

What Changes in Current Practice are likely to improve outcomes?

- Judicious use of blood products to avoid overtransfusion

- Early gastrointestinal consultation regarding a possible diagnostic or therapeutic endoscopic procedure

- Bedside/operating room percutaneous endoscopic gastrostomy placement accelerates hospital discharge and shortens length of stay

Is there a Clinical Algorithm?

| Significant upper gastrointestinal bleeding |
| Hemodynamic Assessment |
| Vascular access
Type & cross, Complete Blood Count, chemistry panel, coagulation assessment |
| History and physical assessment |
| Naso/orogastric tube placement, Diagnostic gastric lavage |
| Gastroenterology and Pediatric Surgery Consults |
| IV Acid Suppression Therapy |
| Assess for Octreotide therapy (load and continued infusion) |
| Upper Endoscopy (bedside or OR) with specific bleeding treatment |

Summary Statement

Rapid endoscopy of the stabilized infant can help in diagnosis and treatment. Gastrostomy tube placement is a safe procedure that can accelerate discharge and allows for removal of a chronically placed nasogastric/orogastric tube, which can help with oral feeding skills.

REFERENCES

1. Benaroch LM, Rudolph CD. Introduction to pediatric esophagogastroduodenoscopy and enteroscopy. Gastrointest Endosc Clin N Am 1994;4(1):121–42.
2. Committee AT, Barth BA, Banerjee S, et al. Equipment for pediatric endoscopy. Gastrointest Endosc 2012;76(1):8–17.
3. Ruuska T, Fell JM, Bisset WM, et al. Neonatal and infantile upper gastrointestinal endoscopy using a new small diameter fibreoptic gastroscope. J Pediatr Gastroenterol Nutr 1996;23(5):604–8.

4. Cote CJ, Wilson S, American Academy of Pediatrics, American Academy of Pediatric Dentistry. Guidelines for monitoring and management of pediatric patients before, during, and after sedation for diagnostic and therapeutic procedures: update 2016. Pediatrics 2016;138(1). https://doi.org/10.1542/peds.2016-1212.
5. Thakkar K, El-Serag HB, Mattek N, et al. Complications of pediatric colonoscopy: a five-year multicenter experience. Clin Gastroenterol Hepatol 2008;6(5):515–20.
6. Thakkar K, El-Serag HB, Mattek N, et al. Complications of pediatric EGD: a 4-year experience in PEDS-CORI. Gastrointest Endosc 2007;65(2):213–21.
7. Gilger MA, Gold BD. Pediatric endoscopy: new information from the PEDS-CORI project. Curr Gastroenterol Rep 2005;7(3):234–9.
8. Hargrove CB, Ulshen MH, Shub MD. Upper gastrointestinal endoscopy in infants: diagnostic usefulness and safety. Pediatrics 1984;74(5):828–31.
9. Lightdale JR, Liu QY, Sahn B, et al. Pediatric endoscopy and high-risk patients: a clinical report from the NASPGHAN endoscopy committee. J Pediatr Gastroenterol Nutr 2019;68(4):595–606.
10. ASGE Standards of Practice Committee, Ben-Menachem T, Decker GA, Early DS, et al. Adverse events of upper GI endoscopy. Gastrointest Endosc 2012;76(4):707–18.
11. Attard TM, Grima AM, Thomson M. Pediatric endoscopic procedure complications. Curr Gastroenterol Rep 2018;20(10):48.
12. Kramer RE, Narkewicz MR. Adverse events following gastrointestinal endoscopy in children: classifications, characterizations, and implications. J Pediatr Gastroenterol Nutr 2016;62(6):828–33.
13. Sierra A, Ecochard-Dugelay E, Bellaiche M, et al. Biopsy-induced duodenal hematoma is not an infrequent complication favored by bone marrow transplantation. J Pediatr Gastroenterol Nutr 2016;63(6):627–32.
14. Byrne WJ, Euler AR, Campbell M, et al. Bacteremia in children following upper gastrointestinal endoscopy or colonoscopy. J Pediatr Gastroenterol Nutr 1982;1(4):551–3.
15. Lipp A, Lusardi G. Systemic antimicrobial prophylaxis for percutaneous endoscopic gastrostomy. Cochrane Database Syst Rev 2013;(11):CD005571.
16. Spach DH, Silverstein FE, Stamm WE. Transmission of infection by gastrointestinal endoscopy and bronchoscopy. Ann Intern Med 1993;118(2):117–28.
17. Rauwers AW, Voor In 't Holt AF, Buijs JG, et al. High prevalence rate of digestive tract bacteria in duodenoscopes: a nationwide study. Gut 2018;67(9):1637–45.
18. Dupont C, Kalach N, de Boissieu D, et al. Digestive endoscopy in neonates. J Pediatr Gastroenterol Nutr 2005;40(4):406–20.
19. Kori M, Gladish V, Ziv-Sokolovskaya N, et al. The significance of routine duodenal biopsies in pediatric patients undergoing upper intestinal endoscopy. J Clin Gastroenterol 2003;37(1):39–41.
20. Volonaki E, Sebire NJ, Borrelli O, et al. Gastrointestinal endoscopy and mucosal biopsy in the first year of life: indications and outcome. J Pediatr Gastroenterol Nutr 2012;55(1):62–5.
21. Friedt M, Welsch S. An update on pediatric endoscopy. Eur J Med Res 2013;18:24.
22. ASGE Standards of Practice Committee, Lightdale JR, Acosta R, Shergill AK, et al. Modifications in endoscopic practice for pediatric patients. Gastrointest Endosc 2014;79(5):699–710.
23. Boyle JT. Gastrointestinal bleeding in infants and children. Pediatr Rev 2008;29(2):39–52.

24. Kleinman RE. Walker's pediatric gastrointestinal disease. 6th edition. Raleigh (NC): People's Medical Publishing House-USA; 2018. p. 1853–62, 1886–904.
25. Pai AK, Fox VL. Gastrointestinal bleeding and management. Pediatr Clin North Am 2017;64(3):543–61.
26. Goyal A, Treem WR, Hyams JS. Severe upper gastrointestinal bleeding in healthy full-term neonates. Am J Gastroenterol 1994;89(4):613–6.
27. Lokesh Babu TG, Jacobson K, Phang M, et al. Endoscopic hemostasis in a neonate with a bleeding duodenal ulcer. J Pediatr Gastroenterol Nutr 2005; 41(2):244–6.
28. Khan K, Schwarzenberg SJ, Sharp H, et al. Argon plasma coagulation: clinical experience in pediatric patients. Gastrointest Endosc 2003;57(1):110–2.
29. Di Lorenzo C, Kaj B, Krishnan K, et al. Case 29-2019: a 14-month-old boy with vomiting. N Engl J Med 2019;381(12):1159–67.
30. Terui K, Saito T, Mitsunaga T, et al. Endoscopic management for congenital esophageal stenosis: a systematic review. World J Gastrointest Endosc 2015; 7(3):183–91.
31. McCann F, Michaud L, Aspirot A, et al. Congenital esophageal stenosis associated with esophageal atresia. Dis Esophagus 2015;28(3):211–5.
32. Romeo E, Foschia F, de Angelis P, et al. Endoscopic management of congenital esophageal stenosis. J Pediatr Surg 2011;46(5):838–41.
33. Amae S, Nio M, Kamiyama T, et al. Clinical characteristics and management of congenital esophageal stenosis: a report on 14 cases. J Pediatr Surg 2003; 38(4):565–70.
34. Takamizawa S, Tsugawa C, Mouri N, et al. Congenital esophageal stenosis: therapeutic strategy based on etiology. J Pediatr Surg 2002;37(2):197–201.
35. Thomson M, Tringali A, Dumonceau JM, et al. Paediatric gastrointestinal endoscopy: European Society for Paediatric Gastroenterology Hepatology and Nutrition and European Society of Gastrointestinal Endoscopy guidelines. J Pediatr Gastroenterol Nutr 2017;64(1):133–53.
36. Bocus P, Realdon S, Eloubeidi MA, et al. High-frequency miniprobes and 3-dimensional EUS for preoperative evaluation of the etiology of congenital esophageal stenosis in children (with video). Gastrointest Endosc 2011;74(1):204–7.
37. Kelay A, Hall NJ. Perioperative complications of surgery for hypertrophic pyloric stenosis. Eur J Pediatr Surg 2018;28(2):171–5.
38. Bos ME, Wijnen RM, de Blaauw I. Gastric pneumatosis and rupture caused by lactobezoar. Pediatr Int 2013;55(6):757–60.

Moving?

Make sure your subscription moves with you!

To notify us of your new address, find your **Clinics Account Number** (located on your mailing label above your name), and contact customer service at:

Email: journalscustomerservice-usa@elsevier.com

800-654-2452 (subscribers in the U.S. & Canada)
314-447-8871 (subscribers outside of the U.S. & Canada)

Fax number: 314-447-8029

Elsevier Health Sciences Division
Subscription Customer Service
3251 Riverport Lane
Maryland Heights, MO 63043

*To ensure uninterrupted delivery of your subscription, please notify us at least 4 weeks in advance of move.

Printed and bound by CPI Group (UK) Ltd, Croydon, CR0 4YY

03/10/2024

01040401-0003